Oh Momma!

Where's the Fat?

Pamela Harrell Jackson

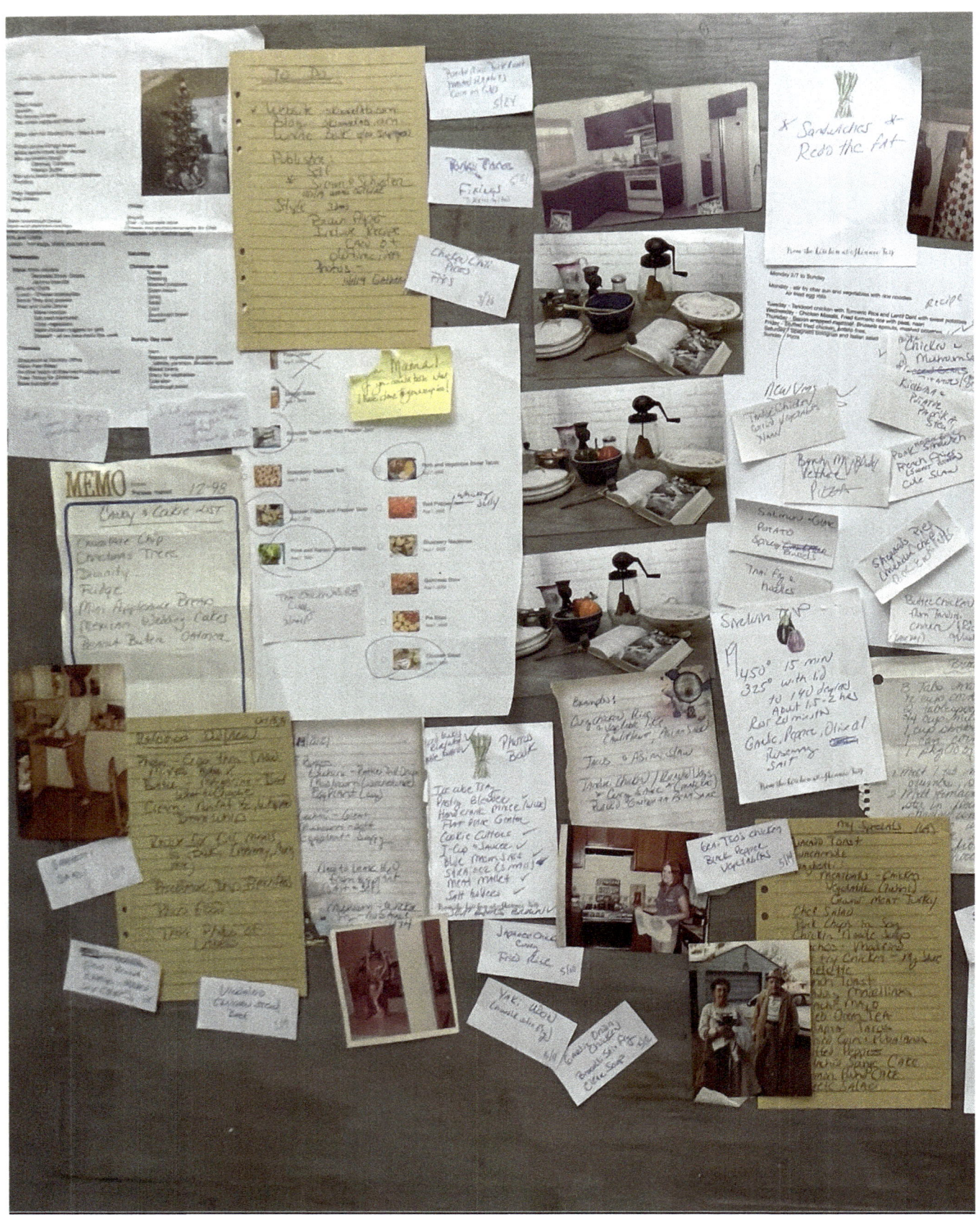

Oh Momma! Where's the Fat?

Copyright 2022 by Pamela Harrell, All Text and Photographs as made a part of the Copyright office records by the United States Register of Copyrights and Director, March 21, 2022.

All rights reserved.

No part of this book may be reproduced or used in any manner without permission of the copyright owner. To request permission, contact the publisher at skinniefats@gmail.com

ISBN: 979-8-9862010-0-9

All Text and Stories written by Pamela Harrell

Edited by Pamela Harrell

Cover art by Pamela Harrell

Photographs by Pamela Harrell

Cover layout design by Kate Camargo

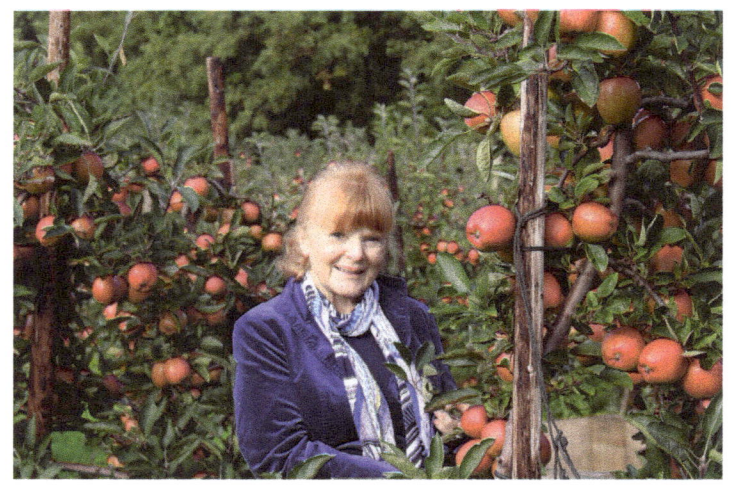

About the Author

Pamela Harrell has been cooking since she was 8 years of age, learning from her grandmother without measurements, but by taste, sight and feel of the food. It was old fashioned cooking with no worries about harmful fats or too much sugar. As an adult, Pamela traveled to Europe where she says she ate and drank her way throughout France and Italy, bringing back experiences and ideas for recipes. After visiting China, Mexico, Scotland and England she added additional flavors and techniques to her style.

Today, Pamela cooks her family's delicious recipes, but has altered them for low saturated fats. She enjoys working with all flavors and ethnics of cooking. She cooks meals for others and has hosted cooking lessons for children called, "Cooking with Gamma". Likewise, she has also provided private cooking lessons for individuals in her kitchen, SkinnieFats. Pamela's recipes can be found on social media platforms under the name SkinnieFats.

Her thoughts on diet are "there are so many diets, and most of my friends and acquaintances who start them, quit them within a month". They are eating foods they would not normally eat. Instead, I like to continue cooking the foods we love, not trying to reinvent the wheel just reducing the saturated fats. It becomes a way of life and fun way to eat with one exception -- saturated fats do not exceed 15 grams per day as recommended by the Heart Association.

Pamela lives with her husband, Robert, and her two dogs, Emmy and Rainey on an island near Charleston, SC.

To my dear husband, Robert, who has been my sounding board, taster, critic and a sideline coach in helping me stay focused and reminding me of my purpose to keep moving forward.

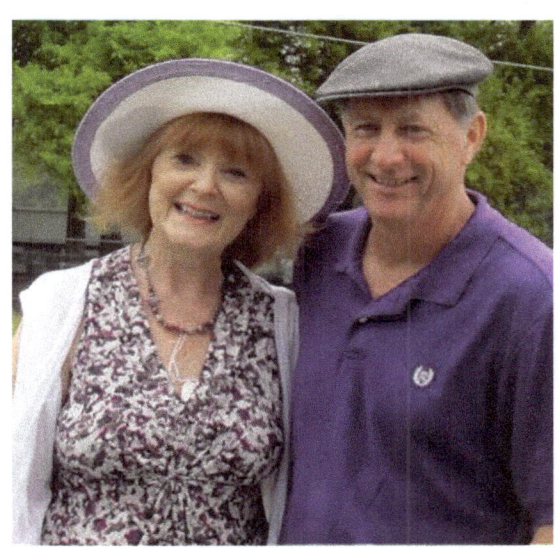

Special Thank You

To all the great and extraordinary women cooks in my family that left me the gift and love of cooking.

To my best friend, Kate, who had virtual coffee with me almost daily to discuss my recipes, give me opinions and be supportive as I continued writing.

To my grandson, Luke, who says my photos make him hungry and told me this book will be family history forever.

To all my granddaughters who I have enjoyed cooking with and teaching their favorite dessert recipes.

And to my son, Nick, who is a great cook himself, and Anabelle, my granddaughter who is the next Harrell family baker.

*

And with a very special thanks to Dr. Looser who saved my husband's life.

*

Pamela

> *Creating healthy recipes is experimenting with foods and flavors. Some are successful and some are not. Then, sometimes you get a whole lot of really good ones.*
>
> *P.L. Harrell*

Contents

Salads 15
Soups & Stews 31
Pasta 47
Pork 65
Chicken & Turkey 83
Vegetables 109
Desserts 131
Fish 155
Beef 165
Burgers 177
Breakfast 185
Beans 195
Seasoning, Marinades and Sauces 201
Common Ingredients 207
Saturated Fat - Reading Labels 207
Converting a Recipe 207
Index 219

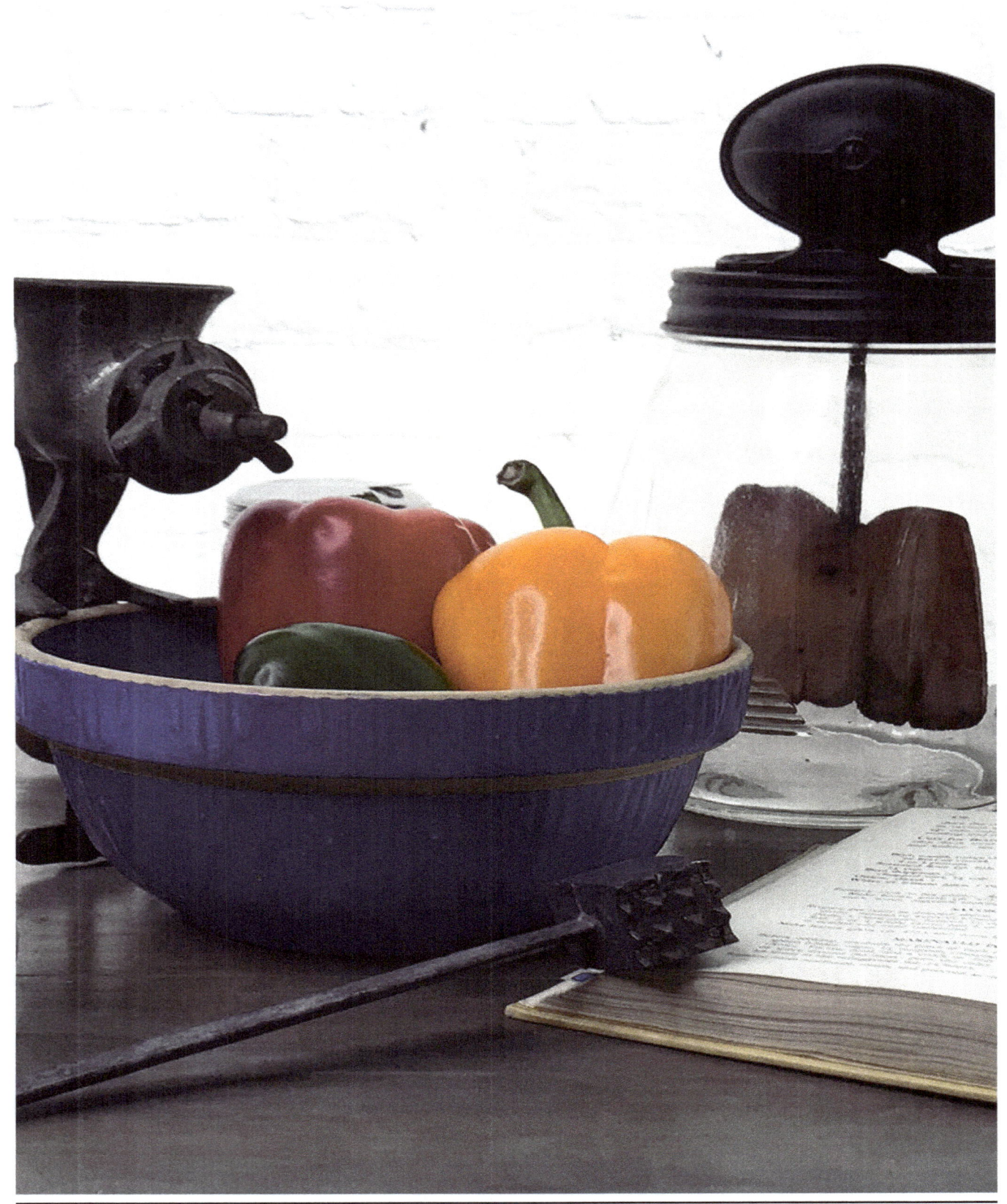

The Skinny on SkinnieFats

When I began revising and creating recipes for less saturated fats, I came up with the terminology, SkinnieFats. I made a comment to my husband that we were going to eat SkinnieFats moving forward, and the name has stuck. The kitchen I create in is called the SkinnieFats kitchen. My blog, Facebook, Instagram and YouTube channels are referred to under the name SkinnieFats.

Oh Momma – Where's the Fat?

My mom, grandmother and all the women in my family who preceded me have passed on. However, during their lifespan, I was able to spend time with all of them and learn from them how to cook and entertain. I learned to cook the 'old fashioned' method - homemade.

I no longer cook like my momma did. I no longer cook like my Mammy did. I no longer cook like all my Aunt's did. Today, I cook with less saturated fats, with different tools and with different ingredients. This cookbook is 'not my mamma's cookbook anymore' but I have taken many of our family recipes and converted them to low saturated fat. All my personal recipes through the years have been converted, and I continue to create recipes with low saturated fat. It has been a challenge. Trial and error, and those recipes that passed my test for cooking and flavor have made it into the first book.

I almost lost my husband to a major blockage on his LAD over New Years, 2019. By January 2, he was grayish in color and very weak. Luckily his doctor caught the signs, tested and scheduled immediate surgery. Instead of me becoming a widow on that day, we had another chance to stay together and enjoy our life.

We both realized that our diets over the years were not as healthy as thought. It was a lot of bad habits made not necessarily by choice, but more by the times in which we grew up.

For me, my father and mother grew up in the depression and during the war had very little to make a meal. My mother never learned to cook as food was too precious for experimenting. When my dad got home from WWII, he made a promise to himself that he would never run out of butter, cream and milk so our family always had plenty of these items always in the refrigerator. Dad taught my mom to cook, and over the years she became a fantastic cook and creator of delicious meals.

My husband's family was similar and lived on a farm in England. If they grew it, they ate it. He, however, was shipped off to boarding school and ate the food provided. When he talks about fried bread in grease for breakfast, it makes my stomach hurt.

So our habits of poor eating started early, and knowing no different, continued through our adulthood. I spent many hours studying the guidelines for healthy heart and everything brought me back to one main component - Saturated Fats. I learned through the American Heart Association, the level of saturated fats we needed on a daily basis. Therefore, I set my goal to 15 grams of saturated fat daily.

Why the Fat?

After my husband's surgery, I cleaned out the refrigerator. I could see tears forming in his eyes as I bagged up all the cheeses, sour creams and full fat creameries and gave them away, along with the steaks, bacon, sausages, hamburgers, hot dog and brats. It was heartbreaking to him, but I was on a mission to make sure we stayed healthy.

It was time to go shopping. I thought, easy enough, but it wasn't. I spent two hours in the grocery store, picking up every item and reading its label to check the content of Saturated Fat. I felt overwhelmed and after having a crying breakdown in the grocery, I went home. I needed a game plan before I went back to the market.

I started looking up "healthy recipes" but was surprised that not everything with "healthy" meant it was heart healthy since many items and recipes contained cheese, full fat milk, creams, and fatty meats. Prepared meals were also the same. So what was I going to do.

I pulled my box of family recipes out of the cupboard and began to go through them. Could I convert them to low saturated fat, and they still taste good. Could I make a pie without lard; make ice cream without cream and milk; make cakes without butter; have a normal Sunday brunch with bacon and eat burgers and French fries again. I realized, I should try to cook them but alter some of the ingredients. Saving the integrity of the recipe and flavors was important, but saving my husband's life was even more important. I was looking through my family recipes and cookbooks that were given to my mother back in the 1940's and my grandmother's recipes. I picked my first experiments to reduce the fat and hoped it would taste as good as the original.

So I began. I wish I had kept track of all the failures as there were many. At one point, I realized some items just could not be recreated with substitutions and be a quality item in my recipes moving forward. However, they could be made new if I could keep the flavor.

I wasn't going to give up. I warned my husband that for the first time since I started cooking at age 8, my meals would be different. Some might not taste as good, but I would make sure at the end of the year, he'd never know the difference. I then went back to the grocery with a list in hand. Luckily, with better preparation, I didn't have a crying meltdown and left the store with all I needed to begin our new meals.

With three years of trial and error, alterations, different methods of cooking and creating new flavors behind me, I now have over 400 recipes to share.

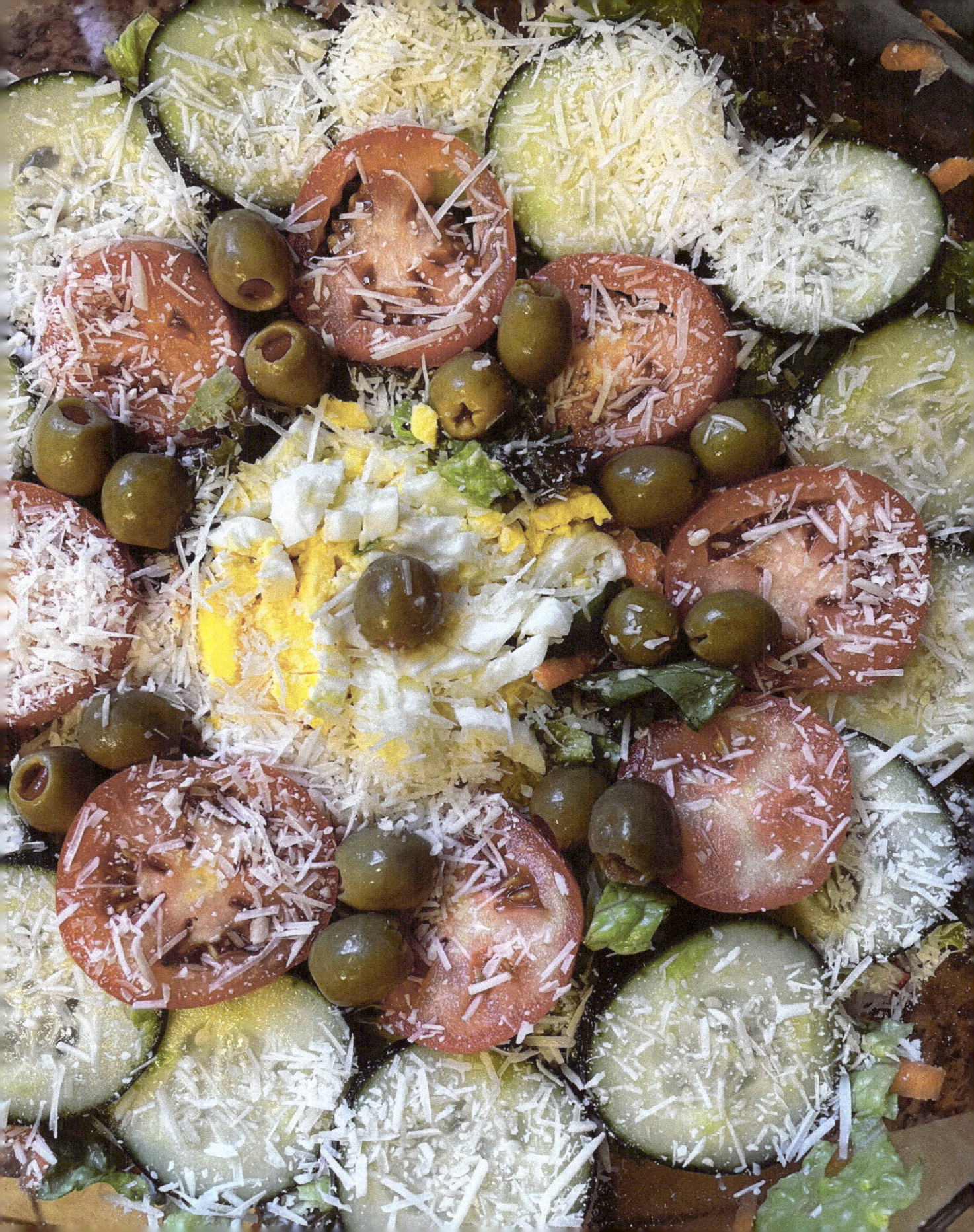

Salads

Chicken & Beets 18
Creamy Broccoli & Apple 19
Seared Pork Strip 20
Taco 22
Cold Slaw 23
Peanut Coleslaw 24
Chef Salad 26
Peanut Butter & Lettuce 27
Niçoise Salad & Tuna 28

There is a Salad for Everyone

Growing up, we had two types of salads: toss salad and endive. We had three types of dressing. My grandmother always and never ventured from her miracle whip and sugar. My dad always had the bright orange, creamy French dressing from the bottle for a toss salad, but had vinegar and oil with sugar for his wilted lettuce salads (endive with hot dressing and bacon bits). Salads were a must at every meal.

Lettuce was never cut with a knife as the old wives tales told stories of knifes touching lettuce and the lettuce turning brown. As a child, of course, a very believable tale. I never thought about it until I was in school and learned about oxidation. We tore lettuce into bite size pieces and the salad was always made in the same bowl. Today, I have the handmade bowl that my Pawpaw mixed and served his wilted lettuce. He was born in 1900 and he made the bowl as a young man. A bowl from Prussia (as marked on the bottom) was my Mammy's dish for her salad. We used those two bowls throughout my childhood as I do now with my family.

Between the fat from the dressings or mayo, pork bacon and the sugar content, I cannot say I ever thought about a salad as anything but healthy. It was lettuce after all. Piling enough dressing on it made it delicious.

Cucumbers were always made with quarter pieces and chopped onion, pepper and soaked in vinegar. Sometimes, I still have the craving but add a few extras like tomatoes and tame the vinegar with a bit of olive oil.

Radishes were some of my favorites, sometimes cut into flower petals on special occasions, but never included in salads. They were on the "trash plate" as my momma called it. My Pawpaw said he never could harvest the radishes in the garden because I would go pull them up, brush them off and eat them before they could be picked. Same with the green onions. My pallet at age 10 was one that enjoyed the spices and heat. The trash plate always had sliced carrots in very even pieces, radishes cut like flower petals, green onions and celery. On very special occasions, a few deviled eggs would grace the plate. The trash plate was an addition to dinner, not a replacement for the salad bowl full of lettuce.

I have evolved from the traditional red/white radishes to also include Daikons. Onions, leeks and shallots fill my pantry. The earthy flavor of shallots, the pungent smell of pickling Daikons and the sweet flavor of leeks enhance flavors in many of my recipes.

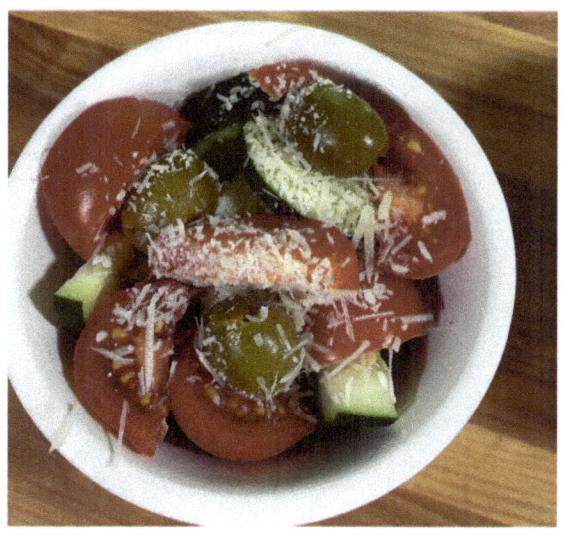
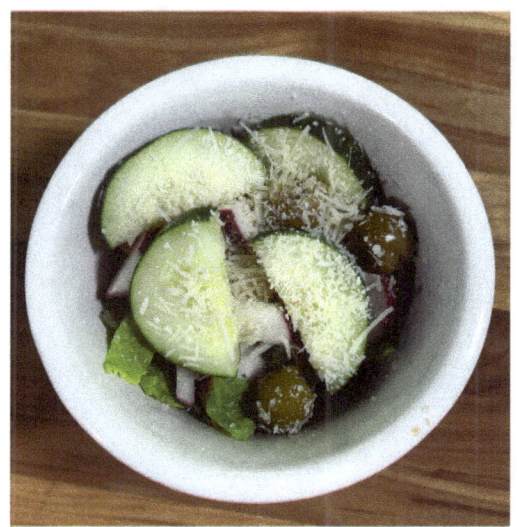

Chicken Salad & Beets

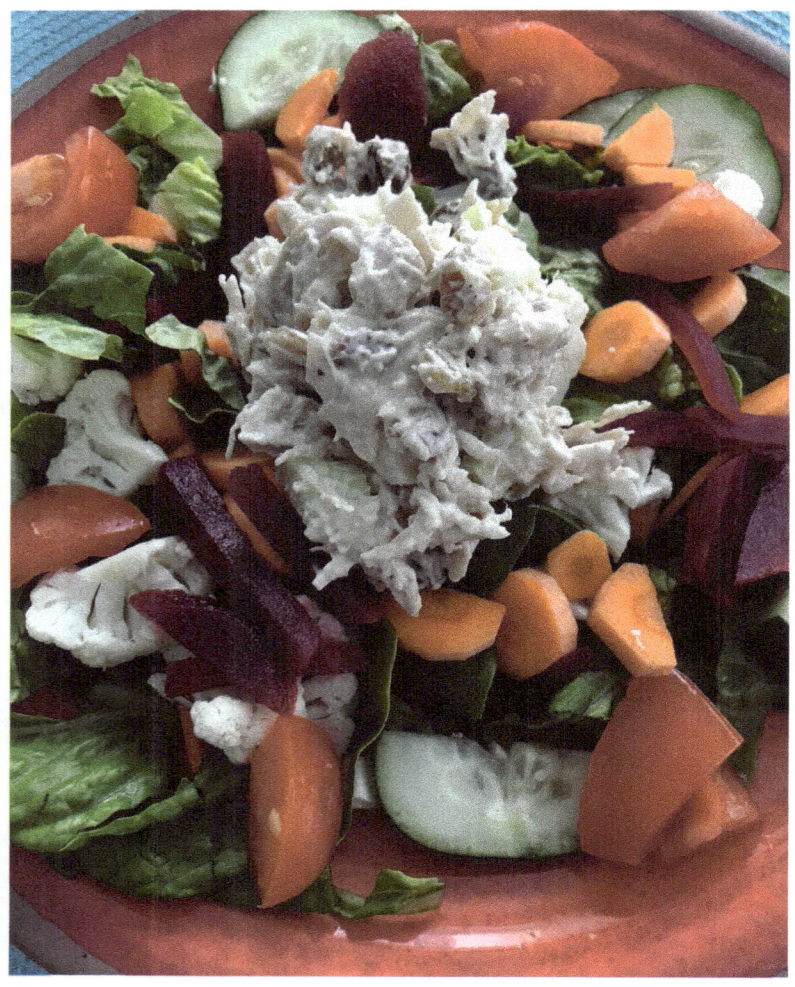

Ingredients (serves 2)

- 1 medium head of Romain, chopped into small pieces
- 1 large carrot, grated
- 1 can sliced beets, drained
- 1small red Roma tomato, sliced
- 1 cup left over chicken (or 1 cup fresh seared chicken breast) - shredded
- 1/4 chopped red or green grapes
- 1/4 cup chopped walnuts
- 1/2 cup olive oil mayonnaise
- 1 teaspoon sugar
- 1 tablespoon Balsamic vinegar
- 1 rib celery chopped
- Salt and Pepper

Chicken Salad in this recipe is one I use quite often and have eaten since I was a teenager - not just on top of salads. It can be stuffed in a pita, put on lettuce leaves and wrapped or eaten on bread or crackers. Adding a teaspoon of curry to the chicken makes a great curry chicken salad,

Method

- Shred the cooked chicken and add the grapes, walnuts, celery, salt and pepper together in a bowl.
- Whisk the mayonnaise, sugar, Balsamic vinegar, salt and pepper together then pour on chicken and mix it very well.
- On a large flat plate or bowl, add the chopped Romain, place tomatoes on lettuce and then add the carrots.
- Scoop some of the chicken salad to the center of the plate. Spoon the drained beets around the chicken salad.

Creamy Broccoli Apple Salad

Ingredients (serves 2)

Salad

- 1 medium head of broccoli, chopped into small pieces
- 1 large carrot, cut into thin strips
- 1 tart apple, cored and chopped
- 1/4 medium yellow onion, chopped fine
- 1/2 cup golden raisins

Dressing

- 1/4 cup low fat mayonnaise (I like the olive oil mayonnaise)
- 1/4 cup non fat sour cream
- 1 tablespoon lemon juice
- 1/4 tablespoon sugar (more or less to taste)
- Dash of salt and white pepper
- Chopped walnuts for topping

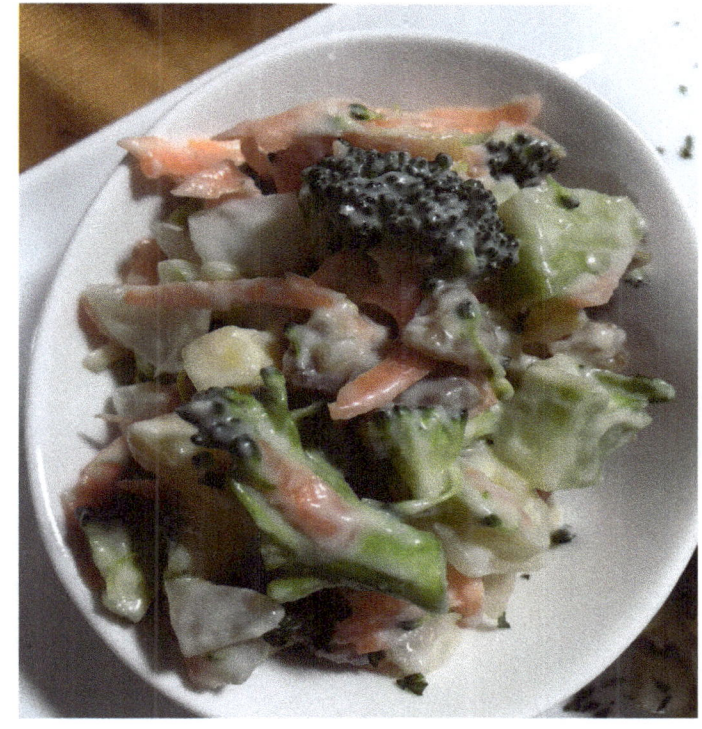

Method

- Put all salad ingredients in a bowl.
- Mix together the dressing ingredients, except the walnuts
- Pour one half of the dressing over the vegetables and mix well. If more is needed, add a little bit at a time and mix to desired consistency.
- Refrigerate for at least 30 minutes prior to serving.
- Sprinkle on walnuts prior to serving

This recipe is modified from my family apple salad recipe which had full fat mayonnaise, lots of sugar and poured over apples, celery and pecans. Now I make it with the apples and add carrots and broccoli and onion as nutritional additions. Sometimes I like to add a few walnuts to the dish.

Seared Pork Strip Salad

One evening, I had a craving for pork chops, which I do not eat often anymore, but really wanted these. I decided to combine the pork with a salad. The pork recipe is one I used for years when I would grill a good bone in chop. The marinade for the pork infuses a great amount of flavor. I like this without dressing, but make or choose a flavorful non fat dressing if desired.

Ingredients

- 2 boneless, lean pork loins
- Romain lettuce, 1 head, chopped in small pieces
- A few leaves of spinach leaves
- 1 can black beans (I like to add a few chopped green chilies, but it is optional)
- 3 carrots chopped
- 1 cup frozen corn, thawed
- 2 medium tomatoes, chopped
- 1 small onion, chopped
- 1/2 cup no fat shredded Cheddar cheese
- Non fat dressing of choice

For The Pork Marinade

- 2 cloves garlic, peeled and chopped
- 1/2 teaspoon chili powder
- 1/2 teaspoon salt
- 1/2 teaspoon pepper
- 1/2 teaspoon ground cumin
- 1/2 teaspoon dried oregano
- 2 tablespoons Olive Oil

Cook The Pork

- Mix all the spices except garlic.
- Rub the spice mixture on both sides of the pork loin chops and marinate 1-2 hours.
- Pour oil in pan and when heated, sear garlic until very light brown. Watch the garlic closely as it will burn easily.
- Add the chops to the pan and cook on each side until brown and tender. Internal temperature of the pork loins (depending on thickness) should reach 165.
- Remove from pan to cutting board. Let rest 5 minutes then slice into thin slices.

Assembling the salad

- Place a generous helping of Romain lettuce in a bowl.
- Add the black beans, sprinkling across the Romain.
- Add the carrots, corn, tomatoes, onion alternately across the beans and lettuce.
- Sprinkle the top with the non fat cheddar cheese.
- Lay the pork strips on top. They will be very tender so lay them carefully.
- Add your favorite non fat dressing, if desired.

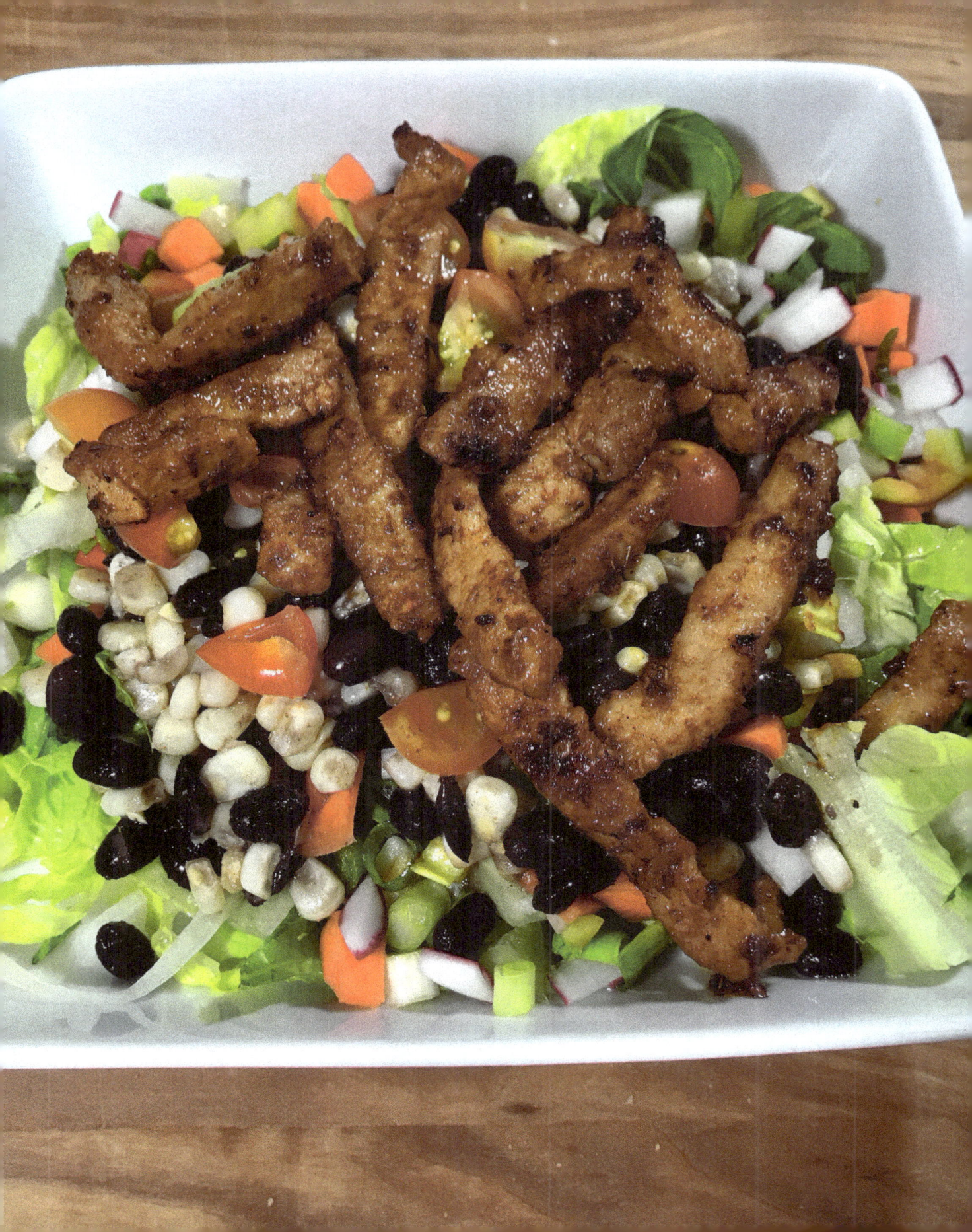

Taco Salad

Ingredients (2-4 Servings)

- 1 head Romain lettuce, chopped
- 1 can seasoned black beans
- 1 can vegetarian refried beans
- 1 large tomato, chopped
- 1/2 cup non fat cheddar cheese
- 1 medium onion, chopped
- 1 bag low fat, low sodium Taco Chips
- Your favorite Salsa and Hot sauces
- 1/4 cup pickled Jalapenos

Assembly

- Start by placing taco chips on bottom of a plate in a single layer.
- In any order you want, assemble the rest of the ingredients.
- Top with hot black beans and/or refried beans
- Top with Romain lettuce.
- Add the onion and jalapenos.
- Sprinkle with chopped tomatoes
- Top with Salsa and hot sauces
- Sprinkle the cheeses all over

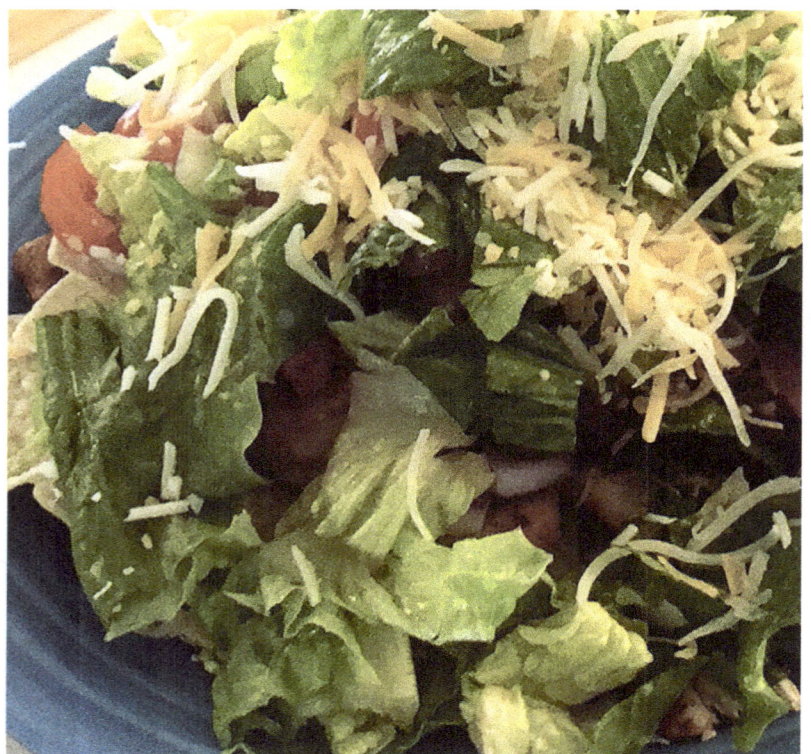

Taco salad is my go to on a night when I get home late, too tired to cook, but still need something full of protein and vegetables. This is the basic beginning of my Taco Salad. Cooked ground turkey or ground chicken add great protein to this salad.

Original Family Cold Slaw

In my Midwestern family, we made and ate Cold Slaw, and it wasn't until I entered college that I learned my family recipe wasn't cold slaw, but coleslaw. However, I still refer to it as cold slaw.

My great aunt Vivian, my grandmother's younger sister, made the best coleslaw. Because we ate a lot of cooked cabbage, when she made it slaw that was refrigerated, she referred to it as Cold Slaw.

It was always my dad's favorite and quickly became all of our favorites. Never did she serve a meal without her "cold slaw"

Prepare the Cabbage & Drain

Make Dressing and let cool.

Add dressing, mix and enjoy.

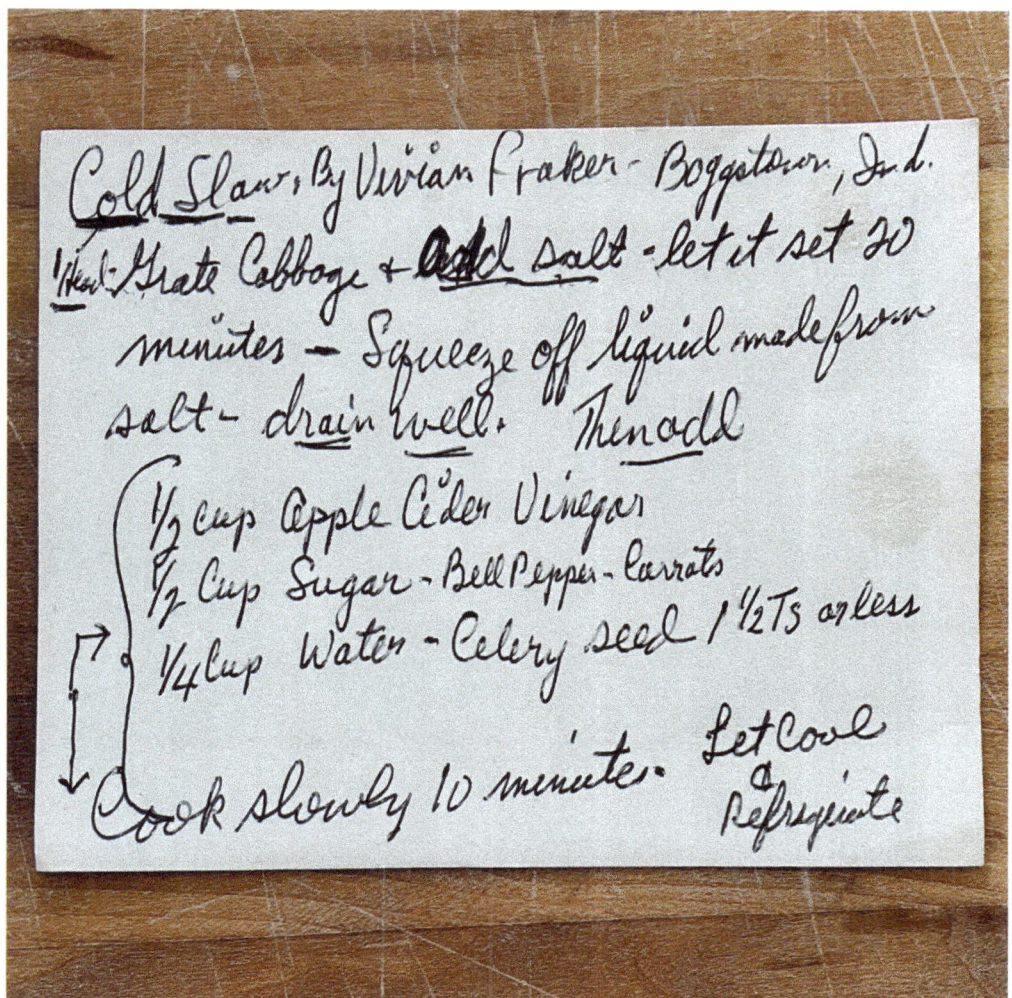

Cold Slaw, By Vivian Fraker - Boggstown, Ind.

1 Head - Grate Cabbage + Add salt - let it set 30 minutes - Squeeze off liquid made from salt - drain well. Then add

½ cup Apple Cider Vinegar
½ Cup Sugar - Bell Pepper - Carrots
¼ cup Water - Celery seed 1 ½ Ts or less

Cook slowly 10 minutes. Let Cool & Refrigerate

Oh Momma! Where's the Fat?

Asian Peanut Coleslaw

Ingredients for Slaw

- 1 head cabbage (about 4-5 cups)
- 1 red bell pepper
- 1 orange bell pepper
- 2 carrots
- 1 medium onion

Ingredients for Dressing

- 6 tablespoons rice wine vinegar
- 6 tablespoons olive oil
- 5 tablespoons low fat, creamy peanut butter
- 3 tablespoons low sodium soy sauce
- 3 tablespoons brown sugar
- 2 tablespoons finely chopped ginger root
- 1-2 small garlic cloves, finely minced

Method for Slaw

- Shave the cabbage in long thin strips, then cut in half.
- Slice the red and orange peppers in narrow strips.
- Grate the carrots.
- Dice the onion into fine pieces.
- Place all in a colander and rinse very well with cold water. Drain well and soak up extra moisture with paper towel.
- Remove to a serving bowl and keep cool until time to serve.

Method for Dressing

- Combine all dressing ingredients in a mixing bowl.
- Using a wise, mix thoroughly.
- Mixture will be creamy and smooth. Do not refrigerate dressing

To Serve

- Pour the dressing onto the slaw.
- Mix thoroughly with a fork so all slaw mixture is covered.
- Serve immediately, or cover and refrigerate to serve later.

The first time I ate warm peanut butter with cabbage was a little restaurant in San Francisco that had a peanut dressing served over Napa cabbage as an appetizer. It was a combination of sweet and nutty.

Today, I make a similar dressing as a topping for my steak or fish tacos. Sometimes, I make it as a stand alone cole slaw for summer cookouts. It is always a favorite. I reduced the saturated fats by using low fat peanut butter and added more seasonings such as peppers and onions for flavor.

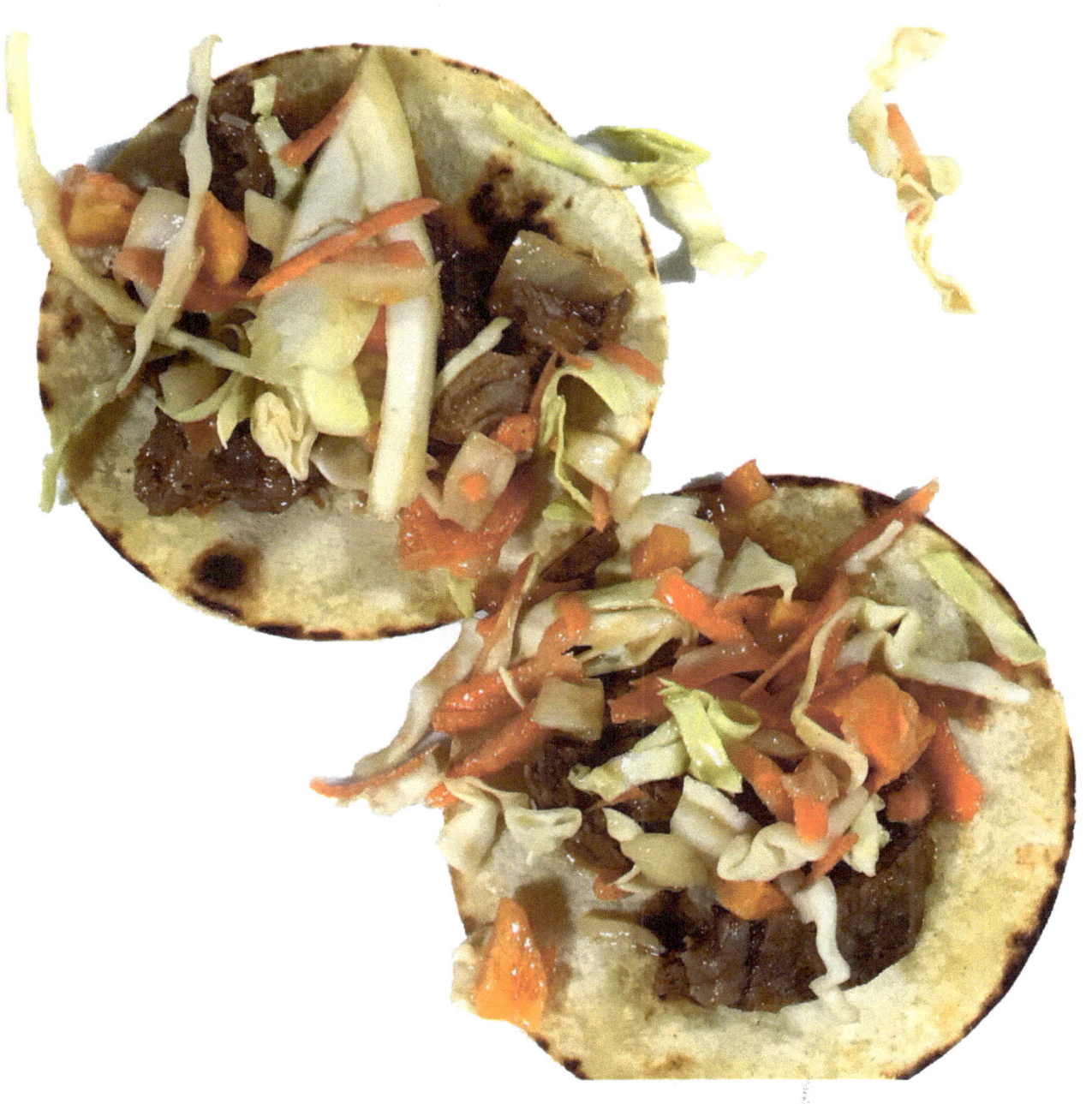

Shown above is the slaw on grilled tortillas topped with top loin stir fried steak strips.

It is also delicious on fish tacos, grilled turkey hot dogs, grilled lean pork or turkey burgers.

I have served it as a stand alone salad side dish at BBQ's.

Go ahead and try it on many different recipes.

My Go To Chef Salad

My go to salad is a Chef Salad, typically made from all the left over fresh produce in my refrigerator that needs to be eaten. Quite the difference from the salads my mammy and dad made except for one thing - the blue bowl that my papaw made in the early 1900's is still used for my salads today.

Anything goes with a chef salad - just remember to use non fat dressing as your topping.

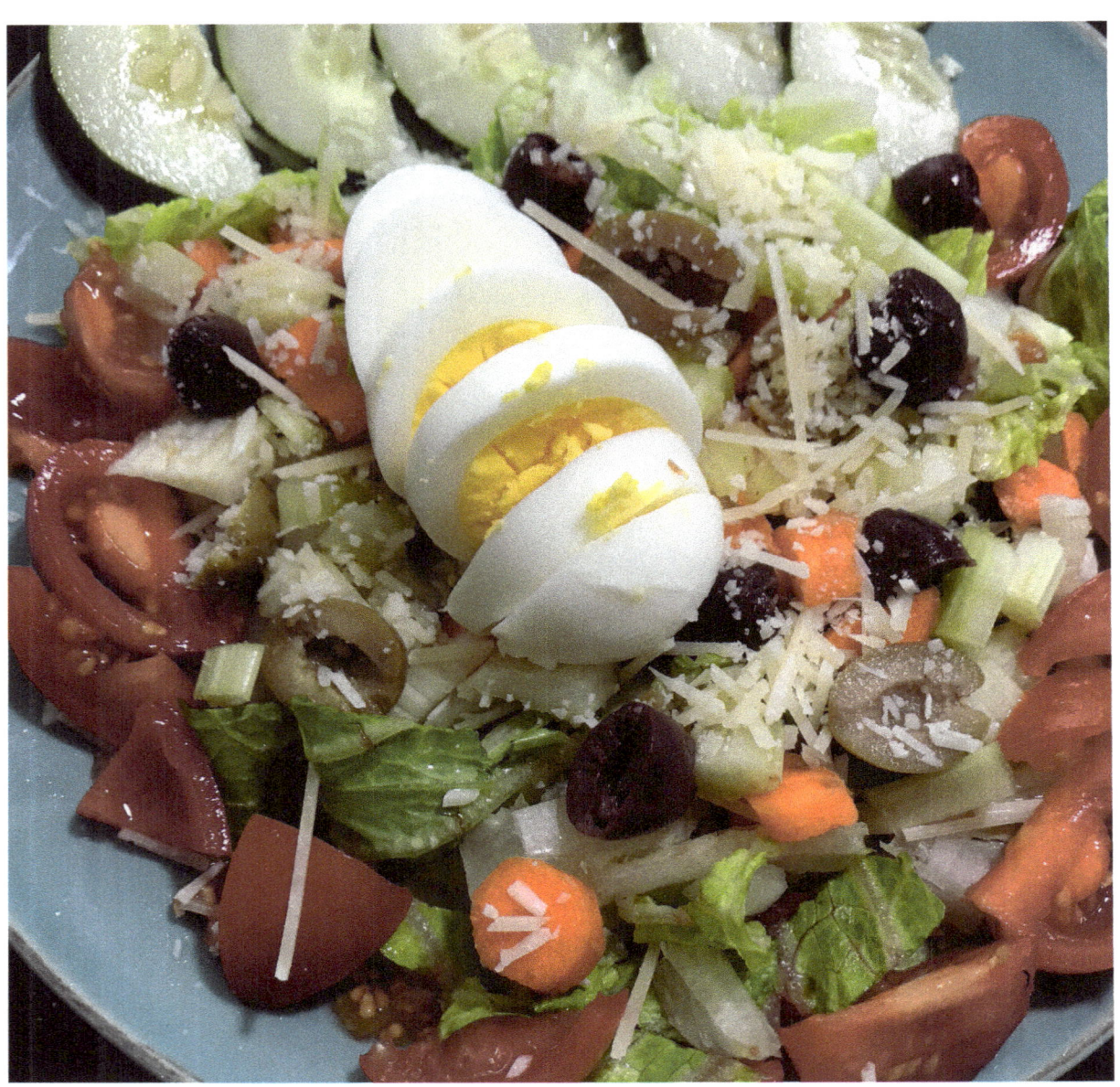

Peanut Butter Lettuce Sandwich

Sunday afternoons were a treat when my dad was not working. Owning his own business kept him away most of the days during the week and even on some weekends. However, during the summer months, we would spend the afternoon eating special sandwiches together while watching golf tournaments.

Not only did I learn a lot about golf and the greats like Arnold Palmer, Jack Nicklaus, Gary Player and all my dad's favorites, but I also learned how to make his very special sandwich.

> *Ingredients Per Sandwich*
>
> *Peanut Butter, Creamy style*
> *White Bread, 2 slices*
> *Quarter wedge of washed and chilled iceberg lettuce*
> *Butter*

Dad would start by buttering one piece of bread for each of us. On the other slice of the bread, he would then layer on the creamy smooth peanut butter, never skimping on the peanut butter, and I remember it being meticulously spread evenly from the middle to all four edges of the crust. When asked about the careful spreading of ingredients, dad replied, "Every bite into the sandwich must have the flavor of all ingredients." Pieces of fresh, cold and crisp wedge of lettuce were placed on the buttered side of bread. The peanut butter piece of bread topped the sandwich. Dad always cut bread in half on the diagonal, in even pieces and put it on our sandwich plates. I would have a glass of milk, and he would have his Tom Collins, and we would watch the golf tournament together enjoying a great Sunday afternoon.

Today, I do not eat a lot of peanut butter due to the saturated fat, but I have been lucky to find a low fat version of peanut butter that is quite satisfying. And while I do not use real butter anymore opting for the low fat margarine spread, I still make these sandwiches and every so often put them in my lunch pail for work.

Niçoise Salad & Tuna

Ingredients (makes two Salads)

- 12 Romain Leaves
- 4 Radishes, trimmed, washed & sliced
- 2 Eggs for medium hard boil
- 6 small Dutch potatoes for boiling
- 6-8 asparagus tips, washed and chopped
- Six slices cucumber, each slice and cut in half
- 10 green pitted olives (green or black)
- 6 green beans, trimmed, but not cut.
- 1 can tuna packed in Olive oil, drained

Method

- Put the potatoes into a pan of water, bring to the boil and cook for 10 minutes until they are tender but still holding their shape. Drain and set aside in a large bowl to cool.
- Add the eggs and green beans to the same water that potatoes were boiled in and cook for 6-8 minutes. Remove from heat, drain and place green beans in a bowl to cool.
- Place eggs in a bowl with cold water, let set a few minutes, then peel.
- Chop up a few radishes, trim the asparagus tips and wash and drain 12 Romain leaves.

Assembly

- Place six Romain leaves on the plate.
- Scatter a few of the asparagus tips on the lettuce.
- Scatter radishes, onions, cucumbers and green beans over the lettuce.
- Add 1/2 can drained tuna to the top of the leaves.
- Cut the potatoes in half and place decoratively on plate.
- Using an egg slicer, slice one egg and place on plate.
- Add a few olives on plate.
- Drizzle with oil and vinegar, and season with salt and pepper.
- Or, drizzle with non-fat Italian dressing.

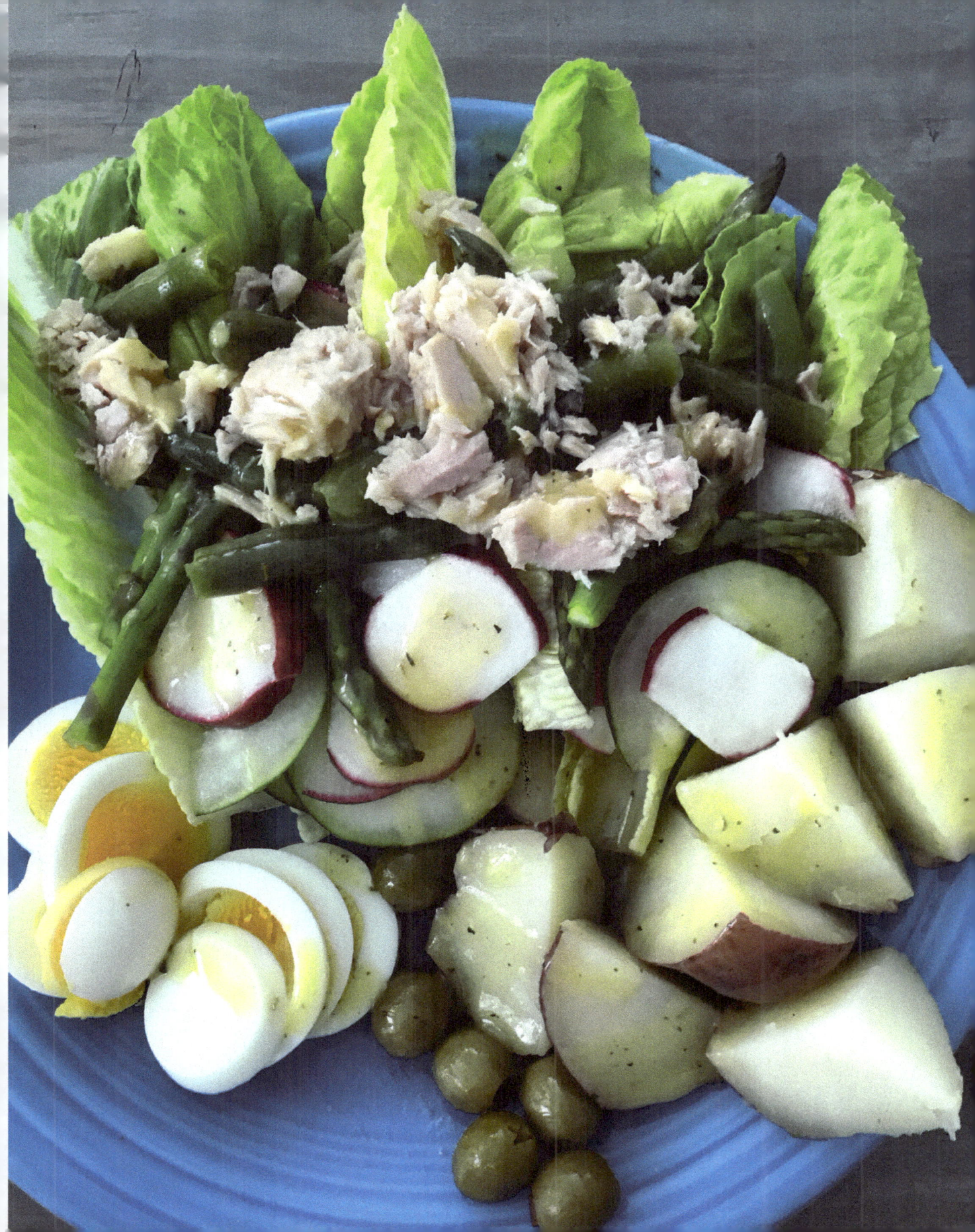

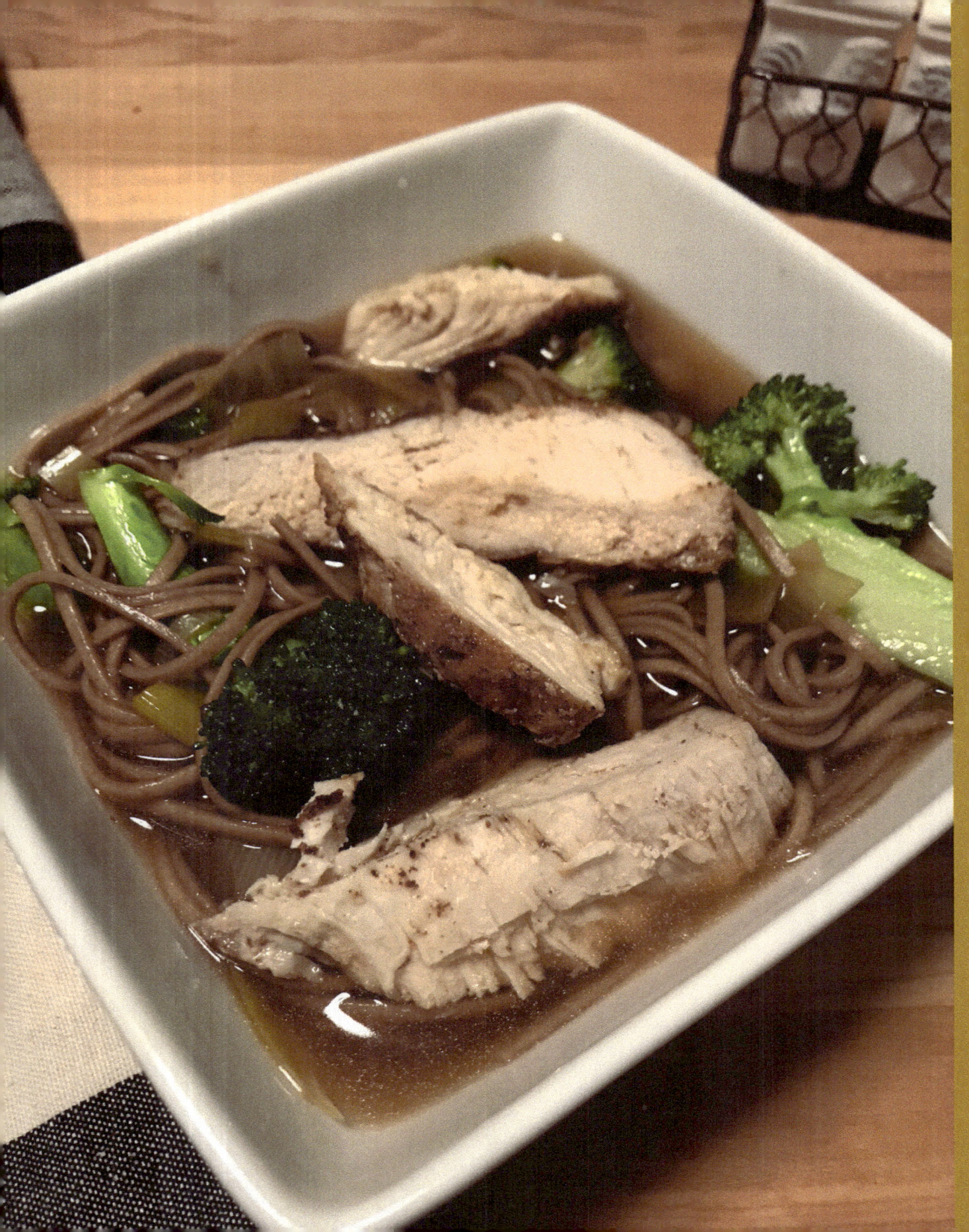

Soups & Stews

Mom's Chili 32

Turkey & Bean Chili 33

Butternut Squash Soup 34

Old Fashioned Chicken Noodle 35

Over the Top Chicken Ramen 36

Kielbasa & Turkey Chili 38

Chicken Potato Stew 39

Curried Vegetable & Chick Pea 40

Potato & Leek 42

Island Chili 43

Ground Turkey & Vegetable 45

Mom's Chili

I love and look forward to the Fall Season. When I was growing up in the mid-west fall always meant soups and stews as major players at the dinner table.

My mom used the same oval cast iron pot for all her stews and soups. It was huge, heavy and had been seasoned over 30 years. It barely fit on the burner of the stove, taking up almost two spaces for cooking. The pot had been my dad's mom's but given to my mom when they married.

One of mom's specialty soups was chili. She called it soup because it was the consistency of soup. It was delicious. Ground beef and kidney beans made up the bulk of the soup, plus a couple chopped onions and a pint or two of my mammy's home canned tomatoes. A few tablespoons of chili powder would be added and a small amount of salt and pepper.

I always knew chili was cooking for dinner as the sweet smell of the soup was noticeable from the sidewalk as I walked home from school.

The chili was never eaten alone. A pot of fresh cooked macaroni noodles would be sitting next to the chili. The routine was a scoop of noodles; then 1-2 scoops of sauce over the top. It was always accompanied with crackers, butter and/or peanut butter.

Today my chili has evolved. My sauces are thicker, and the ingredients vary. I use anything from ground turkey, chopped kielbasa sausage (made from turkey meat), chicken or all beans as the base. Peppers of all varieties are selected which can include poblanos, green, yellow, orange or red peppers, jalapeños, or a few banana peppers - no pepper is off limits in my chili. On some occasions, the chili is served on pasta noodles or a baked potato or just by itself in a bowl.

Turkey Chili & Beans

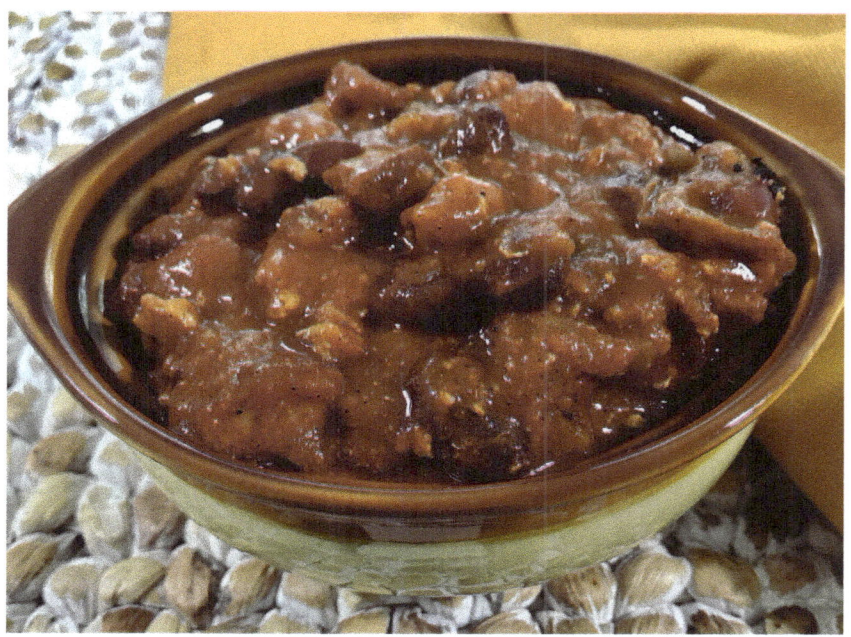

Ingredients (Serves 6)

- 1 pound lean ground turkey
- 1 large can tomato sauce
- 1 medium can tomato paste
- 2 cans water (use tomato paste can)
- 2 cans chopped tomatoes with chilies (mild or hot is your choice)
- ½ cup chili powder
- 1 green and yellow pepper, chopped
- 1 large onion, chopped
- 1 can chili beans with sauce
- 1 can kidney beans, drained
- 1 jalapeno pepper, sliced and seeds removed, chopped fine (optional)
- 1-2 tablespoons Hungarian Paprika
- Black Pepper
- Sea Salt, fine ground
- Olive Oil or Canola oil in a spray can

Method

- Take out a large Dutch Oven or Stock Pot and spray it lightly on the bottom.
- Place ground turkey in the pot and brown over medium heat. Stir to break up the pieces of turkey as it cooks.
- When the meat is light brown, add the onion, green pepper and jalapeno pepper. Stir until onion becomes translucent.
- Add the beans, tomato sauce, tomato paste, water and tomatoes to the pot. Add the chili powder, to taste.
- Add salt and pepper to taste.
- Stir well. Put the lid on the pot and cook on medium heat until it starts to boil.
- Turn heat down to simmer.
- Simmer 1-2 hours, stirring occasionally.

Butternut Squash Soup

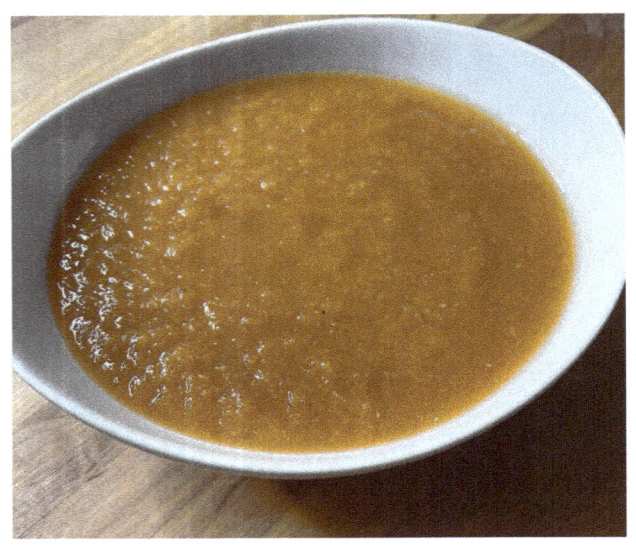

Fall is a time of year when I like to take advantage of the great vegetables available that are fresh. Butternut Squash is very plentiful. Whether I am using it for soup, or adding it in curries or stuffing one, it is always a favorite.

Ingredients (Serves 6)

- 1 medium butternut squash, peeled, seeded and cut into cubes
- 1 medium onion, chopped
- 1 stalk celery, chopped
- 2 medium/large golden potatoes, chopped
- 1 box (32 ounces) vegetable stock
- 2 Tablespoons of olive oil
- 1 teaspoon fresh rosemary or 1/2 teaspoon dried
- Salt (I like the fine ground pink Himalayan)
- Ground White Pepper (you can use black but the flecks will show in the soup)

Method

- Use a heavy pan or Dutch oven and pour in the olive oil and set heat at medium.
- Once oil has heated, add the onion, celery, carrots, potatoes and squash.
- Let the vegetables sear in the oil and stir them as they brown very slightly.
- Pour in the vegetable stock to cover vegetables and bring to a boil.
- Reduce heat to low, cover pot and simmer until vegetables are soft, about 40 minutes.
- Once vegetables are done, use your Immersion blender and blend until the vegetables form a smooth and thick creamy soup. If you do not have a hand held Immersion blender, in batches, transfer vegetables and broth to a blender and blend until smooth. This will take a few batches to get it all done. Return to Dutch oven and keep warm.
- Add the salt and pepper and rosemary once blended. Stir well.
- Serve with a sprinkle of Parsley or Chopped Chives on top.

Old Fashioned Chicken Noodle Soup

Ingredients (Serves 2)

- One large chicken breast
- 2 chopped carrots
- 2 celery stalks chopped
- Parsley to taste (I like medium amount)
- Salt and Pepper
- 1 tablespoons of dried Thyme
- 1 32 ounce or more box of chicken broth
- 1 package pre-made egg noodles (or make homemade)

Method

- Add a tablespoon or so of Olive oil to a pot and heat on medium.
- Add the cut up chicken breast and cook until tender. I like to sear the pieces so there is a bit of brown on the outside.
- Add the carrots, celery, seasoning and chicken broth to the pot, stirring all together.
- Bring to a low boil and then simmer for about 1 hour.
- Add 1 cup of dry noodles to the simmering mix. I like flat medium width noodles, but all of them are good.
- Mix well and let cook per package Method.
- If you like the soup thinner, add more broth.
- If you like it more thick, add a bit more noodles.

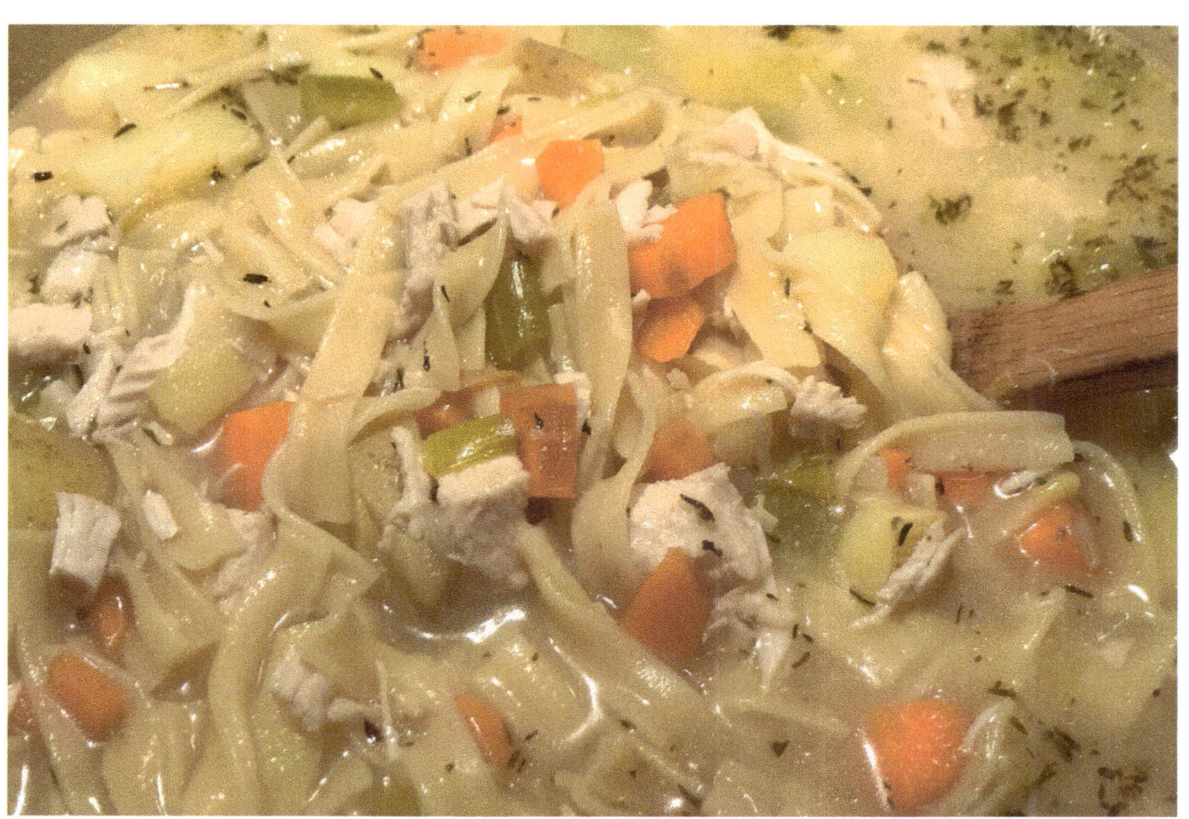

Over the Top Chicken Ramen Soup

Ingredients (Serves 2)

- For the Soup
- 1 medium sliced onion
- 4 ounces sliced shiitake mushrooms
- 1/2-3/4 pounds baby bok choy, sliced (use the whole bok choy)
- 1 pound boneless, skinless chicken breast,
- 1 tablespoon grated ginger root or 1 teaspoon powder
- 4 medium/large cloves of garlic, peeled and chopped
- 1 tablespoon chili garlic sauce
- 2 tablespoons oyster sauce
- 1 tablespoon fish sauce
- 1/2 cup low sodium soy sauce
- 1/4 cup rice vinegar
- 4 cups low sodium chicken broth
- 1 cup water
- 2 packages roman noodles without seasoning

For the Eggs

- 2 eggs
- 1/4 cup low sodium soy sauce
- 1/4 cup rice vinegar
- 3/4 cup water

Toppings (Optional)

- Sliced green onion
- Chopped Cilantro
- Toasted Sesame seeds
- Lime wedges
- Chili Garlic Sauce

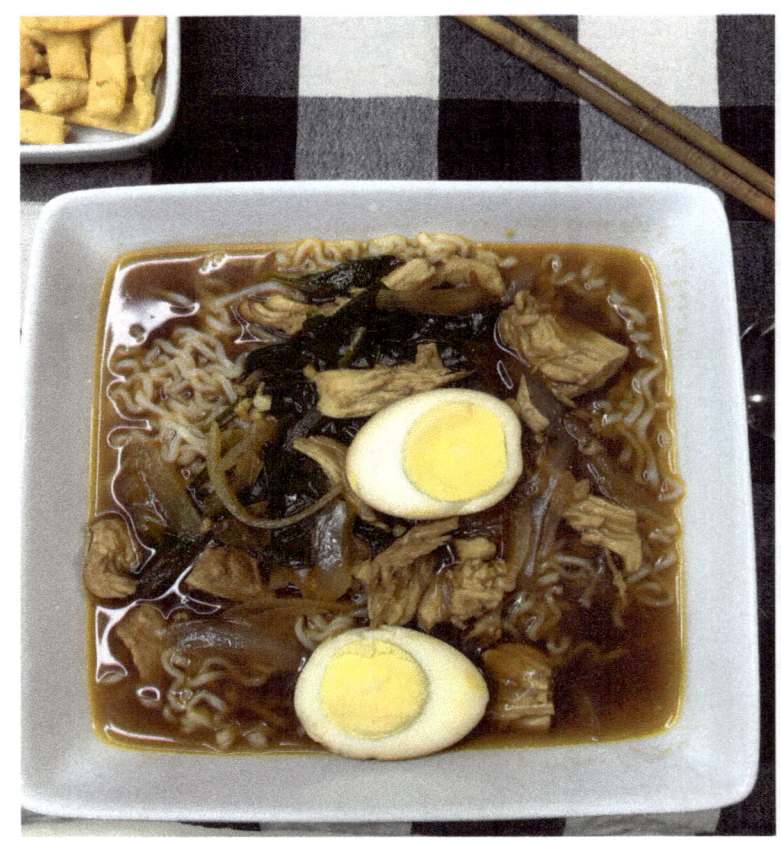

My husband named this soup the first time I created and served it to him. He was so impressed by the mingling of the flavors and how all the ingredients worked together, he said, "This is Over the Top! Be sure you write this one down so you can make it often just like you did tonight."

Method for the Eggs (they will need to marinate 2-3 hours or overnight)

- Place the eggs in a pot and cover with water.
- Bring the water to a boil and boil 7 minutes. Use a spoon to remove eggs from water and let cool.
- Whisk the soy, vinegar and water together in a bowl to make a marinade.
- Peel eggs and place them in the bowl of marinade. The eggs should be covered completely. Chill in refrigerator for 2-3 hours or overnight for more flavor.

Method for the Chicken

- In a shallow skillet, place one tablespoon olive oil and heat. Take the sliced chicken, put in the hot oil and brown it lightly on each side. This will sear and seal the juices into the chicken. Do not overcook chicken or it will become tough. Remove from the pan to a hot plate until time to add to the soup.

Method for Noodles

- Heat a pot with water and once boiling, add the ramen packages of noodles.
- Stir gently to break apart the noodles.
- Let cook 2-3 minutes, then turn off heat and drain the noodles. Do not rinse noodles

Method for the Soup

- Heat a pot or Dutch oven with 1-2 tablespoons of olive oil.
- Add onion and saute until translucent. Add mushrooms, garlic and ginger and let saute another 1-2 minutes.
- Add the chicken broth, sauces and water and stir to combine.
- When the sauce begins to simmer, add the browned chicken pieces. Simmer 15-20 minutes until chicken is cooked through.
- Remove the chicken and shred it using a fork. Add chicken and Bok choy back to sauce.
- Simmer until bok choy is soft - typically 3-5 minutes.
- Remove from heat.

To serve the Ramen

- Place a serving of noodles in a bowl.
- Top with the Soup mixture.
- Slice one of the hard boiled eggs in half and place on top of the soup and add topping.

Kielbasa & Turkey Chili

Ingredients (Serves 4-6)

- 1 pound lean ground turkey
- 1 pound turkey kielbasa, chopped in small pieces
- 1 large can tomato sauce
- 1 medium can tomato paste
- 2 can water (use tomato paste can)
- 2 cans chopped tomatoes with chilies
- ½ cup chili powder
- 1 green pepper, chopped
- 1 large onion, chopped
- 1 cans chili beans
- 1 can kidney beans
- 1 jalapeno pepper, sliced and seeds removed, chopped
- Black Pepper and Salt

Method

- Place ground pork and sausage in a very large Dutch oven and brown over medium heat.
- Add all other ingredients and mix well.
- Bring to boil.
- Simmer 1-2 hours, stirring occasionally.

Serving:

- Serve by itself in a bowl.
- Serve over a baked potato and top with fat free shredded cheddar
- Serve with tortilla chips or low fat crackers of choice

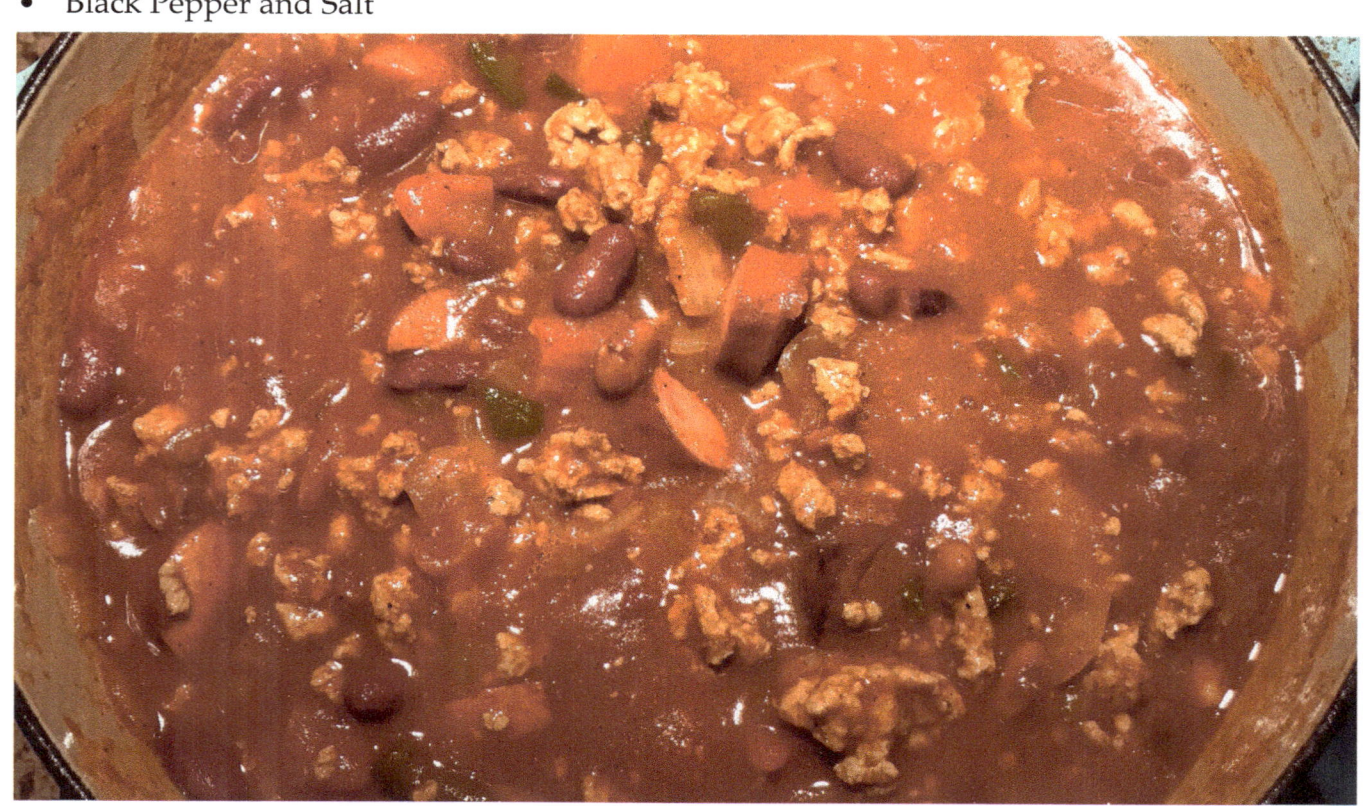

Chicken Potato Stew

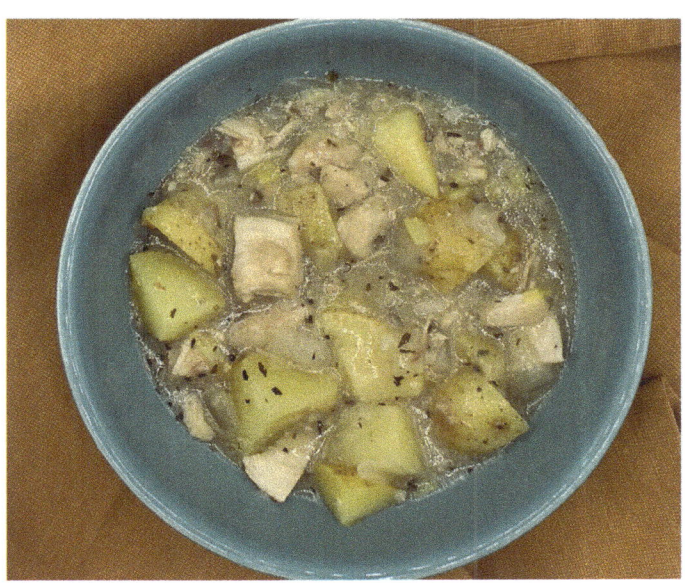

Ingredients (Serves 4)

- 2 chicken breasts cut in bite size pieces
- 2 tablespoons extra-virgin olive oil
- 1 medium onion, chopped
- 2-4 Golden potatoes cut in bite size pieces
- 2 stalks celery, minced
- 1/2 tsp Thyme
- 1/2 tsp rosemary
- Kosher salt to taste
- Freshly ground black pepper
- 4 cups low-sodium chicken (or vegetable) broth
- 2 cups water (if needed). Wait until soup has simmered and then add a little more water if necessary.
- ½ large head cabbage, chopped or shredded. The larger chopped pieces hold up to the long simmer. (Optional)
- 2 tbsp. freshly chopped parsley for garnish (optional)

Method

- In a large pot (or Dutch oven) over on medium heat olive oil and add chicken. Cook until tender. Then add onion, celery and potatoes. Stir for 3-5 minutes.
- Add the spices and cabbage and stir for 1-2 minutes.
- Add the broth, cover and let simmer for 1 hour.
- Remove from heat and serve. Top with parsley if desired.

Easy and Quick comfort food for a cool night. Three ingredients plus low sodium broth. The leftovers do not freeze as well as other soups.

Curried Vegetable and Chick Pea Stew

Ingredients

- 1 tablespoon olive oil
- 1 large white or yellow onion
- 1 teaspoon kosher salt
- 2 medium yellow potatoes
- 1 teaspoon curry powder
- 1 teaspoon ginger
- 3 large cloves garlic, chopped
- 1 tablespoon Mina Harissa Spicy Sauce (optional, but adds good heat and flavor)
- 2 teaspoons Ancho Chili pepper (less if you do not want super spicy)
- 1 teaspoon Garam Marsala
- 1 Teaspoon Cumin
- 1/4 teaspoon Coriander
- 1/2 teaspoon Cardamom
- 2 cups low sodium vegetable broth
- 2 cans chickpeas
- 2 medium carrots, cut in 3/4 inch pieces
- 1 small Broccoli head, cut in bite sized pieces
- 1 12 ounce can diced tomatoes (for a spicy flavor, use fire roasted can tomatoes)
- 1 cup low fat coconut milk
- Parsley for topping
- Chutney for topping

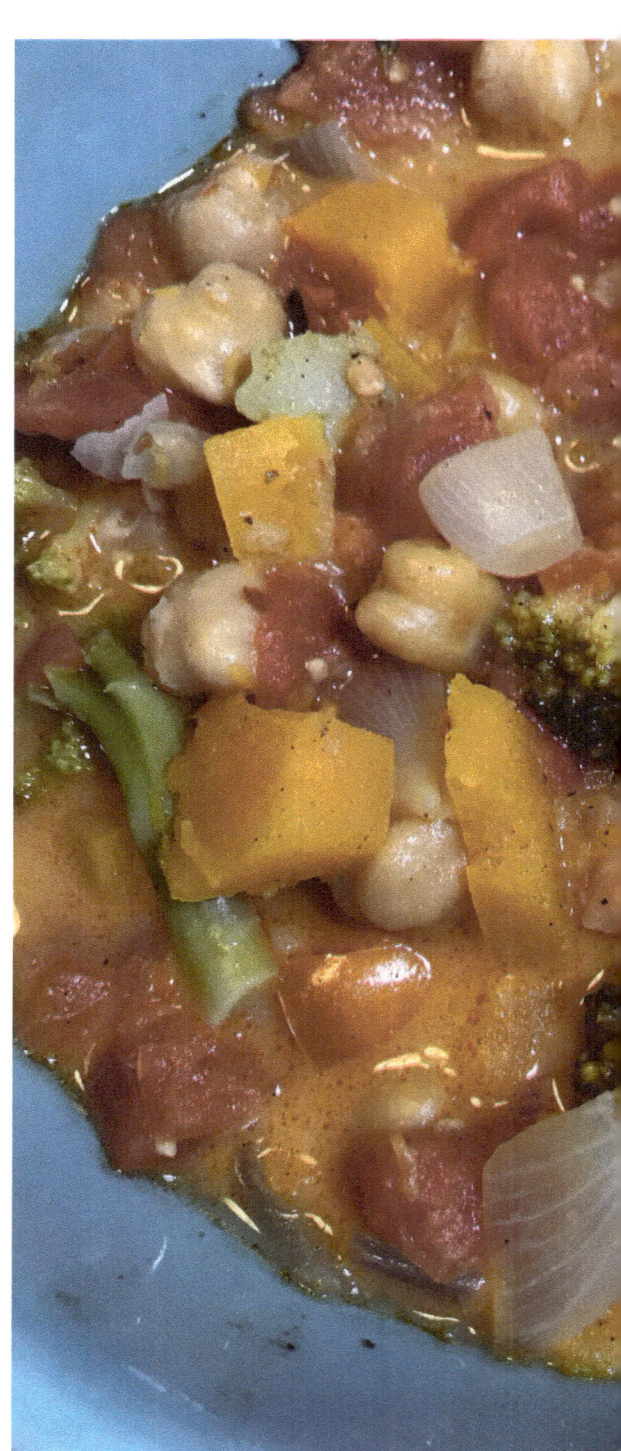

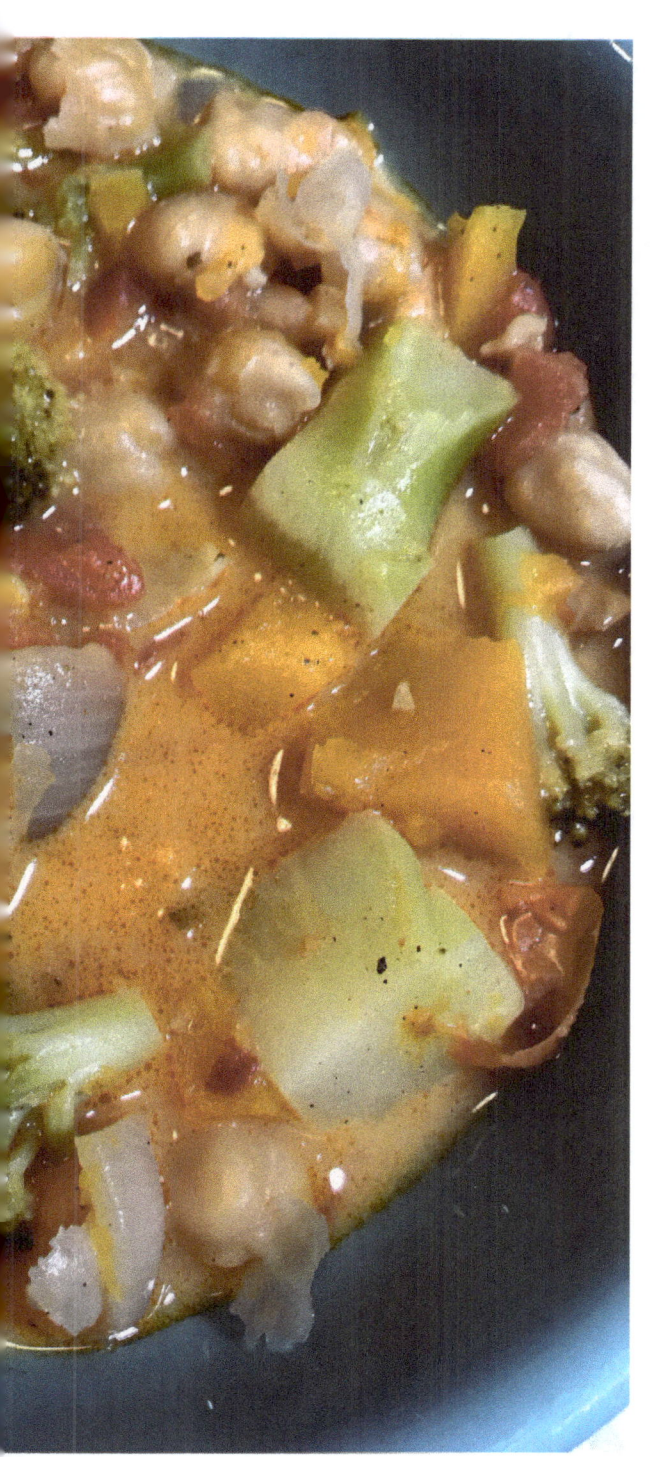

Method

- Place olive oil in medium stock pot or Dutch oven and turn heat to medium.
- Add the onion and stir until it starts to become translucent
- Add all the spices (curry, ginger, garlic, chili pepper, garam marsala, cumin, coriander, Cardamom) and cook about 30-45 seconds.
- Add the potatoes and stir well with spices and onions.
- Add the Mina Harissa Spicy Sauce (optional, but adds good heat and flavor)
- Add the vegetable broth, chickpeas, red and green peppers and the can of tomatoes.
- Cook for 15 minutes on medium low heat
- Add the cauliflower and coconut milk.
- Cook on medium low heat until potatoes and cauliflower fork tender.
- Add more salt to taste and a few grinds of black pepper.
- Serve over Basmati Rice. Top with fresh chopped parsley and a scoop of a fruit chutney on the side.

Potato & Leek Stew

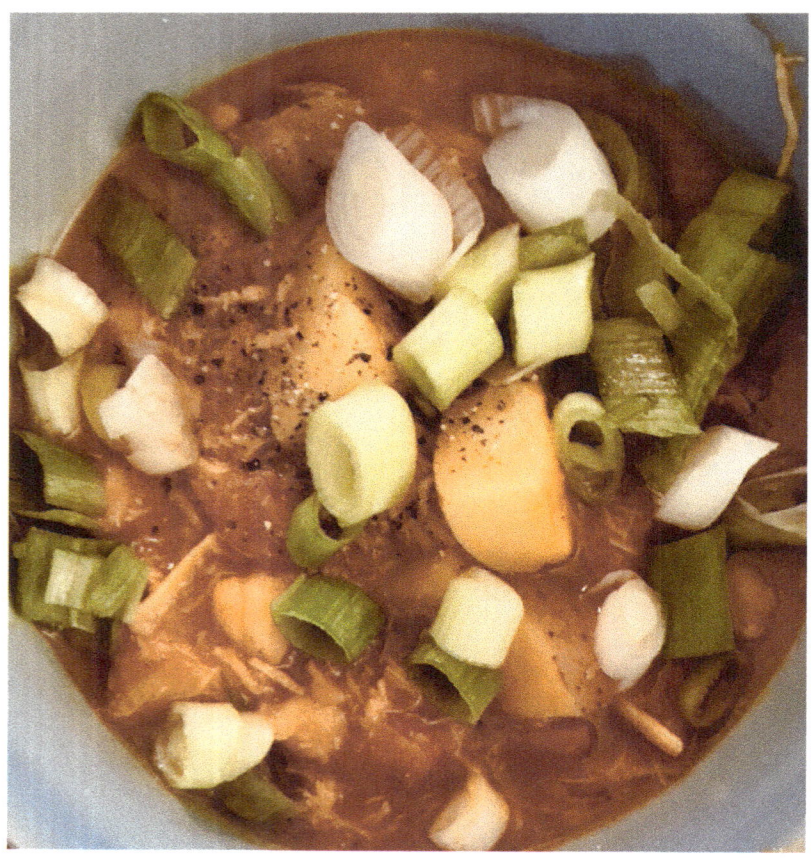

Ingredients (Serves 2-4)

- Left over chicken or turkey, shredded
- 2 leeks, washed thoroughly, cut into strips
- 3 large golden potatoes, cut into bite size pieces
- 1 can chopped tomatoes (I like using spicy chopped tomatoes)
- 2 cups chicken broth
- Salt and Pepper to Taste

Method

- Add all ingredients into a heavy stock pan or Dutch oven.
- Simmer on low heat for 1-2 hours.
- Stir occasionally.
- When potatoes fork tender, stew is done.

Cooking Notes

- This is also a great vegetarian recipe by omitting the chicken or turkey and add vegetable broth instead of chicken.

- To enrich the stew, add another potato, and a teaspoon of thyme with a basil leaf.

I mentioned to my husband a few years back that I now know why a Leek is called a Leek. He was curious, so I said it is because the flavor of the leek, leaks its flavor throughout all stews and other vegetables. It doesn't mask the flavor like cheese on meat, it enhances the flavor. He looked at me and just started smiling, like he knew I made it up at the moment. But I will stay with my story.

Island Chili

Ingredients (Serves 4-6)

- 1 can black beans, drained
- 1 can red beans, drained
- 1 can chili beans
- 1 can dark or light kidney beans
- 2 medium chopped onions
- 1 small can chopped green chilies
- 1-2 fresh Poblano or other Green Pepper, chopped
- 1 fresh Jalapeno de-seeded and chopped (Optional)
- 2 12 oz cans tomato sauce
- 1 can spicy chopped tomatoes
- 1/2 cup chili powder seasoning
- Red pepper flakes to taste
- 1 tablespoon Olive Oil

Method

- Add the olive oil to a Dutch Oven or heavy stock pot and turn heat to medium.
- Add the chopped onion and peppers. Cook until translucent.
- Add all other ingredients and stir well.
- Turn heat to medium low and simmer 1-2 hours.
- Add more chili powder and red pepper for spice, if needed.

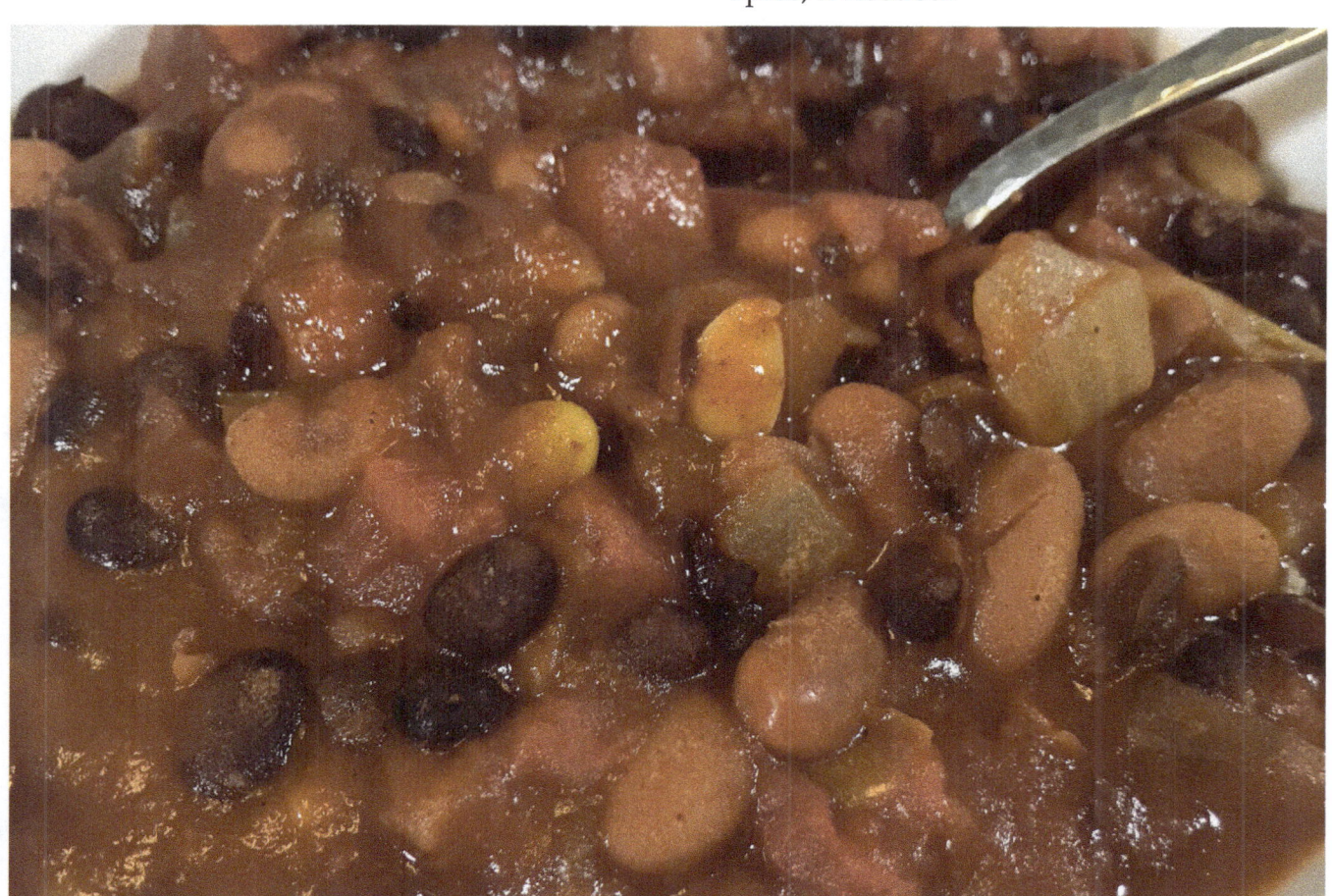

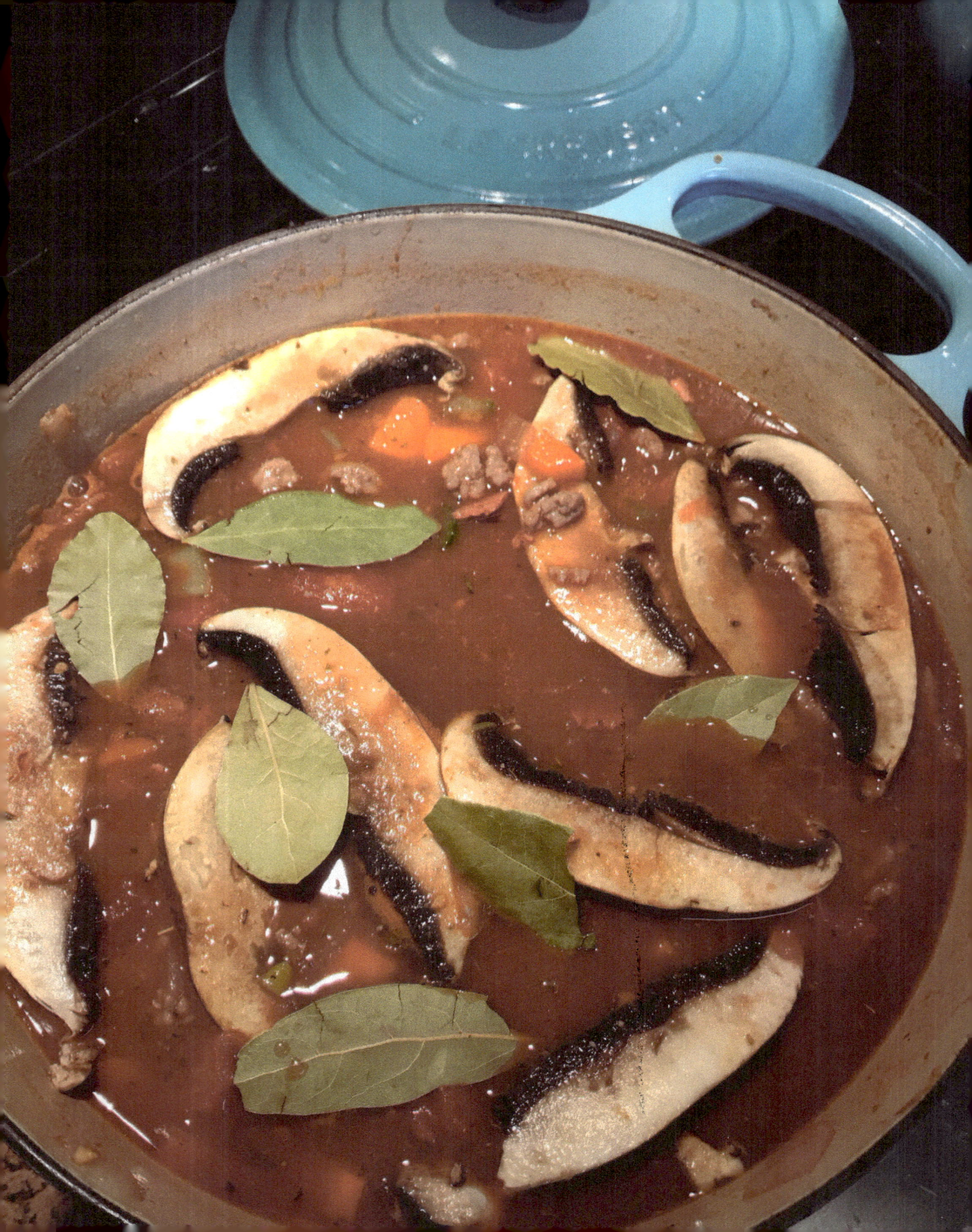

Ground Turkey & Vegetable Soup

When my son was a little guy many years ago, his grandpa would come visit us, and I knew I would come home from work to a huge pot of dad's vegetable soup. He used either hamburger meat (full fat type) or shredded, left over pot roast. The vegetables were plentiful. Dad liked making a guessing game at dinner, and I would have to guess all the seasonings and vegetables. It became a fun time on every visit and allowed us all to test our pallets. One night, though, I kept tasting a flavor and could not figure it out. It was somewhat sweet but not too sweet, and I noticed the tomatoes were not as acidic. To my surprise it was a Jonathan Apple, peeled and chopped which had melded in the tomato sauce. My dad was so pleased that he was able to hide one ingredient from me. Today, I make all kinds of vegetable soups. I do not used beef, but I substitute with lean turkey, chicken or no meat at all.

Ingredients (Serves 4-6)

- 2 pounds lean ground turkey
- 3 large carrots, sliced in bite size pieces
- 1 large onion, diced
- 9-12 slices of shiitake mushrooms
- 7 whole bay leaves
- 1/2 cup frozen baby green peas
- 1/2 cup frozen white corn
- 1 Jonathan Apple, peeled and chopped
- 1 large can tomato sauce
- Salt and Pepper to Taste

Method

- Brown the ground turkey in a Dutch oven or heavy pot that has been preheated with 1-2 tablespoons of olive oil.
- Add the onion to the meat and stir until onion begins to become translucent
- Add carrots, peas, corn, chopped apples and tomato sauce to the pot and stir.
- Place the mushrooms and bay leaves on top of mixture.
- Cook on low heat for 1-2 hours.

What to do with leftovers

This soup freezes well for up to 3-4 months. I like to put it into individual freezer containers and use on a night when it is late, and I need something quick to eat.

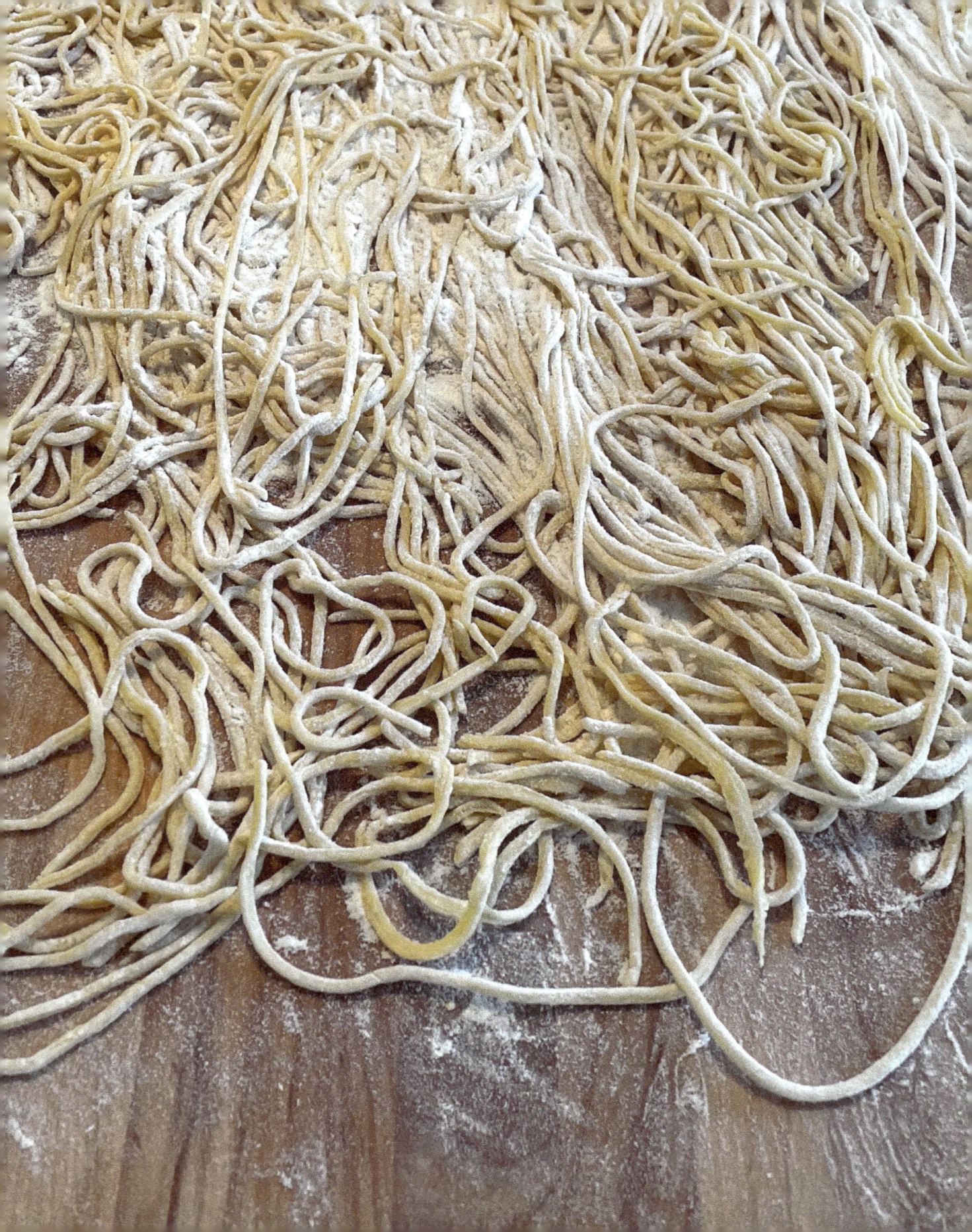

Pasta

Caramelized Cherry Tomato 50

Spaghetti Bolognese Meat Sauce 52

Penne with Vodka Sauce 55

Homemade Pasta 56

Carbonara with English Peas 58

Ham & Pepper Rotini 59

Vegetable Lasagnas (3) 60

Cheesy Macaroni with Tomatoes 62

Baked Vegetable Rigatoni 63

Everything Goes with Pasta

I do not exactly remember the first time I ate an Italian meal made by an Italian, but it had to be my aunt Phyllis who provided the food.

Aunt Phyllis came from a rather influential Italian family. My dad's brother, Uncle Glenn met Phyllis after the war. They had a lavish wedding and settled into the same city where my mom and dad had found a house earlier.

I remember Aunt Phyllis as being beautiful, petite woman, not standing much more than feet one or two. She was full of love to everyone, but also full of rage if you made her angry. Aunt Phyllis was a woman who wasn't afraid to speak her mind, and I admired her spirit. She ran hot and cold, was jealous of her husband working too late or stopping at our home for a meal. However, it was her recipes I learned from in the beginning in my Italian food lessons. Aunt Phyllis was loving and welcoming toward me no matter how long between our visits. Her family became our family and even her brother I referred to as Uncle Mikey. Her dad was Papa, and a bit scary, but a good man.

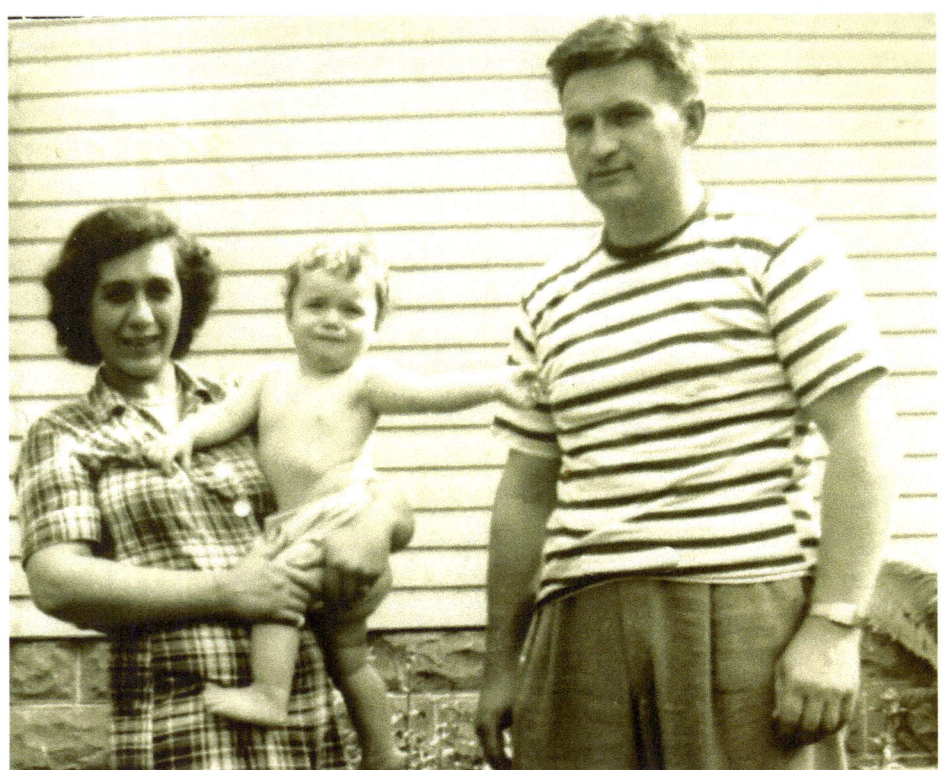

Aunt Phyllis

Back then, we bought dried spaghetti noodles in a box. Even though my family made homemade noodles, they were never used to put a red sauce over or meat over. They were used in soups of chicken broth and nothing more. No one ever thought about using them as spaghetti.

The first red sauce I made was Aunt Phyllis' sauce. Her father had an arrangement with the city's farmer's market and was able to get us something called, "Italian Sausage". We had always used ground hamburger meat or regular pork sausage. I still remember the first time I sampled a bit of this new sausage while it simmered in the tomato sauce. It was sweet, yet it had the flavor of fennel, a bit spicy at times, and the consistency between a hot dog and ground pork. It was delicious and became my favorite along with the great introduction to fennel.

Our sauce would cook all day in the big oval cast iron pot on our gas burner. I could tell it was spaghetti day as I could smell the flavors permeate the air, out the front door, and down the sidewalk as I came home from school. The closer I got to my house, the quicker I walked so I could be one of the first tasters.

Today, I make my own pasta using my family's recipe, and cut it into different shapes and styles. I use it with butter, pesto sauce, tomato sauces and even use them in my stir fry Thai dishes and also replacing the rice in my Chinese dishes. Then there are times, when I am missing all those who have passed before me, that I put a few noodles in a pot of chicken broth and eat them as soup as I did when I was a child.

Caramelized Cherry Tomatoes Spaghetti

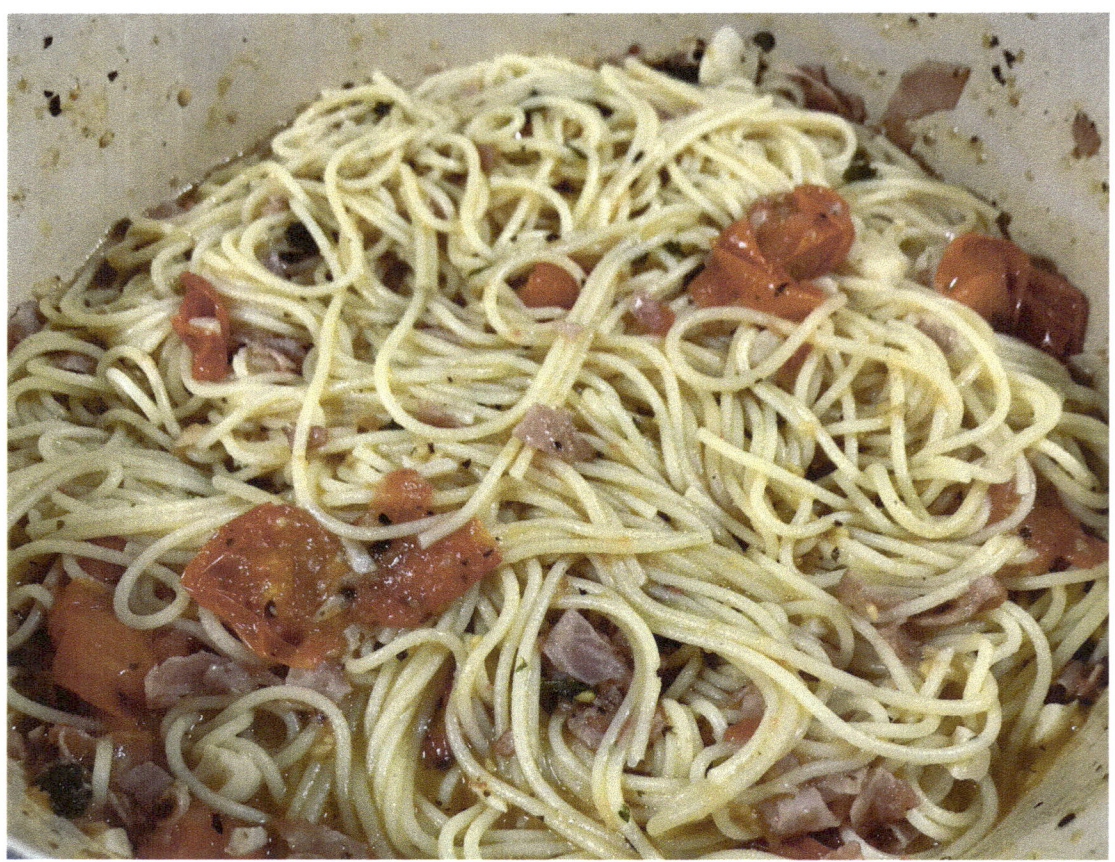

Ingredients:

- One pint of cherry tomatoes. If you are picking them fresh, approximately 15 or so.
- 3 Tablespoons canola or olive oil
- 1/2 cup Italian seasoned bread crumbs
- 1/2 Teaspoon fine ground Himalayan pink salt
- Black Pepper to taste
- 3 cloves elephant (large cloves) garlic, chopped fine
- 6 pieces turkey bacon
- Dash of red pepper flakes (to taste)
- 1/2 cup fresh Italian parsley (if using dry, one tablespoon)
- 1/4 cup finely grated Parmesan cheese
- 1/2 pound Spaghetti

Roasted and caramelized cherry tomatoes that have been breaded in Italian seasoning replaces the ground beef I use to use. It is very low in saturated fat, and high in flavor.

Method:

- Heat the oven to 350 degrees
- Line a baking sheet with parchment paper
- Wash tomatoes and put in bowl
- Pour Olive the oil into bowl of tomatoes and mix until tomatoes are covered
- Pour 1/2 cup Italian seasoned bread crumbs onto the tomato mixture. Mix well so tomatoes are coated.
- Pour out the tomato mixture onto the baking pan, If there are extra bread crumbs in the bowl, just toss them over the tomatoes.
- Place in the preheated oven.
- Let these bake until tomatoes caramelize, but do not let them disintegrate in the oven and do not let them burn. The tomatoes will look shriveled. This can take 20 minutes or so.
- Fill a pot with water to cook the spaghetti.
- Lightly salt the water.
- Once water is boiling, add the spaghetti.
- Use a deep skillet and add a teaspoon of oil to cook the turkey bacon until it is crispy.
- Drain bacon on paper towel and when cool, chop the bacon into small pieces and set aside.
- Add garlic to the skillet and saute until it begins to change color.
- Add two ladles of the boiling spaghetti water to the skillet with the garlic.
- Stir very well and let the water evaporate.
- Lower the heat and stir in the parsley.
- When the tomatoes are done, remove from the oven.
- Add the Al dente spaghetti to the skillet and mix well. Do not drain or rinse the spaghetti.
- Add the tomatoes and bacon to the mixture and continue mixing until all is thoroughly blended.
- If the mixture seems too dry, add a bit more spaghetti water to the skillet
- Turn off the heat, sprinkle with the Parmesan and serve.

Spaghetti Bolognese with Meat Sauce

Ingredients (Serves 2-4)

- 1 tablespoon Olive oil
- 4 pieces Turkey Bacon, chopped
- 1 pound lean ground Turkey
- 3 Turkey Italian sausage links
- 2 medium onions, chopped
- 2 carrots, finely chopped
- 2 celery sticks, finely chopped
- 5 cloves of garlic, finely chopped
- 1 tablespoon dried rosemary leaves
- 2 cans chopped tomatoes
- 2 -3 tablespoons tomato paste (this thickens the sauce)
- 1 tablespoon dried basil
- 1 tsp dry oregano
- ½ cup low sodium beef broth
- ½ bottle dry red wine (I like to add a bit more)
- ¼ teaspoon Hungarian Paprika (or any Paprika)
- ¼ teaspoon ground cinnamon (I like the Vietnamese cinnamon which is stronger in flavor)
- ¼ cup shredded Parmesan for topping

Left over sauce keeps well in the refrigerator a couple days. It can also be frozen for 2 months and reheats well. We always like it the second day as the sauce has had time for the flavors to meld.

Method

- In a Dutch oven, add the 1 tablespoon oil and heat on medium high heat.
- Add bacon and cook until soft brown.
- Remove and chop bacon into smaller pieces.
- Add turkey ground meat and Italian turkey sausages to pot and cook until light brown, then return bacon to pot.
- Add onions and garlic and continue cooking about 3 minutes.
- When meat is almost done, add carrots, celery and dried rosemary leaves. Cook 3 minutes longer.
- Add the chopped tomatoes, oregano, basil, beef broth, red wine, tomato paste and Hungarian paprika.
- Mix all together very well and bring to boil on medium heat.
- Turn temperature down to a low medium (slight boiling) and cook another 30-60 minutes.
- The longer it slow simmers, the more flavors are enhanced.
- About 15 minutes before serving, heat of a pot of boiling water with a dash of salt in the water.
- Add spaghetti noodles (I prefer the thin noodles but any pasta is good with this sauce) and cook per instructions on box.
- Drain noodles. Do not rinse the pasta
- Scoop a portion of noodles into bowl and top with sauce and a sprinkle with cheese.

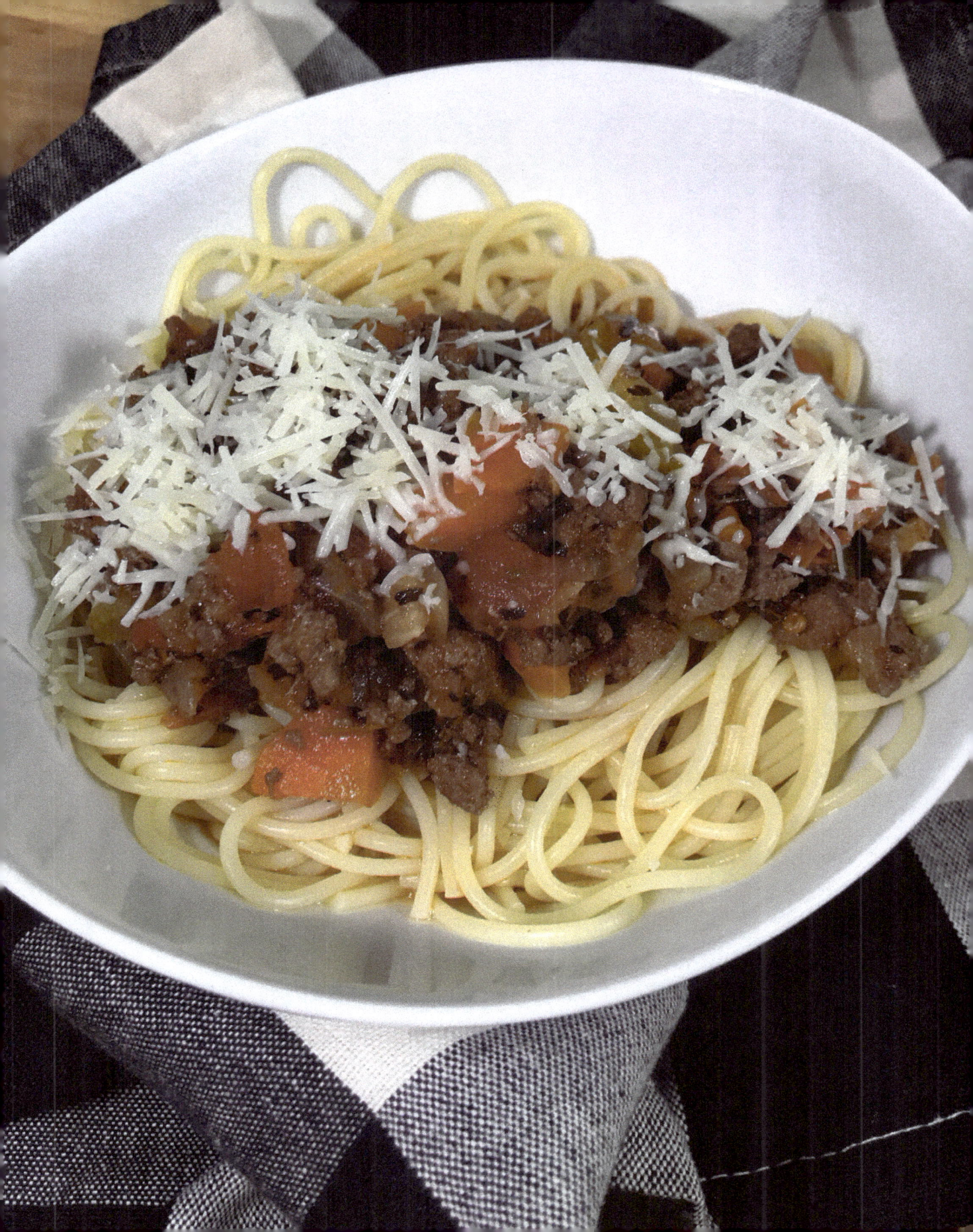

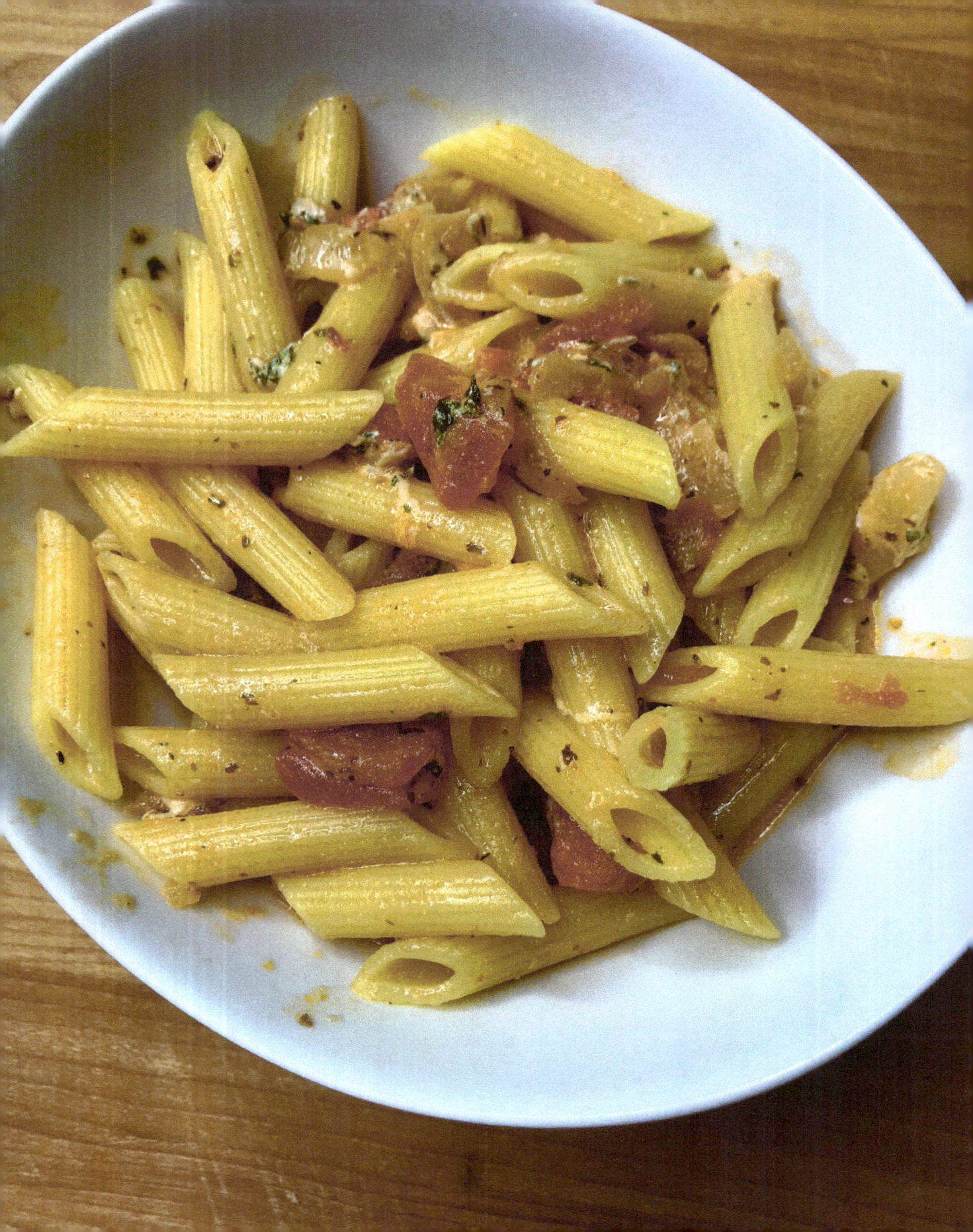

Penne with Vodka Sauce

Ingredients (Serves 2)

- 8 ounces Penne (or Rotini) Noodles
- ¼ cup Non Fat Greek Yogurt
- ¼ cup half and half
- 1 tablespoon olive oil
- 2 small shallots (or 1 medium onion), Chopped in small bites
- 2 jumbo garlic cloves, chopped fine
- One 16 oz can chopped tomatoes
- 1/3 cup vodka
- ½ cup Parmesan cheese, grated
- 1 tablespoons Italian seasoning
- ¼ cup Italian Parsley leaves, chopped.
- Optional: ¼ teaspoon red pepper flakes

I had to try many times to convert my traditional vodka sauce until I perfected this one. Penne with Vodka Sauce is a favorite of my husband's and since he couldn't have it anymore, I wanted to work hard to try and give him a dish that was close to his favorite. Not a lot of good substitutions for heavy yogurt and heavy cream, but surprisingly the non fat Half & Half with non fat Greek Yogurt did the trick.

Method

- Bring a large pot of water to boil and cook the penne until "Al dente", about 7-8 minutes. Drain the pasta and keep 1 cup of the pasta water.
- Mix the yogurt and half and half in small bowl.
- Heat oil in skillet over medium heat. Add shallots (or onions) and dash of salt. Cook until soft. Add garlic and red pepper flakes, cooking another 30-45 seconds.
- Remove from heat and add the can of tomatoes and vodka. Do not pour Vodka in a pan that is over the heat. It could flash fire.
- Place back on burner, add Italian seasoning, and heat on medium to bring to a simmer. Stir often on simmer for about 7-10 minutes.
- Stir in the yogurt and milk mixture and stir constantly for 3 minutes until sauce thickens.
- Add the drained pasta, Parmesan, and parsley. Mix all together, thoroughly.
- If the sauce seems too thick, use the residual pasta water and add gradually until desired consistency is reached.

Home Made Pasta (Noodles)

All the women in my family, both mom's and dad's side, made noodles. That is what we called them. Never did we use the phrase "pasta", just noodles. Typically, noodles would be cooked in a pot of chicken broth, sometimes with left over chicken that fell off the bone during cooking. If we were lucky, we would get noodles on all major holidays, and always a side of mashed potatoes would accompany.

While all the women in the family, going back to my great, great grandmother, used the same noodle recipe, it was my great Aunt Vivian that became the master. She was my dad's aunt, and was born in the early 1900's. She came from a family of women, five sisters (one was my grandmother). Each of my great aunts and grandmother all became fantastic cooks, were all college educated, and each had a career as teachers or owned their own business. I adored all my grandmother's sisters that I remember, but it was Aunt Vivian whom I spent the most time visiting.

Aunt Vivian's noodles were cut by hand so thin and perfect without the use of rulers or guides. She let the noodles dry until not sticky to the touch, rolled the almost dry dough into a long roll, then using a sharp paring knife cut the noodles by hand. Her precision was remarkable. Every cut noodle was the same width as the previous.

In her small Indiana hometown in the middle of corn field mazes she became very well known and liked during Spring and Fall festivals on the town square as the "noodle lady". She would prepare her homemade noodles months in advance putting them in baggies and freezing them to sell at the festival. As word spread, the popularity of her noodles grew and soon people from surrounding towns, cities and states would make the trip to the Spring festival just to buy her noodles.

I use my pasta cutting attachment for my mixer to make homemade noodles, thick or thin and only hand cut special noodles like stuffed shells and twisted spirals. I do not have the precision of Aunt Vivian. However, it is Aunt Vivian's recipe I use and the flavor is wonderful.

> *I have always made the noodles with this recipe, but I couldn't find the recipe and tried to remember if it was water or milk, so I replaced the egg shell of water with an egg shell of non fat Half & Half. The noodles were just as delicious and just a bit creamier.*

© Noodles — Vivian Fraker - Boggstown Ind

Sift 3 or 4 Cups flour in Bowl
Make well in center - ½ egg shell of H₂O
Beat 4 eggs in dish, ad to well - then
with a fork "slowly" beat in flour
until you have a ball of dough that
you can handle — Put some flour
on a surface where you are going

to roll out the dough - B/4 Rolling Knead
dough and work in flour until it
handles easily.
Roll dough out real thin, let it dry
Then Cut - Don't let it dry to much
or it will Crack up when Cutting.
— Cook-Em - Eat-Em.

Carbonara with English Peas

Ingredients (Serves 2)

- 1/2 box dry spaghetti (regular or thin)
- 8 strips of turkey bacon
- 1 1/2 cup frozen English peas, thawed
- 1 chopped Roma tomato
- 3 egg yolks
- 1/4 cup grated Parmesan cheese
- 1/2 teaspoon pepper
- 1/4 teaspoon salt

Method

- Boil a large pot of water and cook spaghetti. When spaghetti is done, and prior to draining from water, remove one cup spaghetti water to a measuring cup to save for later.
- While water is boiling for the spaghetti, add a teaspoon of olive oil to a pan and cook the turkey bacon until crisp. Drain on paper towel and then break it up into small pieces.
- Whisk egg yolks with the Parmesan cheese. Add salt and pepper.
- Add the peas and chopped tomato to the pan that was used to cook the bacon and also add half the bacon. Heat thoroughly then remove from heat.
- Add pasta and 1/2 cup of the spaghetti water to the pan of peas and tomatoes. Mix very thoroughly.
- While stirring mixture, pour the eggs and cheese blend into the spaghetti. Mix very well.
- Serve in bowls and top with remaining bacon and sprinkle with a small bit of Parmesan cheese.

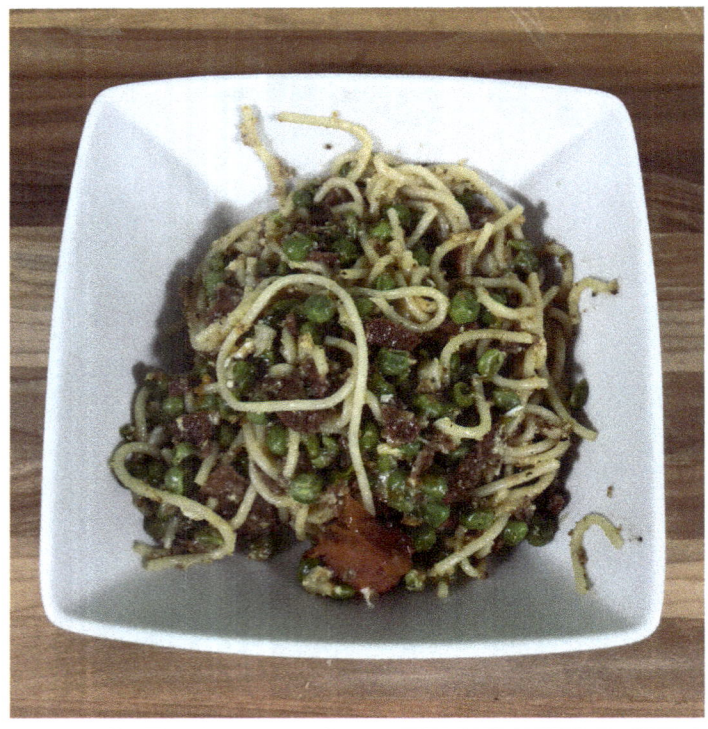

I was told to eat more peas as they contained lots of valuable nutrition and are low in saturated fat, cholesterol, and salt. They are a good source of protein, vitamins, and minerals, including vitamin C.
So what better way to eat more peas than to have them as the main ingredient to a Spaghetti Carbonara. Delicious!

Ham & Pepper Rotini

Select a nice lean piece of ham steak and cut it up for this delicious rotini sauce, or use left over ham from the holidays.

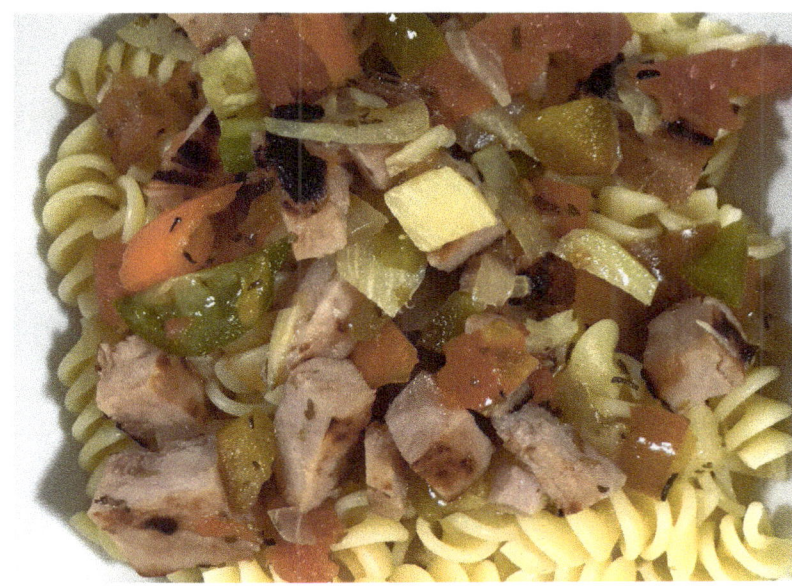

Ingredients (Serves 2 - 4)

- 1/2 - 1 pound left over holiday ham.
- 1 medium onion, chopped
- 1/2 red pepper cut into bite size pieces
- 1/2 green pepper cut into bite size pieces
- 1 can chopped tomatoes, 12-14 ounces
- ¼ teaspoon dried red pepper flakes
- 2 cloves garlic, chopped fine
- 1 tablespoon Italian seasoning
- Salt and Pepper to taste
- 2 tablespoons Olive Oil
- 1 Box spiral dry noodles.

Method

- In a heavy Dutch oven, add 1-2 tablespoons olive oil. Heat on-medium high.
- Add the peppers and onions, and cook until onions become translucent.
- Lower burner to medium and garlic, cooking about 1-2 minutes more.
- Add the can of tomato tomatoes
- Cook on low-medium heat 30 minutes.
- While sauce is simmering, heat a large pot of water until boiling. Add the noodles and cook as per the instructions on the box.
- Drain the noodles when done.
- Place noodles in bowls and scoop a ladle or more of sauce over noodles.
- Have a small bowl of grated low fat Parmesan on the table for garnish when serving.

Three Mini Vegetable Lasagnas

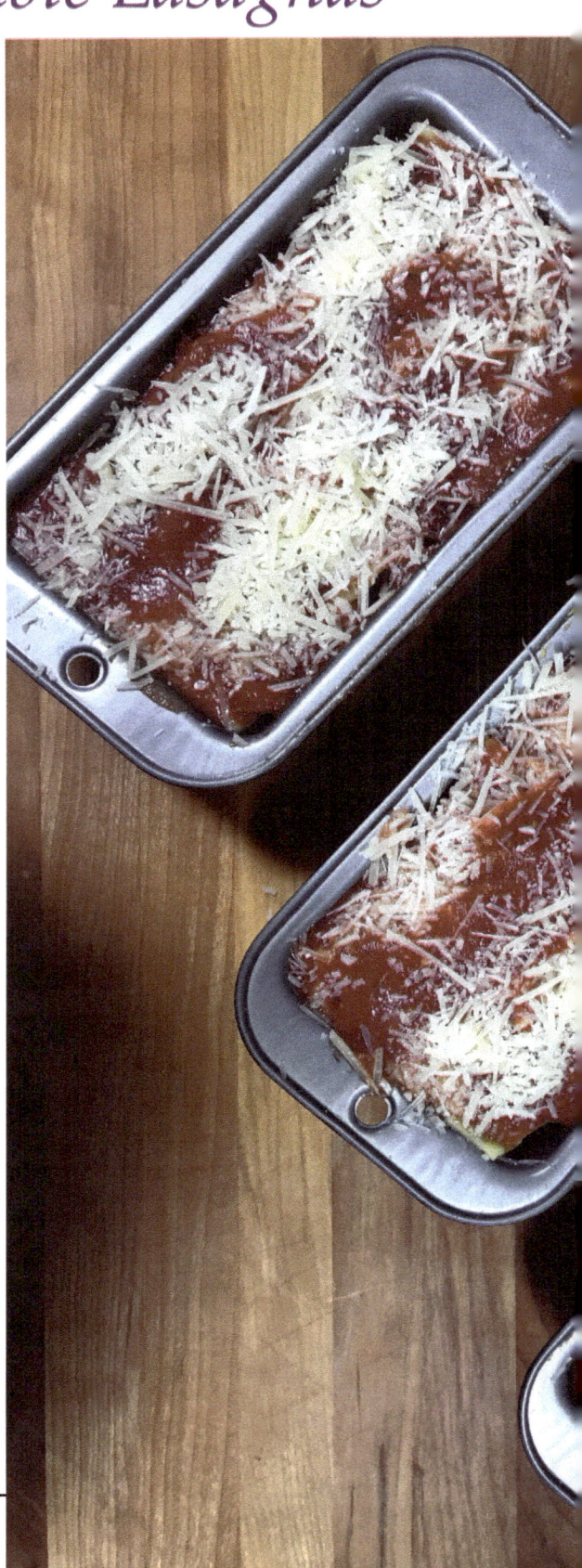

Ingredients (Serves 4-6) Per Mini Tin

- 12 No-Boil Lasagna Noodles
- Salt & Pepper
- 8 Ounces grated part-skim mozzarella cheese
- 2 cups fat free cottage cheese
- 1/2 cup grated Parmesan
- 1 large eggplant
- 4 Portobello mushroom caps
- 1 large zucchini (or two small)
- 1 large can tomato sauce
- 1 red bell pepper, chopped
- 1 small onion, chopped
- 2 cloves garlic, chopped
- 1/4 teaspoon red pepper flakes
- 1 tablespoon Italian seasoning
- 1-2 tablespoons extra-virgin olive oil

Sauce

- Heat oil in sauce pan. Add the garlic, onions, and bell pepper. Stir these until onion becomes translucent.
- Add tomato sauce, red pepper flakes and Italian seasoning. Bring to a slow boil and simmer on low heat while preparing vegetables and cheese mixtures.

Cheese Mixture

- Place the non fat cottage cheese in a bowl.
- Add a dash of salt and few grinds of black pepper.
- Add 2 eggs and stir mixture very well.
- Add the Parmesan and stir well.

Eggplant - Mushroom - Zucchini

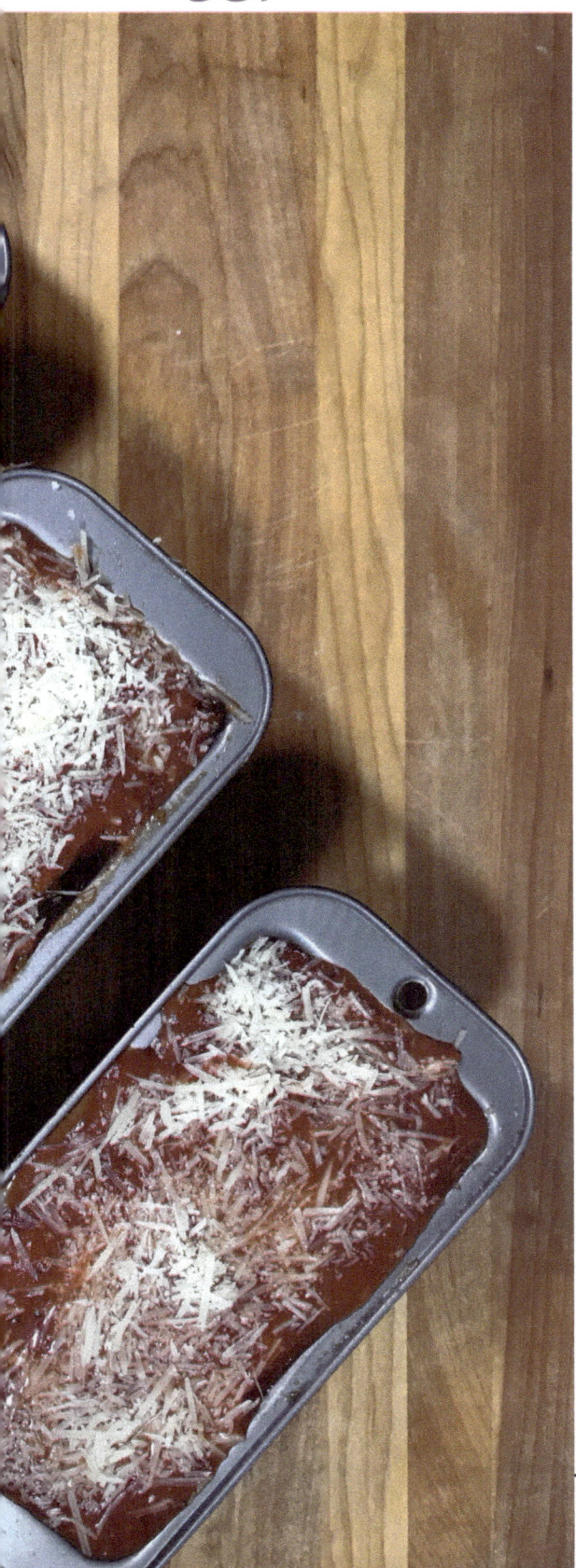

Preparing the Vegetables:

- Eggplant - Slice the eggplant into 1/2 inch pieces the length of the eggplant. Slightly salt the eggplant and place on paper towel to allow the moisture to drain.
- Zucchini - Slice the zucchini on length, rinse and place on paper towel to drain the water.
- Portobello Mushrooms - wash, cut off any stems, lay on paper towel to drain.

Assembly

- Preheat Oven to 425 degrees Fahrenheit.
- Take your three mini bread pans, one for each vegetable, and put in enough tomato sauce to cover the bottom.
- Lay a noodle along the bottom. If the noodle is longer than the pan, just break it off and put on one end. Remember which end, so you will do the next layer opposite.
- Spread some cheese mixture on the noodle
- Add a layer of one of the vegetables and a couple tablespoons of sauce to evenly cover.
- Repeat the above steps with noodle, cheese mixture, vegetable and sauce, finishing with a noodle on top.
- On the top noodle, spread the remaining cheese and then pour the remaining tomato sauce mixture over the tops of each pan.
- Sprinkle the tops with the mozzarella cheese. Cover with tin foil and put in oven to bake for 15 minutes. Remove the tin foil and continue baking until cheese is brown and sauce is bubbly.
- Remove from oven and let set 5 minutes before cutting and serving.

Baked Cheesy Macaroni and Tomatoes

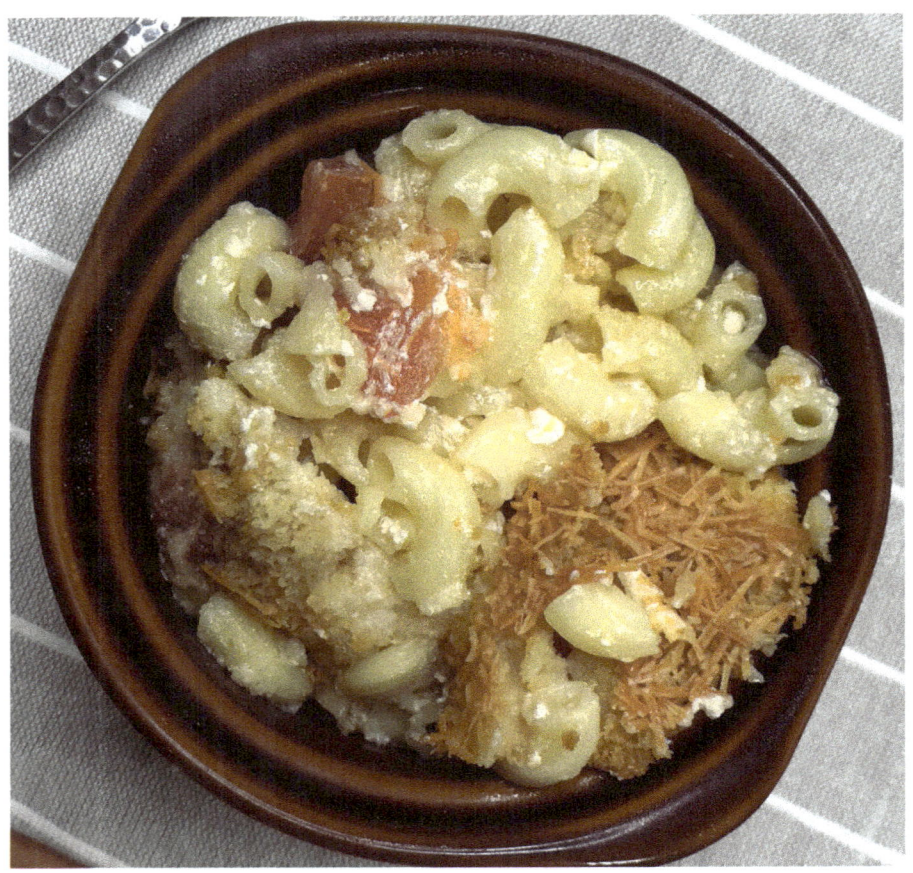

When my husband was in boarding school in England, one dish that he remembers fondly and actually liked to eat was the macaroni and cheese cooked with tomatoes. I knew I would have to try and experiment many times to recreate this favorite because Cheddar cheese has too much saturated fat. Substituting Parmesan for the cheddar gave this dish not only great flavor, but less than 2 grams of saturated fat per serving. He loves it and it has been a hit at many dinners.

Ingredients (Serves 8)

- 1/2 box dried Macaroni noodles
- 3 - 5 Roma Tomatoes, chopped
- 1 cup Non fat half and half
- 4 tablespoons low fat/olive oil margarine
- 1/2 cup shredded Parmesan cheese
- 1/2 cup Panko Bread Crumbs
- Olive Oil in spray can

Method:

- Preheat oven to 350 degrees.
- Bring large pot of salted water to boil and add the noodles. Cook until almost done, drain.
- Pour the noodles into a baking dish
- Add the tomatoes, non fat half and half, 4 tablespoons margarine, 1/2 cup Parmesan cheese
- Mix all together very well.
- If it seems too thick, add more half and half.
- Sprinkle the panko bread crumbs on top and spray with the olive oil.
- Bake in oven 20 minutes until bubbly.
- Sprinkle a little cheese over the panko crumbs and bake until the top becomes brown.
- Remove from oven and let sit 5 minutes before serving.

Vegetable Baked Rigatoni

Ingredients

- 1 box dried Rigatoni Noodles
- 1 Italian zucchini, sliced in bite sized cubes
- 1 onion, chopped
- 2 cloves garlic, finely chopped
- 1/2 red bell pepper, cut into quarter pieces and quarter again
- 1/2 yellow bell pepper, cut into quarter pieces and quarter again
- 1/2 cup English Peas - frozen are the best
- 1/2 cup shiitake mushrooms
- 1 14 ounce can chopped tomatoes
- 1 14 ounce can tomato sauce
- 1/2 teaspoon Italian seasoning
- 2 basil leaves
- 1/2 cup fresh grated Parmesan cheese.

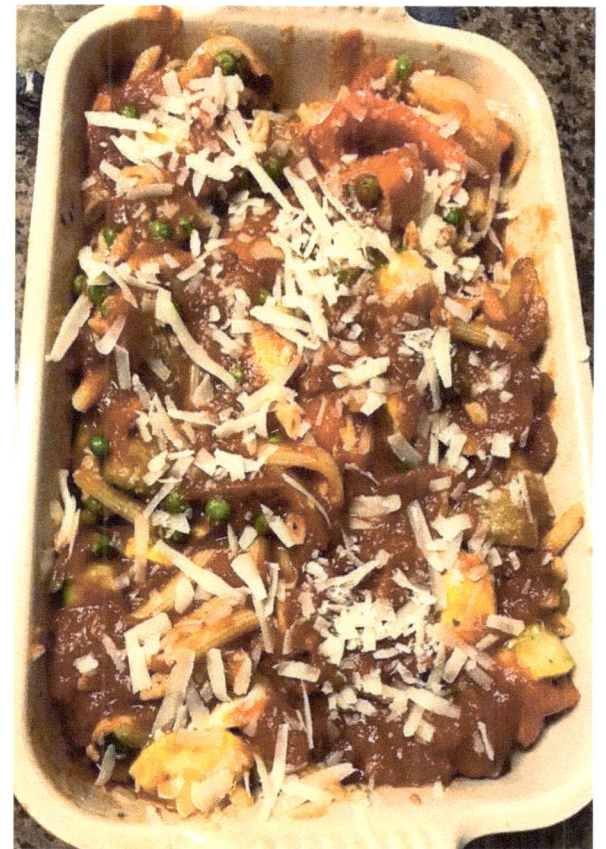

Method

- Preheat oven to 350 degrees.
- Bring large pot of salted water to boil and add the Rigatoni noodles. Cook until almost done, drain.
- In a skillet, heat the olive oil and add the onion, garlic, bell peppers and cook until browned.
- Add the tomato sauce, chopped tomatoes, mushrooms and Italian seasoning. Stir well and cook about 5 minutes.
- Put the pasta in a baking dish.
- Add the Zucchini and English Peas.
- Add the warm vegetables with sauce.
- Mix well.
- Add the bay leaves on top.
- Sprinkle with Parmesan cheese.
- Bake approximately 20 - 30 minutes until cheese has melted. Sauce will be bubbly.
- Remove from oven and let sit approximately 5 minutes.
- Dish up on individual plates and serve.

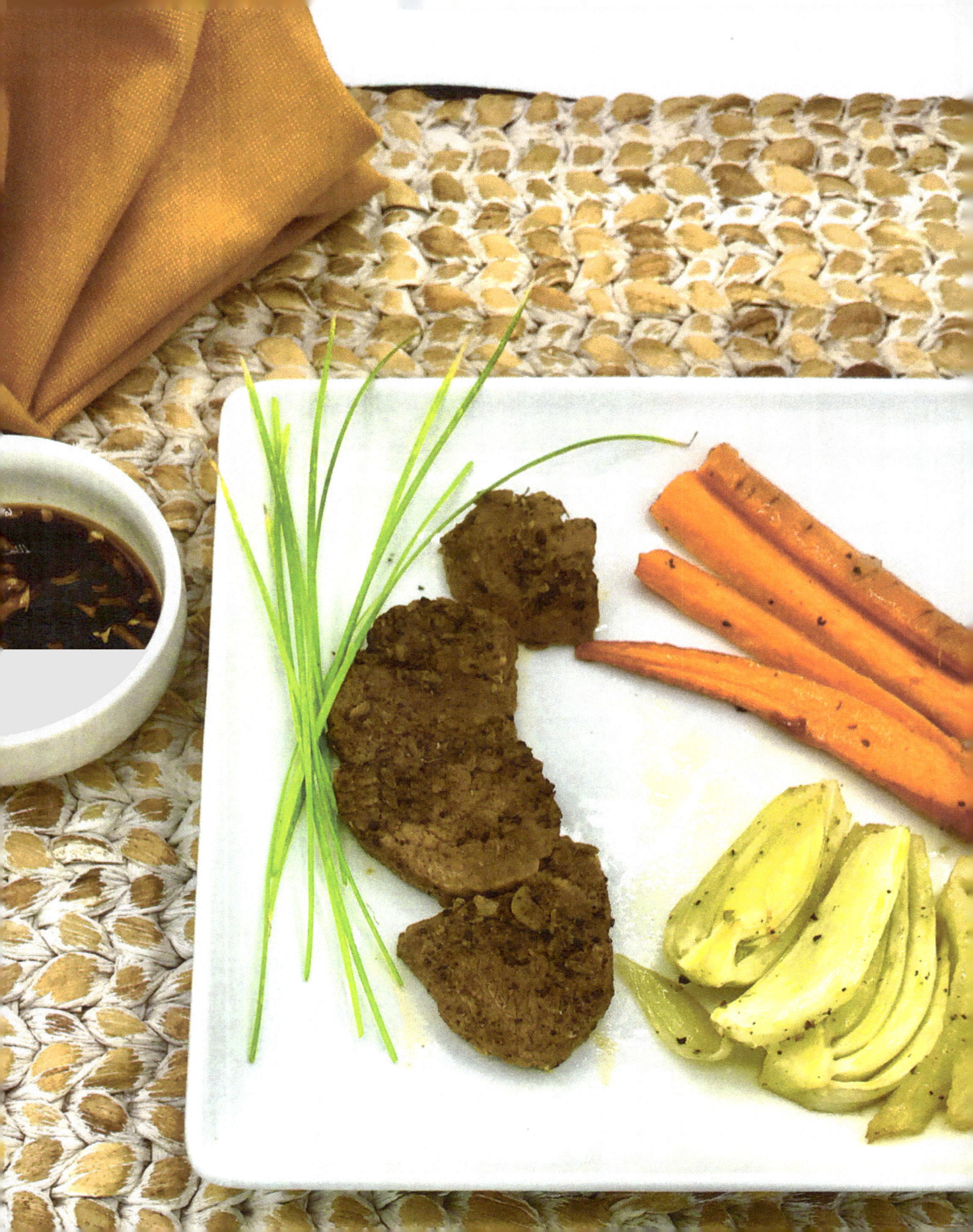

Pork

Best Pork Chop Ever 67
Island Pork Roast 68
Pork Bourguignon 70
Scotch Eggs 72
Soy Baked Pork Chops 74
Hoosier Sandwich 75
Griddle Pork Tacos 78
Spicy Pork & Zucchini Noodles 80
Zucchini Noodles 81

I grew up in what was known as "pork country" where pork was celebrated yearly at festivals. Fried, grilled, Barbecue, baked, breaded on a bun (the Hoosier Burger), stewed or turned into a ham, pork was always my favorite.

When I began this journey into low fat cooking alternatives, I honestly didn't know if I could include pork. I love pork. I was the kid who would eat the meat of the chop, then gnaw on the bone, sucking the gristle and grease from the fat until there was nothing left on the bone. It was so good.

I have found a replacement for the fatty content of the pork which is now in the marinades and rubs I use prior to cooking the meat. I have opted for boneless cuts of lean pork and a serving size is typically four ounces. If I have not had the limit on saturated fat for a day, the size can go up to six ounces.

The Best Pork Chop Ever recipe came from wanting a very well seared, yet tender and juicy pork chop that cuts with a butter knife and melts in my mouth. After several trials, I got it right.

The key is to marinate; use a very high temperature for cooking and time it perfectly until the internal temperature is right at 165 degrees. No skimping on the marinade with these chops!

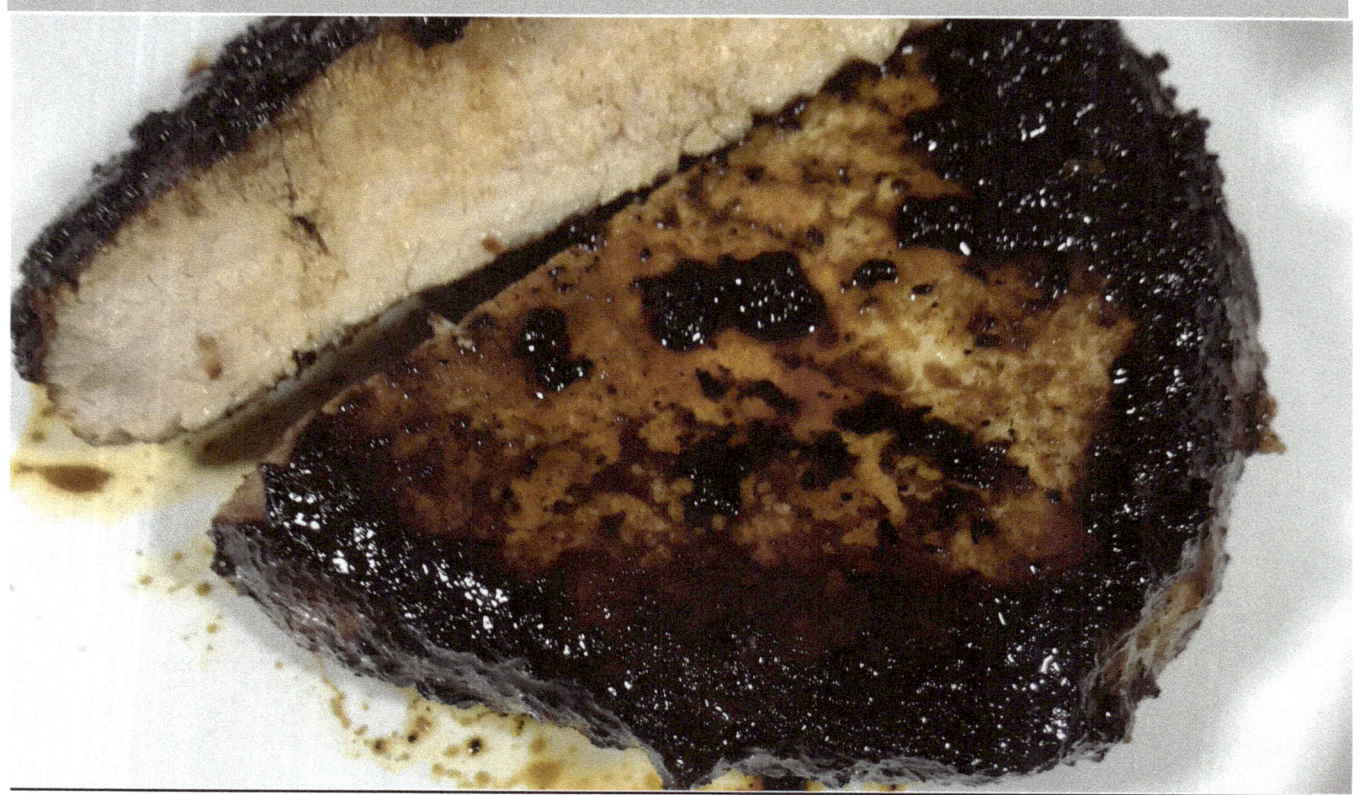

Best Pork Chop Ever

Cooks Note: This is a recipe for 4 chops, increase marinade proportionally if adding more chops. You will need a thermometer to check the internal temperature of the pork as it cooks.

Ingredients

- Boneless pork loin, fat trimmed, and cut into 3/4 to 1 inch thick slices. One chop per person should weigh approximately 4-5 ounces. Use smaller, thicker chops for best cooking. Saturated fat is approximately 5 grams for 4-5 ounce chop.
- 1 elephant garlic, or 3 large cloves of garlic sliced
- 1/2 cup extra virgin olive oil (Use this type of oil as it contains good fat that will not affect the level of saturates in the overall meal)
- 1/2 cup low sodium soy sauce
- 1/2 cup fresh chopped parsley (do not use dried parsley)
- Black pepper - a few turns of the pepper mill
- Dash of Salt

Method

- Place the garlic, olive oil, soy sauce, and parsley in a blender.
- Blend on high until well blended and mixture is smooth.
- Place the sliced pork in a shallow bowl or a large baggie and pour the marinade over chops. Cover and place in refrigerator for minimum of 4 hours.
- Remove the chops from the refrigerator about 30 minutes before cooking.
- Heat an outside flat top griddle on high. The flat top can be cast iron on a grill or an outdoor flat top stove. If you are cooking these indoors, be sure you have a window open to help with the smoke (Yes it will smoke at a high heat, but we want it to smoke so it sears the juices in the chops). Use a heavy duty cast iron skillet on an inside stove.
- Once the griddle is hot, carefully place each chop on the griddle, then spoon some of the marinade over the top.
- Cook for 6 minutes on the first side and then turn the chops over and add more marinade. The chops will take on a dark char look, but they are not burnt - it is the soy sauce causing darkness as it heats. Cook 4 minutes.
- Turn heat down to medium and flip the chops again. Add more marinade.
- Cook about 1-2 minutes and check the internal temperature. If the desired 165 degrees has not been met, flip the chops and cook another 2 minutes.
- As soon as the 165 degree has been reached, remove from heat immediately and place on a warm plate to serve.

Island Flavored Pork Roast

I love the flavors of this roast, and especially look forward to using the leftovers for tacos, enchiladas, soups and salads. When selecting a roast, look for lean pork tenderloin that has less than 4 grams of saturated fat per serving.

Ingredients (Serves 4-6)

- Pork
- 4-6 pound boneless pork loin, fat trimmed
- Kosher salt
- 1 tablespoon dried oregano
- 2 teaspoons fresh ground black pepper
- 1 teaspoon ground cloves
- 1 tablespoon water

Marinade

- 1/2 cup chopped garlic
- 1/8 cup dry cilantro
- Juice from 2 lemons, about 1/4 cup
- Juice from one large orange
- 1/4 cup oregano leaves
- 1/4 cup water
- 1 1/2 cup extra virgin olive oil

Method

Preparing the pork

- Rinse the pork and pat it dry
- Mix the spices and water together to form a paste
- Rub the paste all over the pork.
- Put pork in a large bowl or pan.

Method

Preparing the Marinade

- Put all the ingredients for the marinade in a blender and blend until very smooth.
- Pour the marinade over the pork.
- Cover tightly and let sit in refrigerator 12-24 hours.

Baking the Pork

- Remove the pork from the refrigerator and let it set at room temperature 30 minutes.
- Preheat the oven to 350 degrees.
- Line a heavy duty baking pan with several layers of tin foil; or use a very large Dutch oven with a lid.
- Put the pork in the pan and pour some of the marinade over it. Seal and bake in the oven 3-5 hours. Check each hour, add more marinade and recover to continue baking.
- Pork is done when it easily shreds apart.
- Remove from oven and put on serving board. Let rest 5 minutes before serving.
- Slice against the grain or shred.

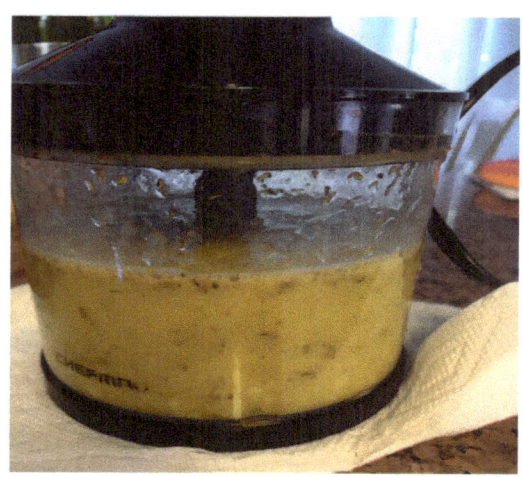
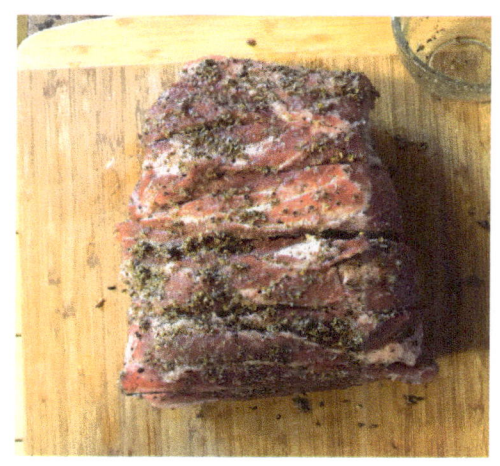

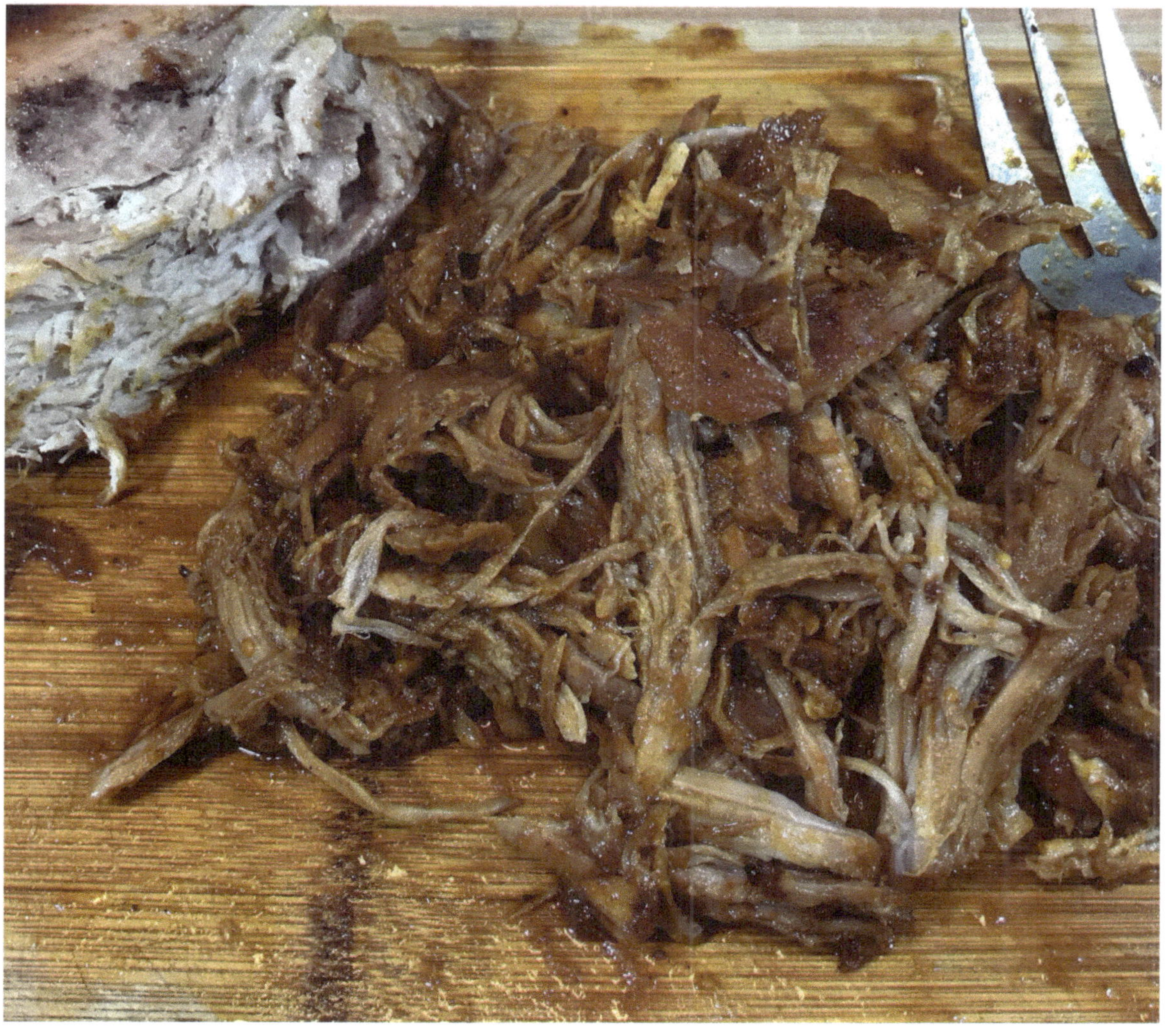

Pork Bourguignon

This recipe was adapted from my family's recipe for Beef Burgundy and beef bourguignon at our favorite Paris restaurant where we have celebrated a couple anniversaries. Instead of Beef, I selected a lean, boneless pork loin and cut it into squared pieces. It contains no trans fats like beef and has less saturates. It is just as good as the beef with its thick sauce. Served with a heaping scoop of mashed potatoes - it will melt in your mouth.

Ingredients (Serves 6)

- 1.5 lb Boneless Pork Loin (fat trimmed) or Beef Top Sirloin (leanest cut and fat trimmed)
- 1/2 lb Turkey Bacon
- 1 small package Portobello Brown Mushrooms
- 3 Tablespoons Canola Oil
- 1 Large Onion (white or yellow) sliced
- 2 Large cloves of garlic or 4 small cloves, chopped
- 2 sprigs fresh thyme or 1 Tablespoon dry
- 1 Bay leaf
- 12 oz Shallots (sliced)
- Salt & Milled Black Pepper (to taste)
- 2-3 Tablespoons flour (unbleached white or bleached white)
- 15 fluid ounces red Burgundy (you can also use a Cabernet)

Method

- Slice the pork loin into 1 inch thick slices, then cut each of the slices into 1 inch square shaped pieces.
- Heat the oil in a heavy pot (I like using my Creuset Dutch oven - but any pot that can also be put into the oven)
- Once oil is heated, add the pork pieces and brown on all sides. Turn pieces often.
- Remove the meat to a warm tray once nice and brown on all sides.
- Add onion and garlic to pot and bring it to a caramel color.
- Return the meat to the pan.
- Sprinkle in the flour a bit at a time. You want enough flour to soak up the juices of the meat and onions.
- Add the wine gradually and continue stirring until well blended.
- Add the seasonings
- Cover the pan and place in the oven at 350 for 1.5 - 2 hours. Meat should fork tender.
- When the casserole is about 15 minutes from the 2 hour baking, Prepare a separate pan with a tablespoon of oil and heat.
- Add the shallots and bacon to brown them lightly.
- Remove the meat from the oven.
- Add the shallots and bacon to the casserole.
- Add the sliced mushrooms to the casserole.
- Place back into the oven and cook for one more hour.

Beef Burgundy

4 servings

1 1/2 lbs. Beef Round Steak
(1/2 inch thick)
2 tbsp. flour
2 tbsp. Butter
1/4 cup onion
2 tbsp. parsley
1 small clove garlic
1 small bay leaf
1/2 tsp. salt
Dash Pepper
303. can whole drained mushrooms
1/2 cup Burgundy Wine
1/2 cup water

Cut steak into bite-size cubes; shake with the flour to coat, be sure all flour is used. Melt butter in skillet; brown steak pieces on all sides. Remove from heat. Add onion, parsley, garlic, bay leaf, and salt & pepper. Stir in mushrooms, burgundy & water. Heat mixture to boiling. Reduce heat & simmer, covered about 1 hour or till meat is tender. Remove Bay leaf.

Scotch Eggs

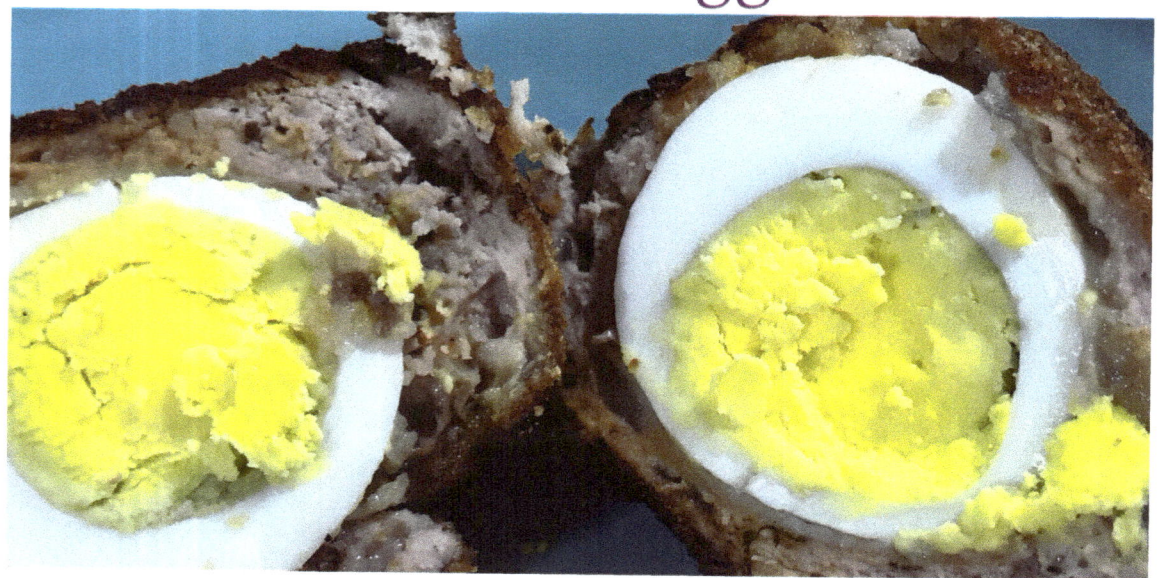

Ingredients (serves 4)

- 4 medium eggs
- 3/4 pound lean ground pork (see Cook's Tip)
- 1/2 teaspoon salt
- 1/2 teaspoon pepper
- 2 teaspoons Thyme
- 1 teaspoon sage
- 1 teaspoon brown sugar
- 1/2 teaspoon allspice
- Dash of Nutmeg
- 1/4 cup chopped fresh parsley
- 1/4 teaspoon onion powder
- 1/8 teaspoon cayenne or Himalayan Paprika
- 1 small onion, chopped fine
- 1/2 cup all purpose flour seasoned with salt and pepper.
- 1 beaten egg
- 1/2 cup Italian flavored fine ground bread crumbs or fine plain Panko crumbs.
- Spritzer of Olive Oil or Canola Oil

Method

- Place 4 medium eggs in a pot and cover with water, bringing to a boil. Let boil for 5 minutes and remove from heat. Place eggs in a shallow bowl with cold water and peel the eggs. Set eggs aside to cool.
- Mix the ground pork with all the seasonings. Mix very well with your hands to get everything thoroughly seasoned throughout the meat.
- Divide the meat mixture into 4 pieces and flatten on a board prepared with a piece of parchment paper so the patties are easy to lift.
- Put the seasoned flour on a small plate.
- Take one egg at a time and roll it in the flour until it is covered.

- Place an egg on a pork patty and wrap the sausage all around the egg until it is covered completely.
- Dip the sausage covered egg in the beaten egg mixture.
- Dip the egg covered sausage in the bread crumbs/Panko crumbs covering completely.
- Repeat steps above for each of the eggs.
- Preheat the air fryer at 400 degrees for the required time (each air fryer is different)
- Once eggs are coated, they are ready for the air fryer. Spray the air fryer pan with a light coating of canola oil.
- Place each egg in the air fryer, giving space between the eggs.
- Spritz with a light coating of oil
- Cook at 350 for 7 - 10 minutes.
- Open air fryer and if sausage has browned, continue with steps below; otherwise cook another 3 - 5 minutes before
- When sausage has browned, turn eggs over to other side.
- Spritz with a light coating of oil.
- Continue in air fryer at 350 for 7 - 10 minutes.
- When done, remove eggs to a platter and let cool slightly before serving.
- Drizzle with your favorite sauce (red pepper hot jam, chutney, mustard BBQ sauce or eat plain.

> *If you have problems finding lean ground pork, do not worry. Buy 4 lean, boneless pork chops, cut fat away and cut into chunks. Put in your food chopper and grind it up. Then add the seasonings and continue with the instructions.*

Soy Baked Pork Chops

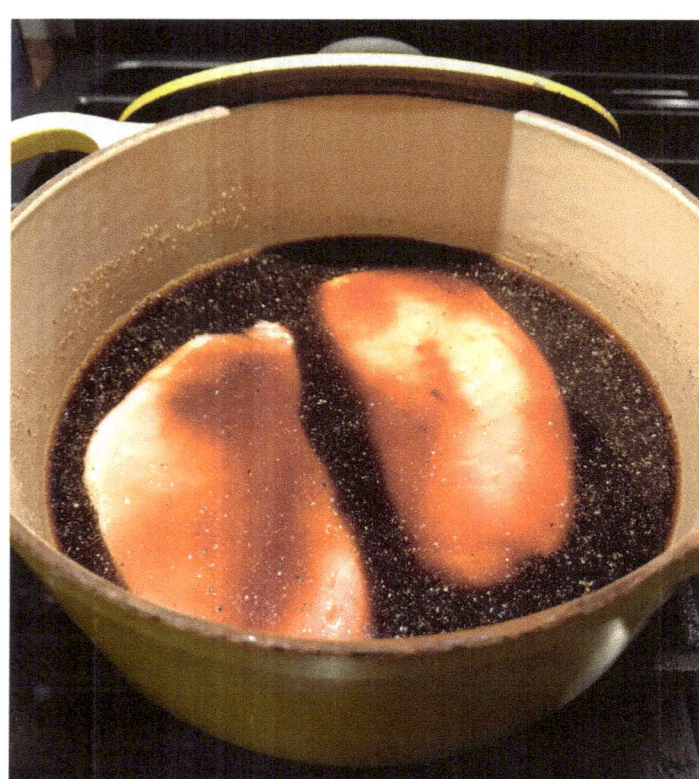

Ingredients: (Serves 2)

- 2-4 Center cut lean pork loin boneless chops
- 2 cloves garlic, chopped fine
- ½ cup low sodium soy sauce
- ½ cup water
- 3 tablespoons brown sugar
- ½ teaspoon fresh grated ginger
- Fresh milled black pepper
- Olive Oil for cooking

Method

- Heat a heavy duty Dutch oven with a tablespoon of Olive oil.
- Place the pork chops in the heated oil and quickly sear each side. The chops should have a nice light brown color to all sides.
- Turn off heat. This Dutch oven will be used to bake the chops.
- Mix the garlic, soy sauce, water, ginger and brown sugar together thoroughly.
- Pour the sauce mixture over the chops.
- Place a tight fitting lid over the pan and bake in a pre-heated 350 degree oven, on the middle rack, for 30-45 minutes (thickness of chops determine cooking time)

Serve

- These chops are wonderfully served with baked or roasted potatoes, steamed or fried rice.

I started experimenting with sauces and seasoning for pork. I poured some soy sauce in a pan with some garlic, water and brown sugar. I added two boneless lean pork loin chops and baked in oven for almost an hour. The result was extreme flavor. The left over sauce thickened as it cooked and was used as a gravy over the mashed potatoes. It is now one of our "go to" evening meals when I want quick and delicious.

Hoosier Sandwich

Ingredients: (Serves 2)

- 2 Center cut lean pork loin boneless chops, thin cut
- 1 cup all purpose flour on a flat plate
- 1 cup panko crumbs on a flat plate
- 2 beaten eggs in a bowl
- Iceberg lettuce cut in thick chunks, or several leaves of Romain
- Kosher dill whole pickles sliced in half I use dill pickles now but either dill or sweet are delicious on this sandwich
- Roll of choice (I like Small French or Italian Rolls)
- Low fat olive oil mayonnaise to spread on the bun/bread.

Method

- Take each pork chop and place between pieces of plastic wrap on top of a wooden board.
- Use a rolling pin and pound the chops until they are flattened. Typically they end up twice the size that you began with so it overlaps the bun/bread
- Heat a large skillet with 2-3 tablespoons of Olive oil. Use medium heat to begin.
- Dredge the chops into the flour, then the egg, then the panko crumbs.
- Place the chops in the hot oil.
- Cook on one side until brown, then flip and cook on the other.
- The pork is done when it is white in center and juices run clear.
- Prepare the buns with low fat mayonnaise spread on each side, then top with a pork chop Put a few pieces of lettuce on the chop and then top it off with a large slice or two of pickle.
- Serve with air fried French fries.

Hoosier sandwiches come from Indiana. It was pork country when I was growing up. At a local Drive Up, if you ordered a pork sandwich, you were served a flattened pork chop, breaded and deep fried on a regular hamburger bun with mayonnaise, lettuce and a big slice of sweet pickle

A 40 Year Taco Adventure

The first time I ate Mexican food was with a friend. I was 16 and we were driving to check out this new restaurant called Taco Bell . It had opened its doors just weeks before. We had no idea what a Taco Bell was or what type of food, but we were teenagers and adventurous.

We didn't call restaurants like Taco Bell or McDonald's fast food as we do now, they were restaurants. We didn't call our A&W Root beer stands or MugNBun stands restaurants, but called them drive ins. And, we called Steak N Shake the cruiser shack. You can probably guess why.

Anyway, we hoped into my car and drove to the Taco Bell. It was a very impressive building setting a bit higher on the hill as there was a dip for an underpass on either side. Bright colors and impressive signage were displayed. When we got inside, we gazed in amazement at the picture menu on the wall and descriptions of each. I had no idea, absolutely none, on what I should order but the list was short. I figured I could work my way through them all.

<u>The menu items we selected from included:</u>
Frijoles, mashed pinto beans served in small container with cheese on top
Tostadas, about the same as today's item
Taco Burger (sometimes called chili burger) which was seasoned ground beef on a bun and very similar to a modern sloppy Joe mix with a Mexican twist.
Burritos - Red sauce burrito was a basic beef burrito, wrapped in flour tortilla and sauce and cheese oozing out.
Taco - a basic beef taco with lettuce sour cream and cheese.
Burritos - Green Sauce which was similar to a salsa verde we eat now.

I wanted to try all of it but settled first on the Taco Burger. I thought it was the safest selection. The flavors were unforgettable and so delicious. They were similar to mom's Spanish hamburger, but better! Each visit thereafter, I would try something new until I had run through the menu.

When I drove to St. Louis to visit my friend, she had learned to make homemade tacos while in California and was eager to show me the recipe. We bought corn tortillas as flour tortillas were not for tacos at that time. In a skillet filled about 1/4 way with Crisco (a less fat version of Lard) and heated until it smoked, one corn tortilla at a time would be dropped into the oil and fried about

1-2 minutes on each side, then laid on a plate with paper towels to somewhat drain the oil. This process would be repeated until 12 or more tortillas would be fried. Ground hamburger came next, no seasoning added; followed by a serving of shredded lettuce and cheddar cheese and refried beans, sometimes chopped onion. Hot sauce of some sort was always available.

Today, I make tacos with all types of ingredients, corn tortillas and flour tortillas, raw and cooked onion, peppers, chicken, ground turkey, fish, or pork. I have added black beans in addition to refried beans. I like fried jalapeños or poblanos or Serrano peppers to chop up and sprinkle on the tacos. I even have a special pickled red onion to have on Asian tacos, and peanut cole slaw for fish tacos.

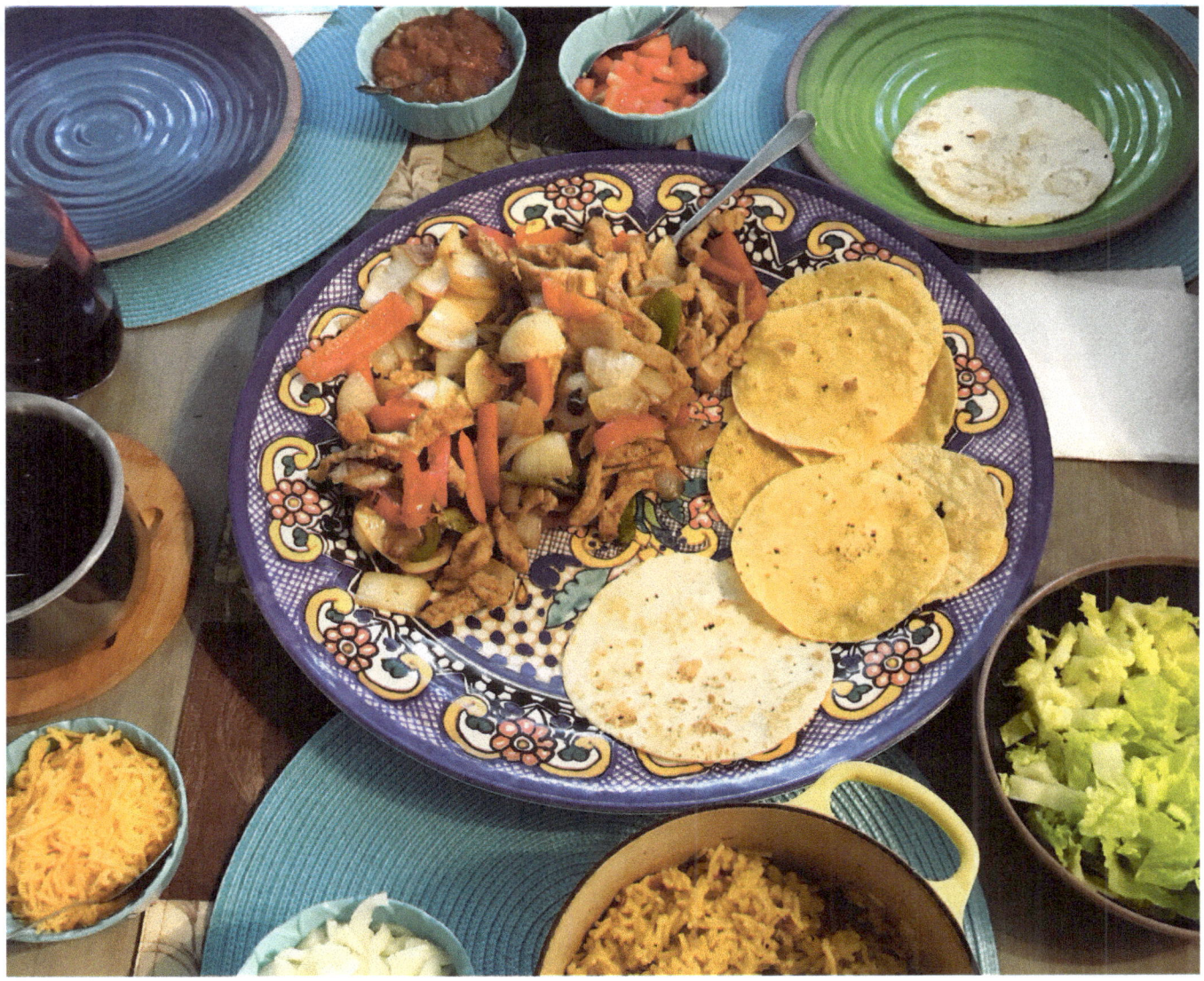

Griddle Pork Tacos

When I got my outdoor flat top griddle, one of the first meals I cooked on it was Griddle Pork Tacos, a similar style to Street Tacos. The meat cooked quick and I was amazed how the extreme high heat locked in the juices and made the meat very tender.

Ingredients (Makes 6-8 Tacos)

- 2-4 lean pork chops, trimmed and sliced in long lengths
- 1 large green bell pepper, sliced
- 1 medium onion, chopped
- 1 jalapeños or Poblano pepper chopped
- Olive Oil for searing on flat top
- Flour tortillas and Corn tortillas (You can also use pre-made taco shells)
- Your choice of salsa, hot sauces or pico
- Non fat, shredded cheddar cheese
- Chopped Roma tomatoes
- Chopped Romain lettuce

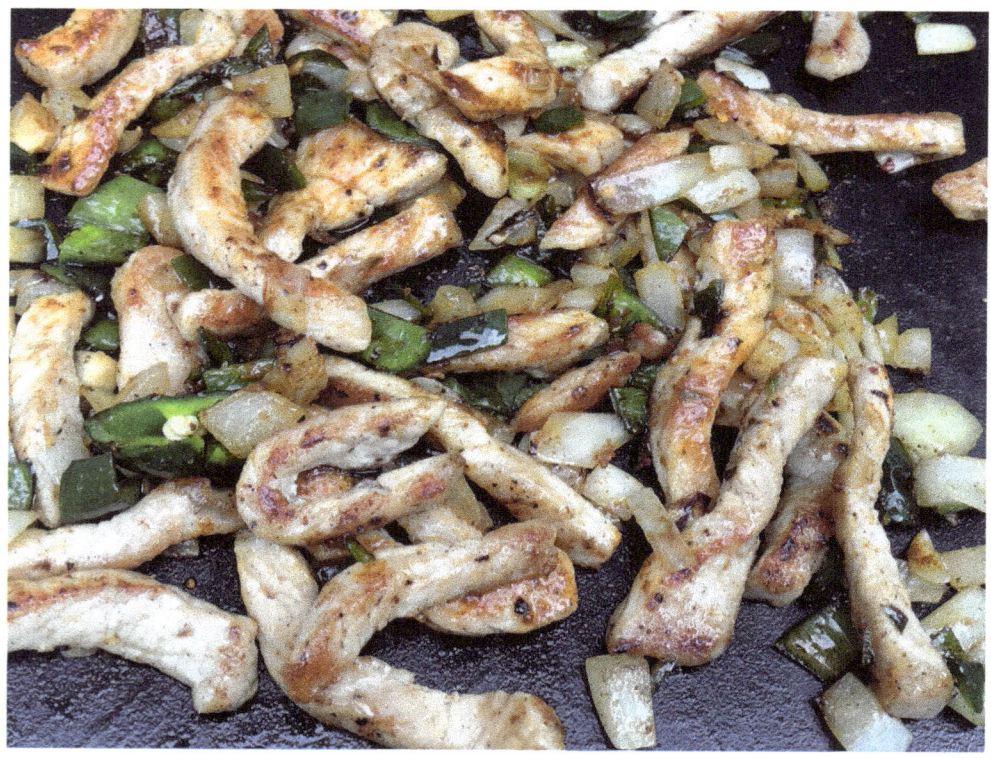

Method

- Heat an outdoor flat top griddle, or use a large cast iron flat skillet on stove top. Heat on high heat.
- Add olive oil to cover surface.
- When oil is hot, add the pork. Cook while turning and flipping until pork is brown on outside.
- Remove to warm plate.
- Add more Olive oil (if needed) and cook peppers and onions until almost done. Onions become translucent and peppers turn darker green.
- Add the pork back to the griddle, mixing everything together to heat through.
- Remove to plate for serving, cover and keep warm.
- Place tortillas on griddle and brown on each side.
- Remove from griddle and put on plate with meat.
- Serve with a choice of toppings.

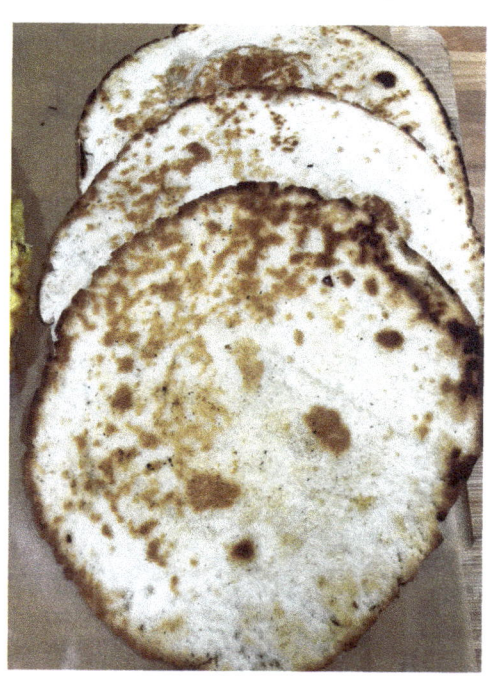

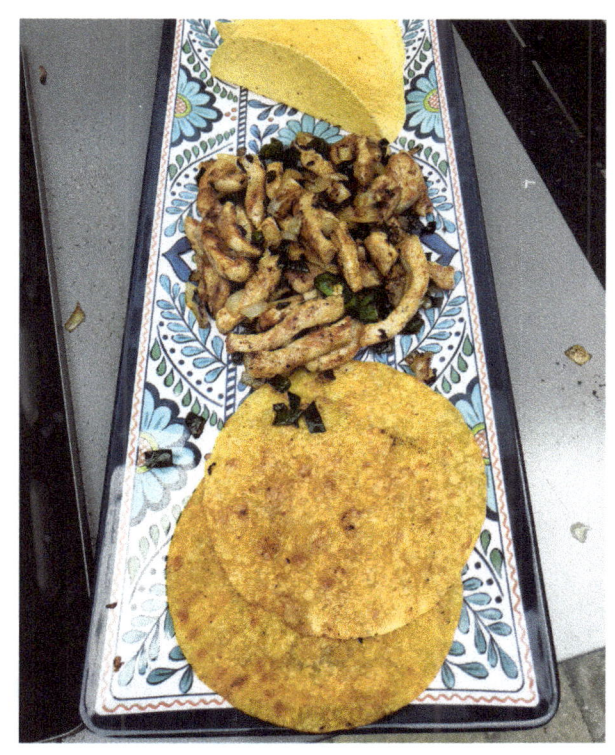

Spicy Pork and Zucchini Noodles

Ingredients (Serves 2-4)

- 1 tablespoon hoisin sauce
- 1 tablespoon low sodium soy sauce
- ½ tablespoon oyster sauce
- 2 tablespoons sweet chili sauce
- 2 tablespoons Olive oil
- 2 boneless, pork chops, cut into thin slices
- 1 tablespoon Thai Red Chili Paste
- 2 tablespoons honey
- 2 shallots, chopped or 1 onion
- 2 cloves garlic, minced
- 1 green bell pepper, sliced
- 2 medium zucchini, spiralized (see recipe on next page)
- Salt and Pepper

Method

- Heat a large skillet or wok on medium heat.
- Add hoisin, soy, oyster sauce, sweet chili and stir together. Cook 2 minutes until sauce is warm. Remove and put in bowl, setting aside.
- To the wok, add the Olive oil and heat on medium heat.
- Season pork with salt and pepper.
- Cook pork in wok or heavy cast iron skillet until brown on all sides.
- Mix Thai Red Chili paste and honey together and add to pork. Stir well and cook for 1-2 minutes. Remove pork and sauce to a plate, setting aside
- Add the shallots, garlic and green bell pepper to the wok. Cook until they become soft. Add the hoisin sauce mixture and heat 1 minute.
- Return all the sauced pork back in the Wok and add the Zucchini Noodles.
- Cook 1- 2 minutes, stirring constantly, until the zucchini noodles soften. Plate in bowls and serve.

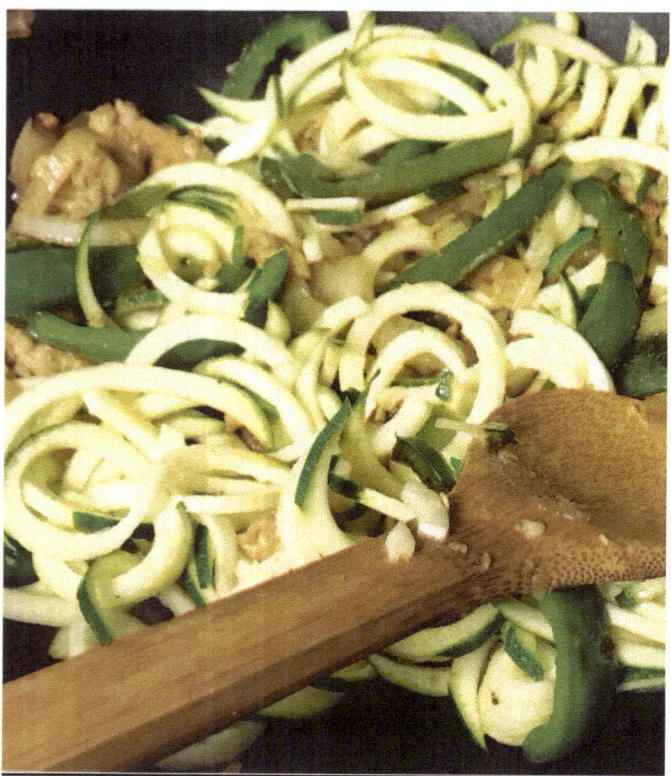

Zucchini Noodles

To prepare the Zucchini Noodles take 1-2 large Zucchinis with peeling on and spiralized either by hand machine or a mixer attachment. Put them in a strainer and rinse the noodles well.

Lay the noodles out on a bread board covered with parchment paper to dry. Once they are dry, they are ready to cook.

The key to working with Zucchini spiralized noodles is to not cook them long. 1-3 minutes is all that is needed.

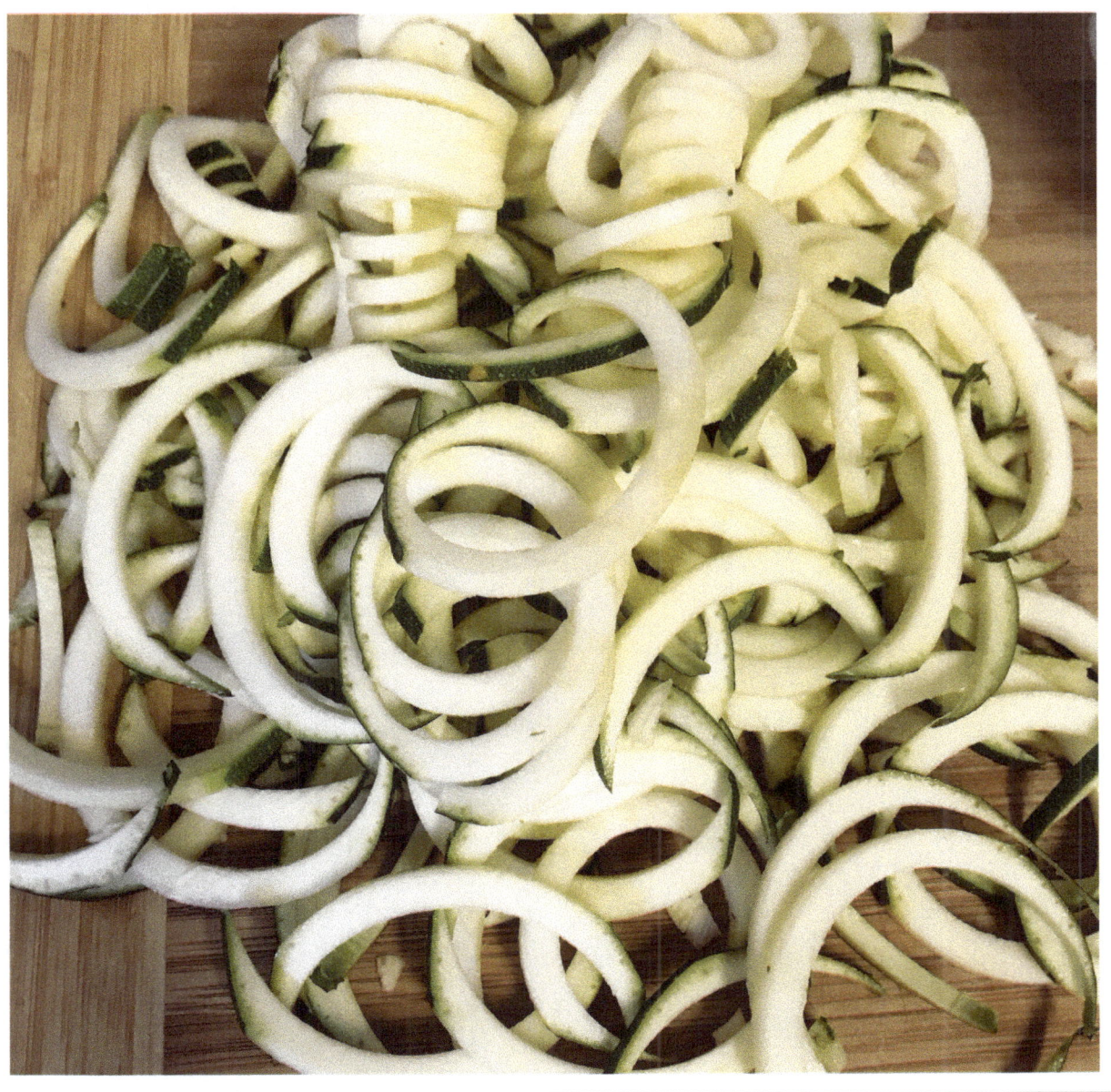

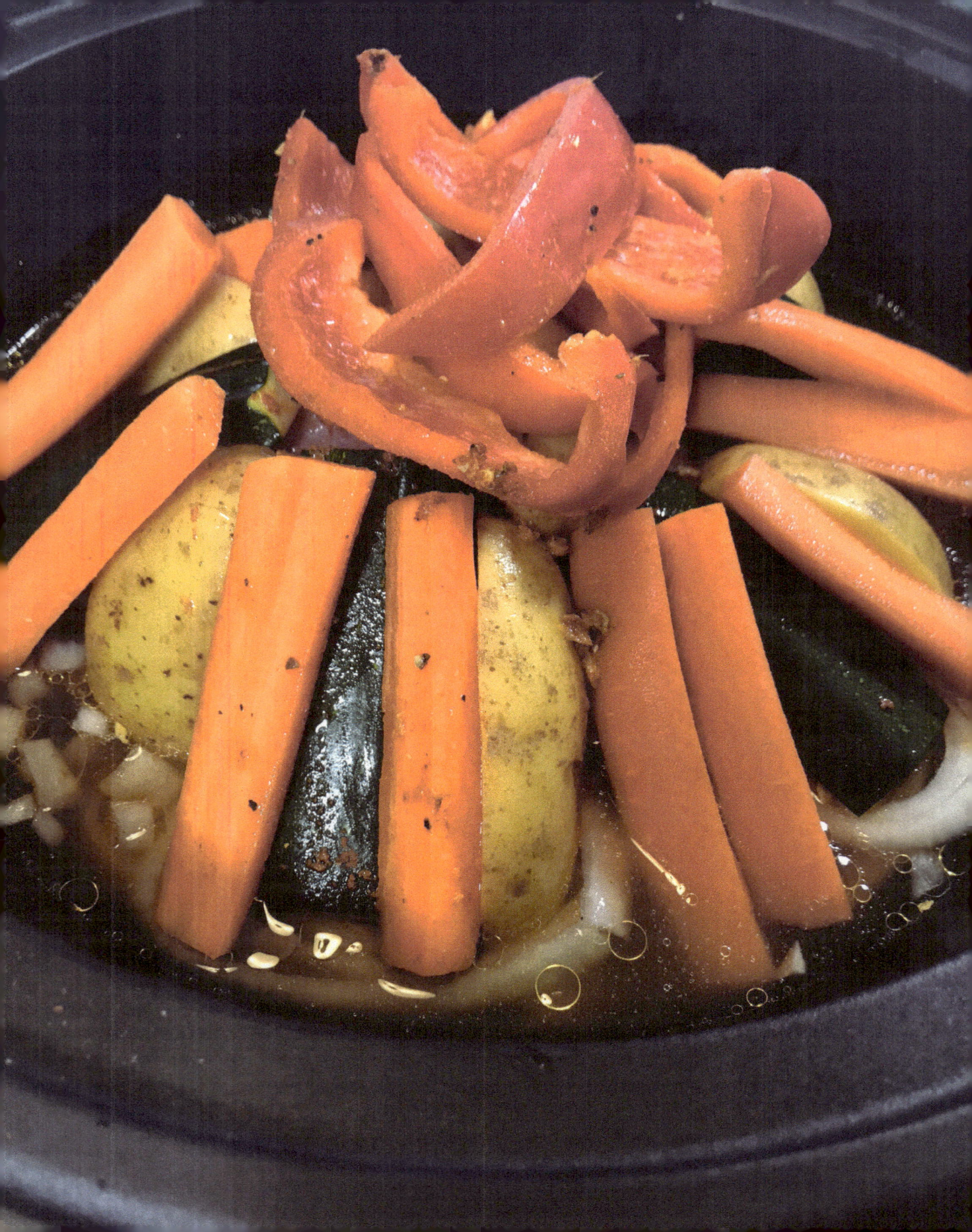

Chicken & Turkey

Fried Chicken 86

Asian Griddled Chicken 87

Hurricane Chicken (Coq au Vin) 88

Tandoori Chicken & Vegetable Bake 90

Upside Down Meatloaf Wrapped In Bacon ... 92

Italian Meatballs 94

Bourbon Chicken & English Peas 95

Cocktail Meatballs 96

Black Pepper Stir Fried Chicken 97

Shepherd's Pie 98

Grilled Mediterranean Chicken 100

Spicy Chicken Meatballs 101

Kung Pao Chicken 102

Spatchcock Grilled Chicken 104

Chinese Chicken & Broccoli 105

Chinese Chicken Dumplings 106

There's Only One Fried Chicken

"There's only one fried chicken - - and that's your mother's on Sunday", was quoted to me by my dad and probably more than once.

We ate a lot of chicken. My papaw raised them and my mammy would prepare them for cooking.

My mammy never ate chicken in any form, except fried chicken. It was a Sunday favorite and my mom and my mammy knew how to fry some great chicken. Each of them used a cast iron skillet filled with lard. The whole chicken would be cut up and the wish bone was always the coveted piece to get. When the lard started to smoke, mammy would drop the flowered chicken into the oil and brown it, both sides and put a lid on it and cook at a lower temperature until tender. The lid came off towards the end so the chicken could brown even more. Even the liver and gizzards and heart were not spared and would be cooked last and put on the platter for serving. Sunday afternoon lunch was always something to look forward to. Big plates of mashed potatoes, a salad, buttered sweet corn and pinto beans that had cooked all morning would be the sides.

It was in the 1960's when down the road on a main drag in our town, a restaurant called Kentucky Fried Chicken was opened. It was different than the Mug N Bun and A&W Root beer or the diner in the drug store. It only served chicken, and it was only fried chicken.

When I rode my bike in front o the restaurant, I noticed that it was always busy. The interesting thing was people didn't eat in the restaurant, but carried out dinner to take home. It was in a box or a round tub and the smell of the chicken was strong and flavorful, even from where I sat on my bicycle on the sidewalk. I was very curious about the food.

So, on one Sunday afternoon, I asked my dad, "Can we try some chicken from the new place down the street." He looked directly at me and said, "Why would we pay money to buy chicken someone else cooked when your mom makes perfectly great fried chicken every Sunday afternoon."

It took awhile for me to realize, well, maybe he was right, but my curiosity still had the best of me. I saved my allowance for a few weeks, rode my bike to the restaurant without telling anyone and ordered me some chicken. I had to try it and just didn't want to wait any longer. The chicken was hot, delicious and tender, but I thought the side items needed a lot of work. I had never eaten instant mashed potatoes, even though I could tell the restaurant worked hard to disguise the flavor, but I could tell. I had never eaten slaw like they made because we always ate vinegar slaw. However, it didn't stop me from eating the chicken with the seasonings and enjoying every bite.

I never told my dad about my secret mission to visit Kentucky Fried Chicken or that I used my allowance on such frivolity. Thirty years later when dad came to visit the family, we were going out for a picnic on July 4th. We stopped at Kentucky Fried Chicken and picked up a bucket and some sides. Potatoes, beans, slaw, rolls and lots of gravy were included. We all enjoyed the day and the food and even dad thought it was pretty darn good chicken.

Today, I make fried chicken in the air fryer, and it is pretty darn good too, but not quite like my mom's and mammy's with the bones in tact and the grease still clinging to the breading. I like experimenting with recipes and flavors for chicken from stir fry, roasting, curries, stews, soups, savory pies and salads. It is very low saturated fat overall, so I cook with it often.

Fried Chicken (in Air Fryer)

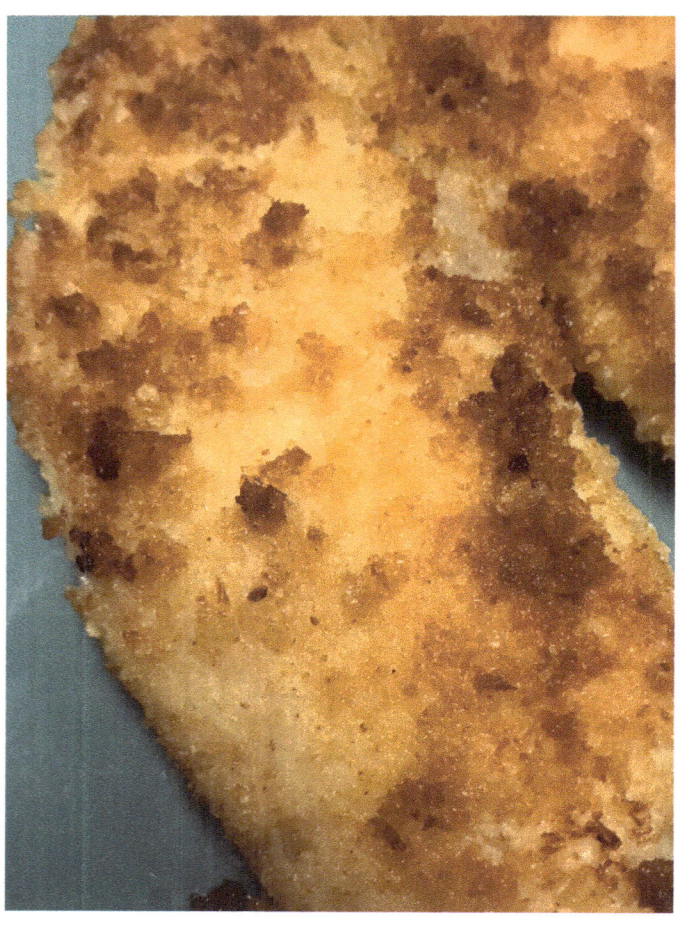

Ingredients (Serves 4)

- 4 boneless, skinless chicken breasts (4 ounces for each serving)
- 1/2 teaspoons kosher salt
- 1 teaspoon paprika
- 1 egg well beaten in separate bowl
- 1 cup flour in separate bowl
- 1 cup bread crumbs in separate bowl
- Olive oil spray

I have seen some air fry notes that recommend putting parchment paper on the bottom of the air fryer. I do not do this, unless the items I am frying are small enough to fall through those tiny holes in the bottom. Just spray lightly the bottom of the grate before placing the chicken in the basket. Works perfectly. Use tongs to flip the chicken as it will become very tender.

Method

- Heat an air fryer to the manufacturer's recommendations
- Wash chicken and pat dry
- Put the three prepared bowls on counter (flour, egg, breadcrumbs)
- Take each piece of chicken and dip in flour, then egg, then breadcrumbs
- Lay the chicken in the grill pan of the air fryer after it has preheated
- Spray olive oil on top of chicken. Sometimes to be a bit different and add flavor, I sprinkle some Italian seasoning or other seasoning after spraying the oil.
- Insert air fryer basket and cook 10 - 12 minutes at 350. The time may be a bit longer depending on the thickness of chicken breasts.
- Open air fryer and turn chicken over, spraying olive oil on top of chicken
- Continue cooking for 10-12 minutes. Chick is done when it reaches 165 degrees at its thickest point, juices are clear and meat is white throughout.
- Remove chicken to serving plate.
- Let rest 3 minutes before serving.

Asian Grilled Chicken

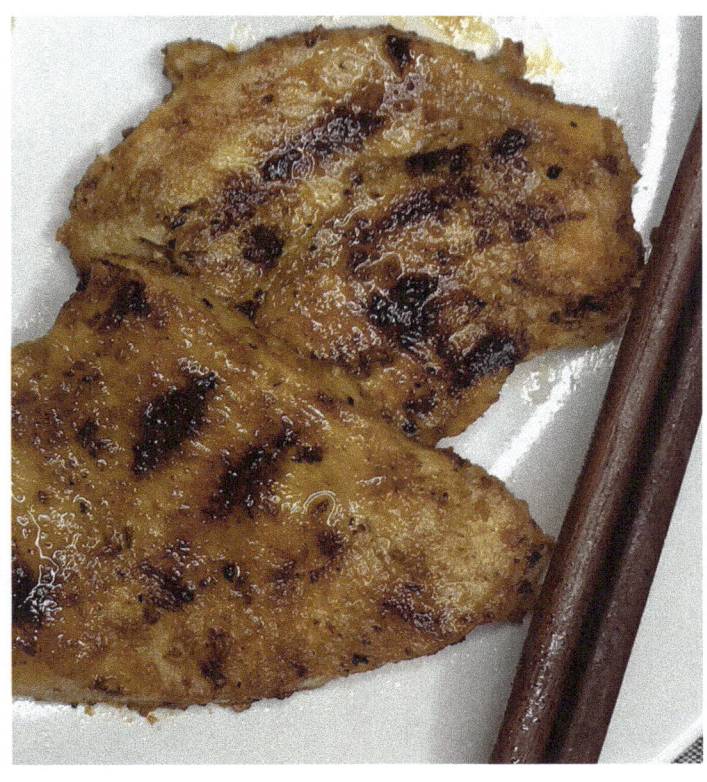

Ingredients (Serves 2-4)

- 2 boneless, skinless Chicken breasts, 4 ounce serving per person
- 1 small onion, chopped
- 2 cloves garlic, peeled
- 2 teaspoons Five-Spice Powder
- 1 teaspoon Allspice
- 1 teaspoon Dried Thyme
- 1/2 teaspoon ground nutmeg
- 1/2 cup low sodium soy sauce
- Salt
- Pepper
- 1 tablespoon of Canola Or Olive Oil
- 1 teaspoon dried chipotle peppers (or Smokey paprika, or dried crushed chili peppers)

- Method
- If the chicken breasts are very large, slice down the middle to make two pieces.
- Place all other ingredients into a blender and mix until very well blended.
- Put chicken into a freezer bag and pour mixture over.
- Seal the bag and place in refrigerator to marinate for 6 hours.
- Every hour or so, turn the bag over so the chicken is evenly flavored by the marinade.
- Remove the chicken from the refrigerator about 15 minutes before cooking.
- Heat a griddle with olive oil or canola oil on medium high heat.
- Remove the chicken from the bag and let extra sauce drip back into the bag.
- Place pieces of chicken on the griddle. They should sear a total of 8-10 minutes, 4-5 minutes per side, depending on the thickness of the chicken breast.
- Basted with some of the left over marinade every few minutes and flip to other side. Keep repeating this process until chicken is done. If the chicken starts getting too dark, reduce the heat.
- Chicken is done when juices run clear or internal temperature reaches 165 degrees. The meat should be white through and through.

Hurricane Chicken

Hurricane Chicken became a nick name for Coq au Vin when we lost power for 5 days during one of our worse hurricanes on our island . The gas stove automatically locked the electric ignition and could not even be lit with a match. We had a gas grill outside and it did not have an electric ignition so we could light it with a lighter. Our neighbor was able to connect us with an extension cord to his generator, so we could keep our refrigerator going, but I still had to cook. I wanted to use what I could without losing too much food as it looked like we were going to be in the dark for a long time. Trees blocked our road and it was the only way out   I took a package of chicken breasts and turkey bacon out of the refrigerator and said to my husband, I am going to cook Coq au Vin and call it Hurricane Chicken. I used my heavy Dutch oven and cast iron skillets to make the entire meal on the grill. It is now our "go to" every hurricane season.

Coq au Vin

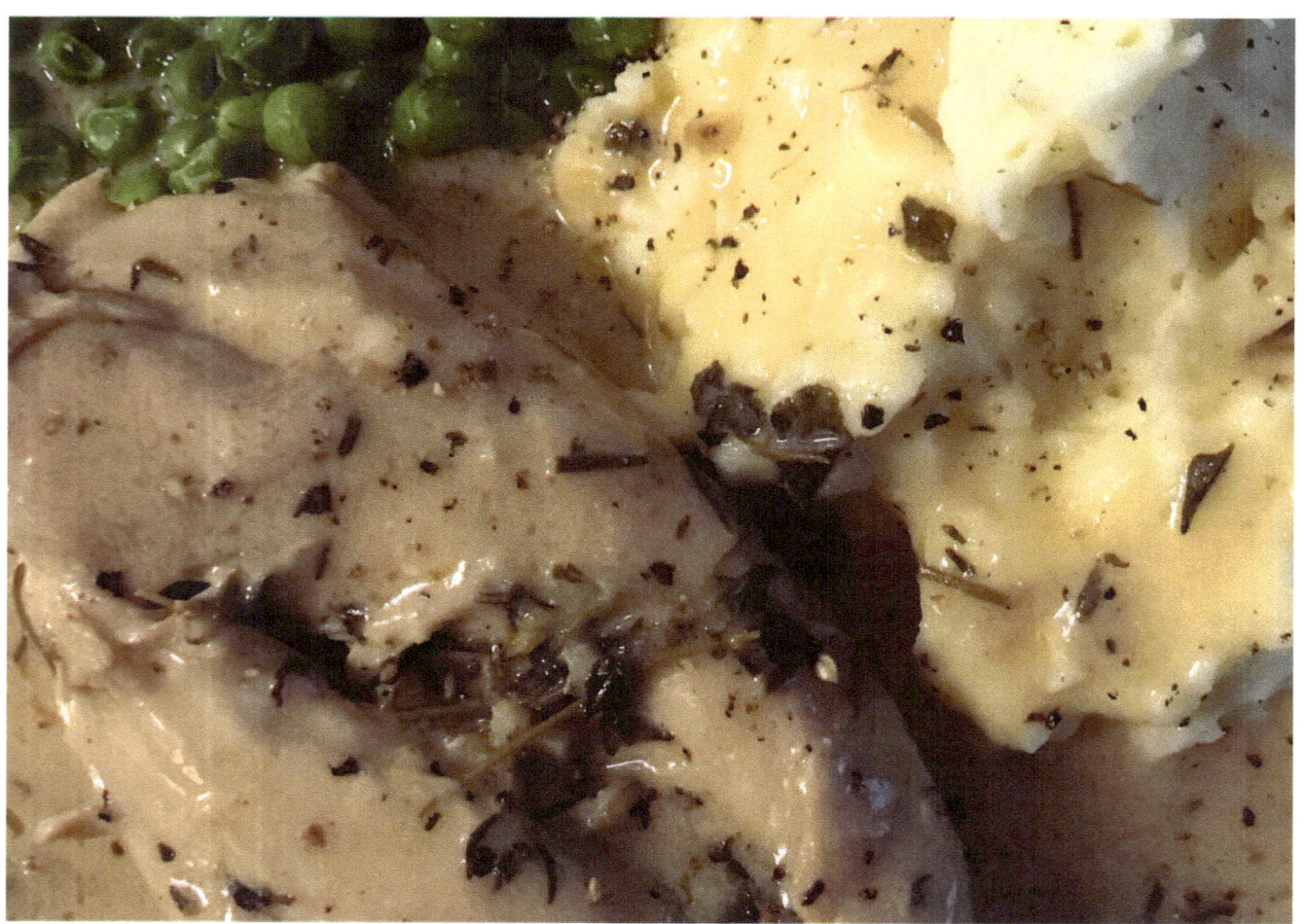

Ingredients (Serves 4-6)

- 2 Tablespoons Extra Virgin Olive Oil - or Canola Oil (less fat in Canola Oil)
- 8 Slices Turkey bacon
- 1 Large Onion - yellow or white - chopped
- 3 Boneless Chicken Breasts
- 2 Jumbo Garlic Cloves, diced
- 1 Small package fresh Portobello mushrooms - sliced thick
- 1/4 cup Brandy
- 1 Bottle Dry Red Wine - Burgundy or Cabernet
- 6-8 Fresh Thyme sprigs or 3 Tablespoons dried
- 2 Bay Leaves
- 1 Tablespoon tomato paste
- 1 Cup low sodium Chicken broth
- 1-2 Tablespoons flour
- 2 Tablespoons low fat Margarine
- Salt & Milled Pepper
- Optional - 1/2 pound carrots sliced in 1-inch pieces

Preparation

- Heat oil in a heavy pot or Dutch oven that is set to medium heat.
- Add the bacon and cook until browned, then remove to a plate. Let it cool before chopping into smaller pieces.
- Season chicken with salt and pepper.
- Add chicken pieces to pot and brown on all sides, approximately 5-7 minutes.
- Remove chicken pieces to the plate with the bacon.
- Once all chicken pieces have been browned, add onions to pan and cook until brown. If you are adding carrots to the recipe, add these with the onions.
- Add the garlic and cook, stirring constantly so sit does not burn.
- Add the Brandy and stir in the Bacon.
- Add the chicken and any juices from the plate or bowl where they rested.
- Add the wine, chicken broth and tomato paste. Stir together very well.
- Add the Thyme sprigs and bay leaves on top of the mixture.
- Cover the pot with a tight lid and put in the preheated 325 degree oven for 40 minutes

While the Coq au Vin is in the oven:

- Heat a skillet with the 2 Tablespoons low fat Margarine
- Add the sliced mushrooms and stir slowly until they begin to brown. Sprinkle 1 tablespoon of flour in the pan and mix very well.
- Remove the Coq au Vin from the oven and add some of the wine sauce to the mushroom mixture being careful to mix well to make a smooth lump free consistency..
- Add the mushroom mixture to the Coq au Vin
- Simmer on top of the stove 10-15 minutes then serve.

Tandoori Chicken & Vegetable Bake

Ingredients: (Serves 4)

- 2 pounds skinless and boneless Chicken breast or thighs
- 1 cup no fat Greek Yogurt
- 3 cloves Garlic, minced
- 1 tablespoon grated fresh Ginger
- 1 tablespoon Hungarian Paprika
- 1 teaspoon Turmeric
- 1 teaspoon Garam Masala
- 1 teaspoon Cumin
- ½ teaspoon ground Cloves
- 2 teaspoons salt
- 1 teaspoon black pepper
- 1 tablespoon lemon juice
- 8-10 Small Petite Red Potatoes
- 8 Brussels Sprouts
- 1 Red Pepper cut into pieces
- 2 small carrots sliced
- 1 small onion cut into chunks

Method

- Mix all spices and lemon juice with yogurt in a large bowl.
- Wash and pat dry the skinless and boneless chicken breast
- Cut each chicken breasts in two pieces, lengthwise
- Place all chicken pieces in the bowl of yogurt and spices and mix well.
- Add all the cleaned vegetables to the bowl.
- Place a lid on the bowl and refrigerate for at least 1-2 hours. While the mixture is marinating, be sure to give it a good mix occasionally.
- Preheat oven to 350 degrees. Spray the bottom and sides of a heavy duty baking dish with non-fat cooking spray. You will want to use a large dish so the pieces do not overlap. I like to use stoneware baking dishes as they bake evenly.
- Remove the chicken from the marinate and lay each piece in the baking dish careful not to overlap the pieces.
- Spread the vegetables around the casserole dish.
- Cover the top tightly with tin foil.
- Bake 30 minutes until chicken is almost white through and through.
- Remove the tin foil top and cook an additional 10-15 minutes to let chicken brown and vegetables to get soft.
- Remove from baking dish to platter and serve with your choice of chutney.

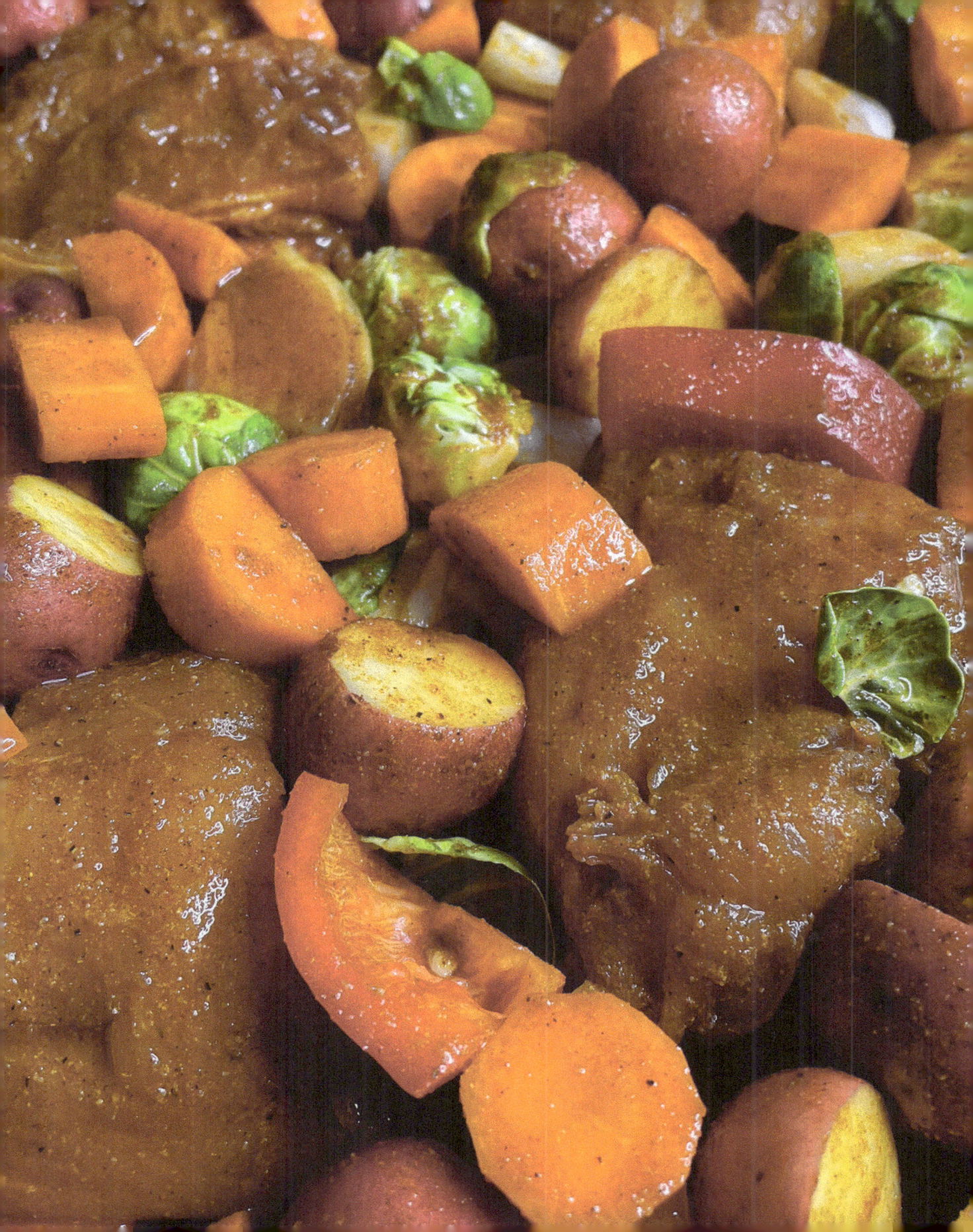

Bacon Wrapped Upside Down Meat Loaf

Ingredients (Serves 6)

- 1 - 1/2 pounds ground turkey meat
- 2 eggs
- 1 cup breadcrumbs (a bit more if the meat seems soggy)
- 1 yellow onion diced
- 1/2 green pepper chopped
- 1/2 orange pepper chopped
- 1 cup ketchup, more or less depending on consistency of mixture
- 1/2 cup brown sugar
- 2 cloves of garlic, minced
- 1 teaspoon Italian seasoning spice
- 1/2 pound turkey bacon

Method

- Preheat oven to 350 degrees
- Mix turkey, eggs, breadcrumbs, onion, peppers together.
- Add 1/4 cup ketchup, garlic, and Italian seasoning.
- Mix all together very well.
- In a loaf pan, add the ketchup to cover the bottom of the pan.
- Sprinkle the brown sugar on top the ketchup covering the entire bottom of the pan.
- Take long slices of the Turkey bacon and drape across the narrow length of the pan so it lays on the bottom and up the sides.

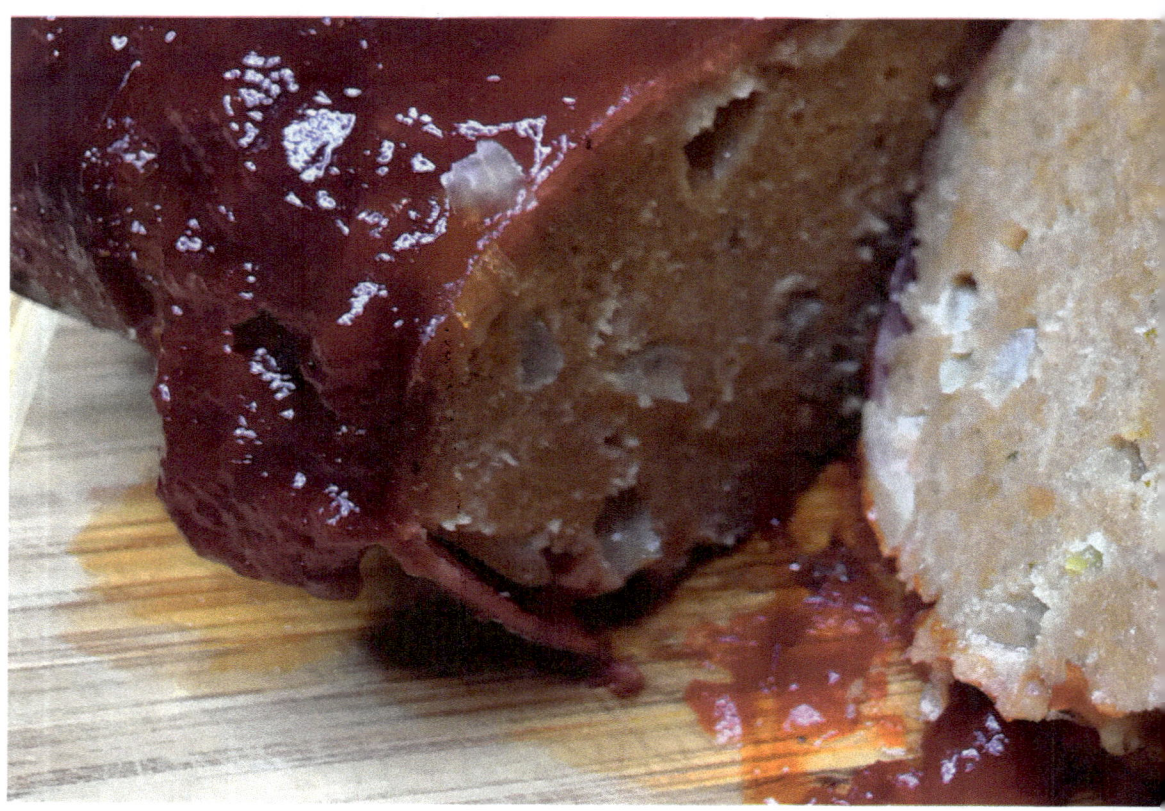

- Repeat this process all the way down the long length of the loaf pan.
- Shape the meatloaf mixture in a loaf the length of the pan.
- Place shaped meat loaf mixture on top of the turkey bacon.
- Bring the sides of the bacon to the top of the meatloaf. It is okay if it doesn't fit all the way since the meatloaf will be turned out and the top in the pan becomes the bottom on the plate.
- Cover the loaf pan with tin foil and bake in a 350 degree oven for 45 minutes to 1 hour.
- Take off the tin foil and let brown for 10-15 minutes. The internal temperature should be no less than 170 degrees.
- Remove the meatloaf from the oven. While it is still warm, turn it out onto a serving platter that is the length of the loaf pan. The bottom of the loaf is now the top.
- Let cool before slicing.

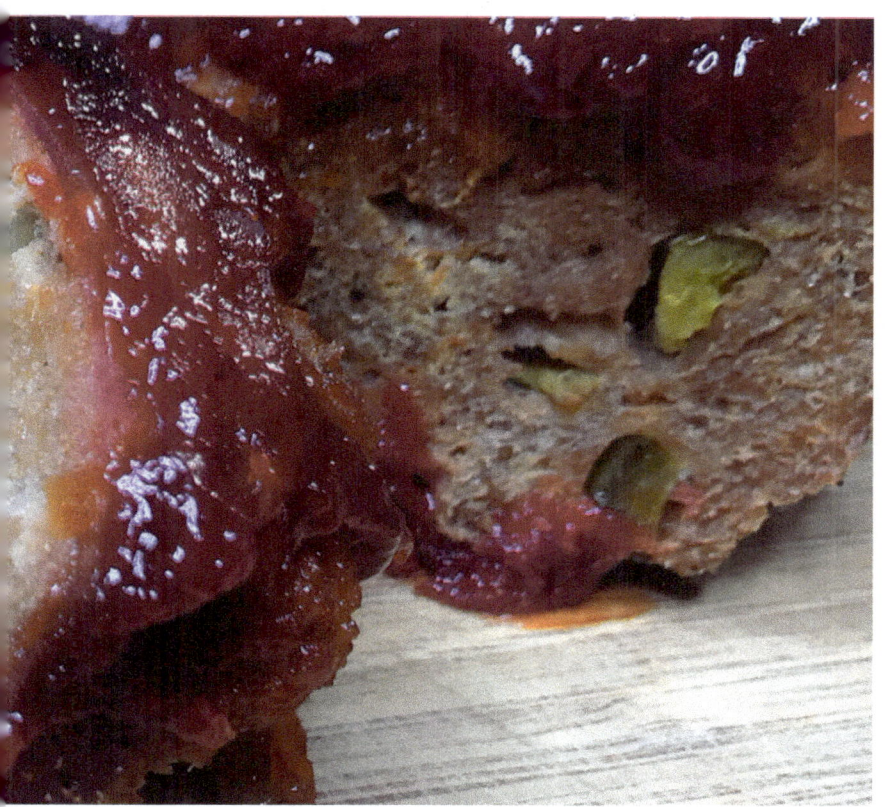

Meatloaf night was special. Mom would combine pork and ground beef together with onions, salt and pepper. She would shape a big loaf and put it in the pan with ketchup all over it so it dripped down the side. Then she would top it with 4 or 5 pieces of thick cut bacon. Slow cooking for 2 hours or more created a crispy topping. Dinner always included mashed potatoes and mom's famous corn.

Oh Momma! Where's the Fat?

Italian Meatballs

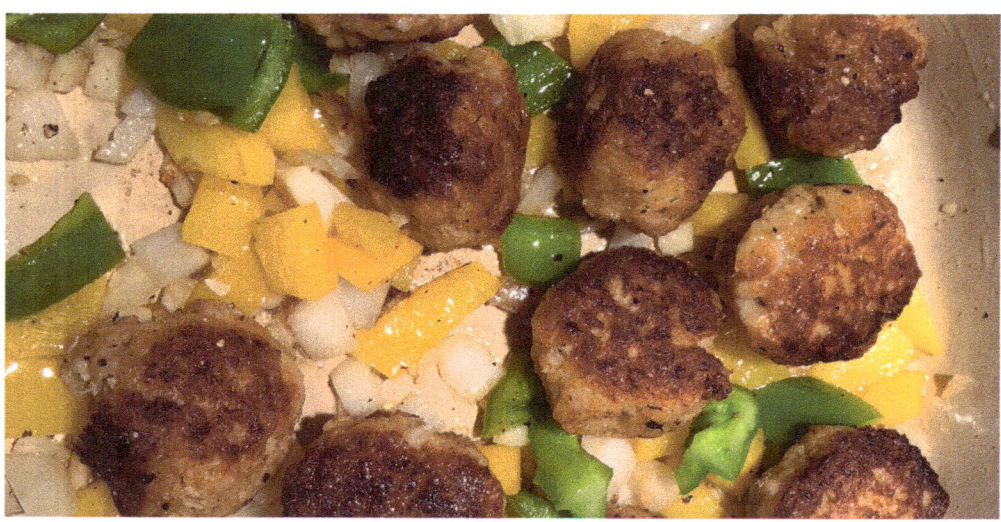

Ingredients (Makes approximately 12)

- 1 pound of ground turkey or chicken meat
- 1 onion, chopped fine
- 2 cloves of garlic minced
- ½ to 1 cup breadcrumbs seasoned with Italian Seasoning mix
- 1 egg, slightly beaten
- Salt
- Pepper
- ½ teaspoon crushed Fennel
- 1 teaspoon oregano and basil

Method

- Combine all ingredients in a large bowl.
- Using your hands, mix all together thoroughly.
- Place a sheet of parchment paper on a long cookie sheet.
- Form the meatballs into 1 inch diameter balls and place on the parchment paper
- Repeat this process until all the mixture has been formed
- Take a large heavy duty pan and put in enough Olive oil to cover the bottom
- Heat on medium heat
- When oil is hot, place meatballs in the pan
- Keep a watchful eye on them and turn them to brown on all sides
- When done, remove to warming tray

I love meatballs with my spaghetti. When I was younger, we made these with Italian sausage. Today, these meatballs can be made with ground turkey or ground chicken for a meatball sandwich or spaghetti.

Bourbon Chicken & English Peas

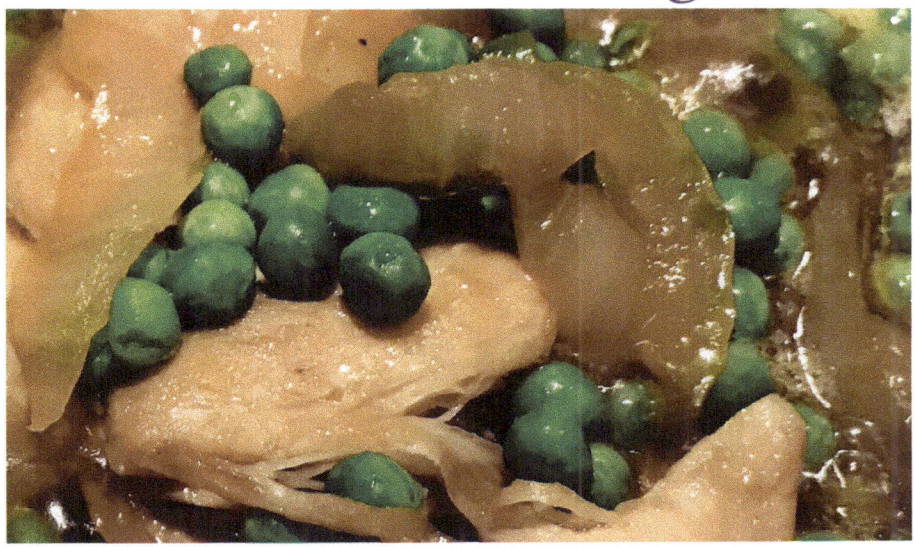

Ingredients (Serves 4)

- 4-6 boneless, skinless chicken thighs
- 2 Tablespoons low fat margarine
- 2 tablespoons extra virgin olive oil
- Salt and Pepper
- 6 small cloves garlic, minced
- 1 large onion, sliced in whole circles and cut in half
- 1 cup bourbon (your choice of brand)
- 2-1/2 cup low sodium chicken broth
- 1 cup frozen English peas (baby or tiny peas work quite well
- 1 tablespoon dry parsley or 2 tablespoons fresh chopped parsley

Method

- Rinse chicken thighs, pat dry with paper towel and season with salt and pepper
- In a heavy pan with lid, heat 1 tablespoon margarine and olive oil on high heat.
- Place chicken thighs in pan and sear on both sides until golden brown approximately 5-7 minutes then remove to a warm plate.
- To the pan add the remaining margarine and saute garlic and onions until soft.
- Remove pan from heat and then add the bourbon and chicken stock.(Remember alcohol can catch fire quickly and easily. Removing the pan from the burner and pouring bourbon in away from heat/flame will be safest.)
- Add pan back to burner and simmer stock for 5 minutes.
- Add the chicken back to the pan and simmer another 15-20 minutes with lid on pan for the first 10 minutes. Watch the sauce that it doesn't get too dry, but it should thicken just a bit.
- 5 minutes before serving, add the peas to the chicken and sauce and let heat thoroughly.
- When the peas appear done, garnish with parsley and serve.

Cocktail Meatballs

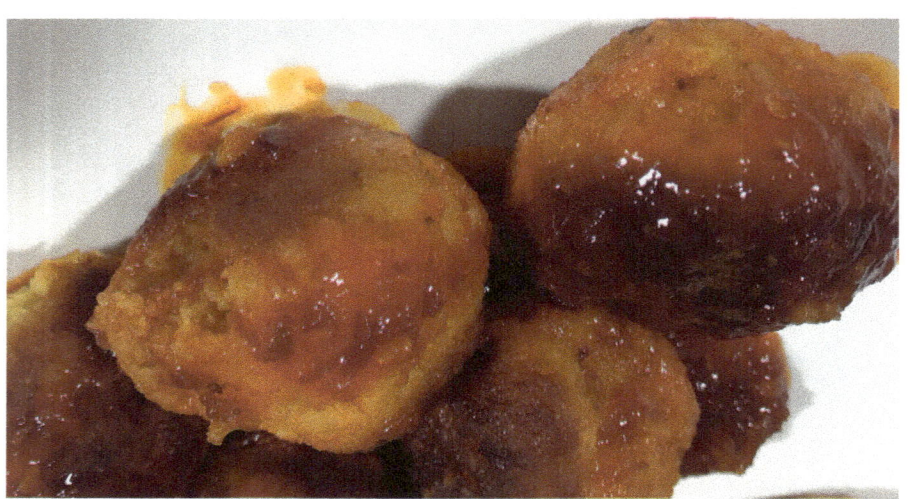

Ingredients (Makes approximately 18)

- 1 & 1/2 pounds of ground turkey
- 1/2 cup dry bread crumbs (i like Panko)
- 1 egg
- 1/4 cup half and half
- Dash of ground cloves (I like the flavor of cloves, so I use 1/4 - 1/2 teaspoon in the meat and a dash in the sauce)
- 1 tablespoon ketchup (if mixture seems to stiff, add a bit more ketchup)
- 1 bottle chili sauce of choice
- 4 ounce jar of regular grape jelly
- Olive Oil
- Salt and Pepper to taste

If this makes too many meatballs just for you, take the remainder meatballs and freeze them for up to 30 days. Take out of freezer, thaw and follow recipe at browning meatballs. Always nice to have some around.

Method

- Mix meat, bread crumbs, egg, milk, cloves, ketchup and some salt and pepper together.
- Shape into meatballs (small)
- Brown meatballs in skillet with small amount of oil.
- While browning, mix jelly and chili sauce. If you like lots of sauce, double the sauce and jelly.
- Once meatballs are brown, put in a slow cooker or Dutch oven.
- Pour sauce mixture over and cook very low (simmer) for 30-45 minutes.
- Be careful they do not burn. Stir them occasionally.
- Pour in a warmed bowl and serve, allowing your guest to dip them up.

Black Pepper Chicken

Ingredients (Serves 2)

- 1 large boneless, skinless chicken breast (this feeds two people), sliced in bite-sized pieces
- 1 Small red sweet pepper, sliced thin
- 1 Medium onion, chopped
- 2 stalks celery, chopped
- 2 cloves garlic, minced
- 2 tablespoons sesame oil
- 1/2 cup low sodium soy sauce
- 1 tablespoon flour
- 2 tablespoons white rice wine vinegar
- 2 tablespoons oyster sauce
- 1 teaspoons ground black pepper
- 1 teaspoon ginger

Method

- Heat 1 tablespoon sesame oil in wok or large heavy skillet.
- Add the chicken to the pan and stir often as it browns and cooks.
- Chicken will be white through the middle when done.
- Remove chicken to a plate
- Add the other 1 tablespoon sesame oil to pan.
- Add vegetables and stir consistently until vegetables are soft, about 5 minutes.
- Stir the soy sauce, flour, vinegar, oyster sauce, ginger and black pepper together. Whisk until smooth and well blended.
- Add chicken back to pan; add the sauce to pan.
- Stir and cook another 2 minutes. The sauce will thicken slightly.
- Remove from heat and serve over cooked rice, noodles or barley.

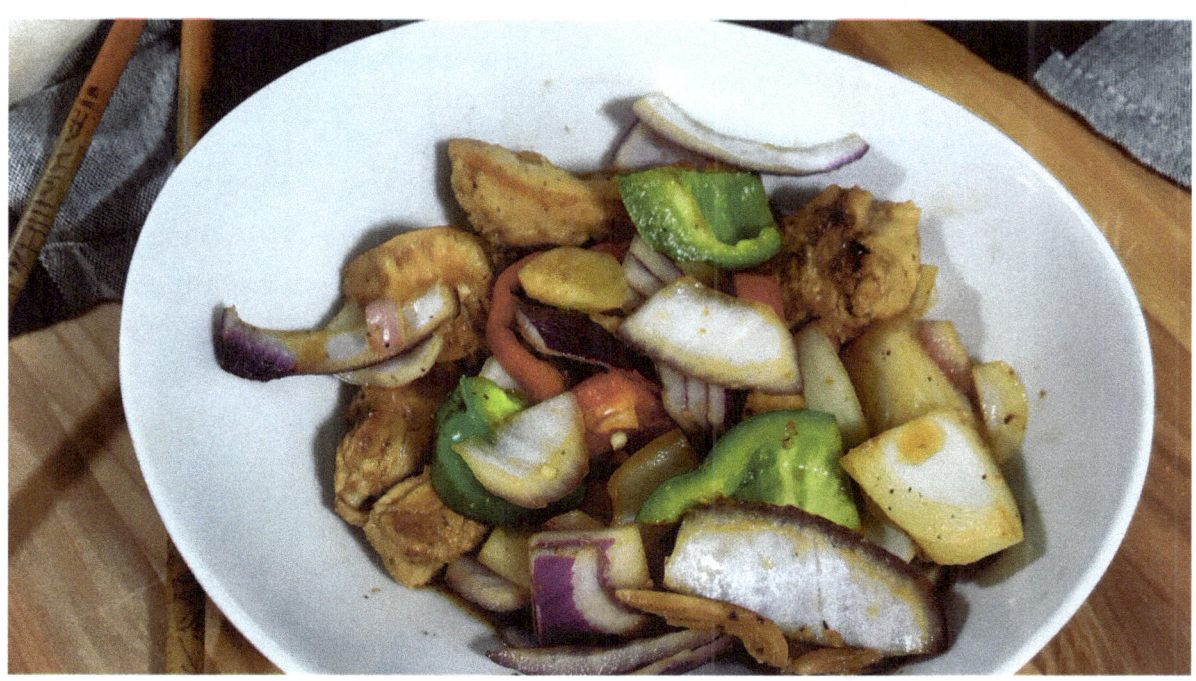

Shepherd's Pie using Ground Turkey

Mashed Potato Topping

Ingredients

- 6-8 Golden potatoes
- 1/2 to 1 cup Non Fat Half & Half
- 4 Tablespoons Low Fat Margarine
- Salt and Pepper

Method

- Peel and cut your potatoes into large pieces.
- Boil them in a large pot over high heat until tender. Make sure to add a generous amount of salt to flavor the potatoes.
- Drain the potatoes and return them back into the pot.
- Melt the margarine milk mixture in a small saucepan, then pour on top of the potatoes.
- Mash the potatoes using a hand masher until they're light and fluffy.
- Taste test to see if it needs more salt or pepper.

Turkey and Vegetable Filling

Ingredients

- 1 pound lean ground turkey
- 1 medium onion, diced
- 1-2 carrots diced
- 2 stalks celery diced
- 2 tablespoons Tomato paste
- Worcestershire sauce
- 1/2 teaspoon Rosemary
- 1/2 teaspoon Thyme
- Salt and Pepper
- Frozen Peas
- 1 cup chicken broth
- 1 cup dark red wine

Method

- Preheat your oven to 350 degrees Fahrenheit.
- Saute the onion and garlic in a large oven-safe saute pan.
- Add the diced carrots, celery, and turkey.
- Cook for 8-10 minutes or until the meat is browned. Make sure to break up the meat using your spatula.
- Add the chicken broth, tomato paste, Worcestershire sauce, rosemary, thyme, salt and pepper. Simmer for about 5 minutes, until the sauce is slightly thickened.
- Add the frozen peas and stir together.
- Pour the mixture in a baking dish
- Use the back of your spatula to flatten the meat mixture into an even layer.

Finish the Pie

- Spread the mashed potatoes on top of the meat and use a spoon or spatula to flatten the edges. Bake the Shepherd's pie for about 25-30 minutes, until it's slightly golden. Cool 10 minutes before serving.

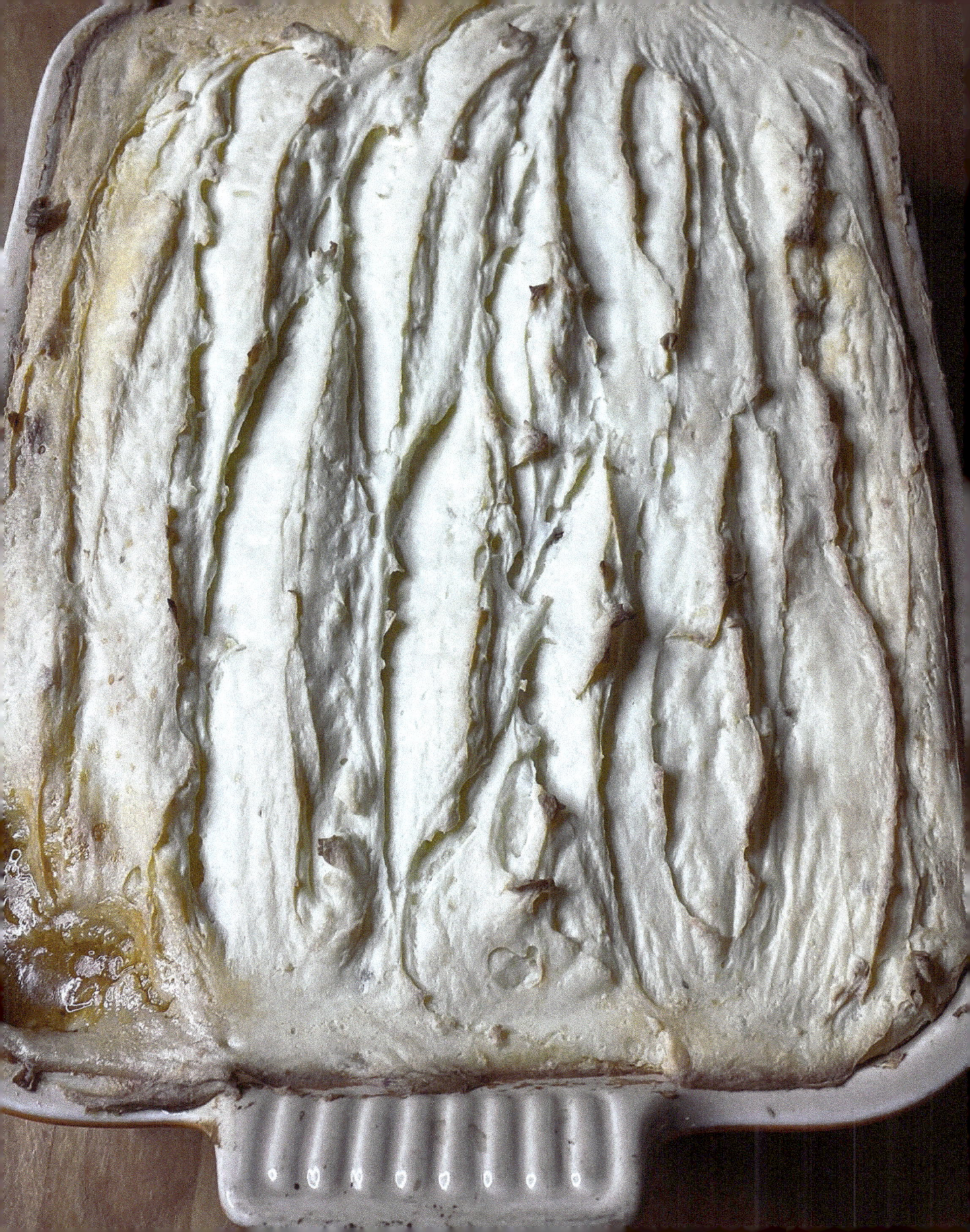

Grilled Mediterranean Chicken

Ingredients (serves 2)

- 2 small boneless and skinless chicken breast
- 1/2 cup olive oil
- 1/4 cup water
- 1 clove garlic, minced
- 1 tablespoon Italian seasoning mix
- 1/2 teaspoon pepper
- 1/4 cup fresh, chopped parsley

Method

- Combine the oil, water, garlic and Italian seasoning with pepper and parsley. Mix well.
- Place chicken breasts in a baggie and pour the marinade into the baggie
- Seal and refrigerate for 2-4 hours
- Remove chicken from refrigerator 10 minutes before grilling.
- Heat the grill or a griddle on top of the stove. Brush generously with oil.
- Place chicken on the grates. Save the oil from the marinade to use as basting the chicken when grilling.
- Cook 4-5 minutes on one side, brush generously with marinade as chicken cooks.
- Flip chicken over and cook another 4-5 minutes brushing with marinade.
- Chicken is done when the juices are clear and meat is white in the middle.

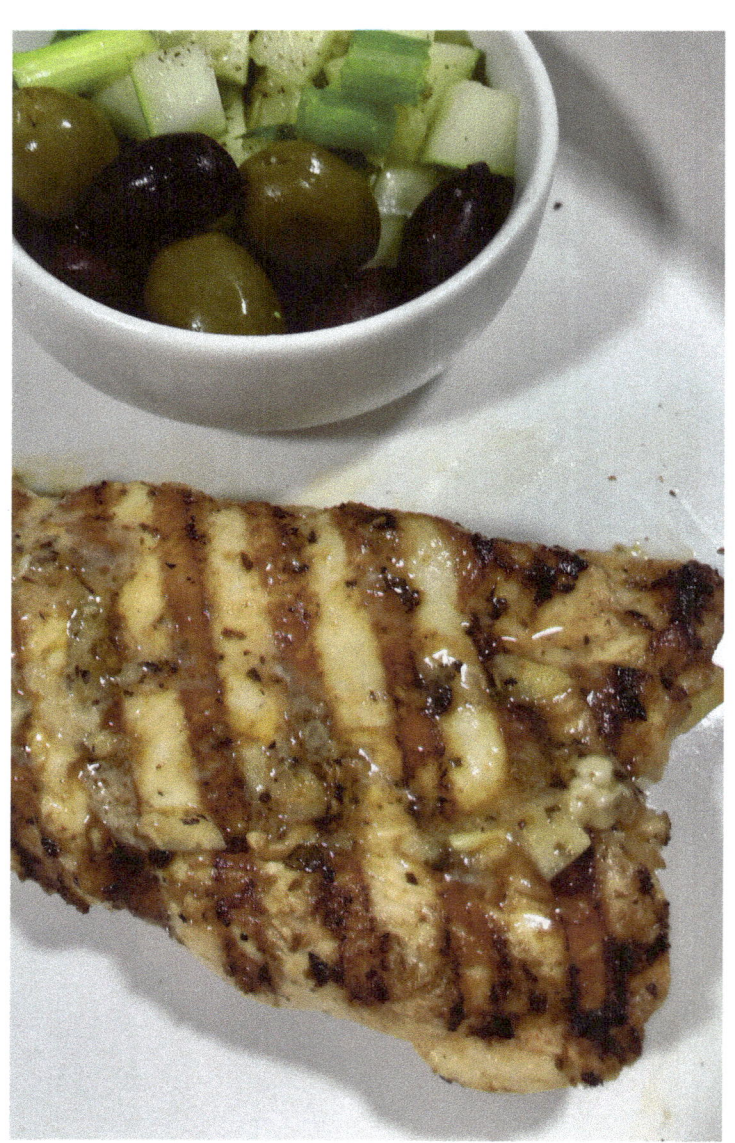

Spicy Chicken Meatballs

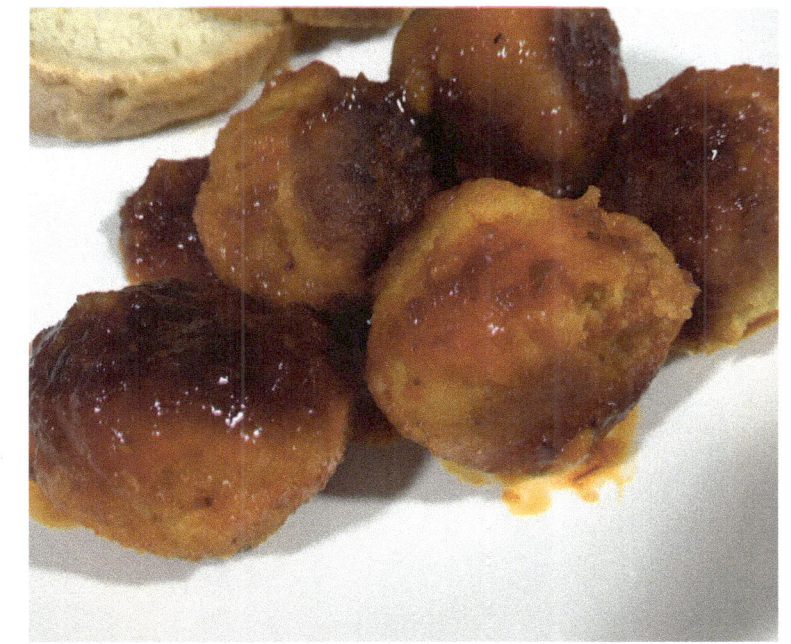

During college I made these meatballs when some of my tutor students came over for a meal. I use to make them with hamburger - it was cheap. The meatballs were always a favorite.

Today, I use ground chicken, and to be honest, I think they are even better than the original ground beef.

Ingredients (Makes 12-18 meatballs)

<u>Meatballs</u>
- 1 pound ground chicken
- 2 medium garlic cloves, minced
- 1 small onion diced
- 1 teaspoon salt
- 1 teaspoon black pepper
- 1 large egg
- 3/4 cup Panko breadcrumbs (unseasoned)
- 1/2 teaspoon Hungarian paprika or Smoked Paprika

<u>Sauce</u>
- 1/4 cup hot sauce (use your favorite brand)
- 1/2 cup light brown sugar
- 2 tablespoons apple cider vinegar
- 1/4 red pepper flakes
- 1/4 cup water

Method

- Preheat oven to 475 degrees.
- Mix the chicken ingredients together and form small round balls.
- Place the meatballs on a piece of parchment paper on top of a cookie sheet.
- Bake 10 minutes and turn meatballs over, then bake another 10 minutes. Chicken meatballs are done when brown all over and inside is white.
- Mix the sauce ingredients in a saucepan on low heat until bubbling.
- When meatballs are done, put in a serving bowl.
- Pour the hot sauce over the meatballs and mix well.
- Serve as a side dish or on sourdough bread or a baguette

Kung Pao Chicken

I have taken a basic recipe that I use to cook and made it low fat by using less oil and more flavor with spices. Chicken breasts that are boneless and skinless are less fat. When I cook with my Wok, only 1 tablespoon of oil is needed. If I want more flavor, I use 1/2 tablespoon of Sesame oil. The meat and vegetables are not swimming in oil, and it is just as good.

Ingredients (4 servings)

<u>For the Marinade</u>
- 1 - 1/2 pounds boneless, skinless chicken breasts, cut into 1-inch chunks
- 1/4 cup soy sauce
- 1 tablespoon dry sherry
- 1 tablespoon cornstarch

<u>Sauce</u>
- 1 - 1/2 teaspoons toasted sesame oil
- 1/2 teaspoon kosher salt
- 1/4 teaspoon freshly ground white or black pepper
- 1 tablespoon Chinese black vinegar (substitute with rice vinegar)
- 1 tablespoon hoisin sauce
- 1 tablespoon granulated sugar
- 1/4 teaspoon ground ginger
- 1 tablespoon Thai chili-garlic sauce (Spicy)
- 1/3 cup water

<u>For the stir-fry</u>
- 1 tablespoons canola oil
- 1 medium bell peppers, red and green, medium diced
- 2 medium celery stalks, thinly sliced on a slight diagonal
- 1 whole carrot chopped
- 1 small can chopped water chestnuts
- 2 cloves garlic, minced
- 1 tablespoon peeled and minced fresh ginger or 1/4 teaspoon dried ginger
- 1/2 cup roasted peanuts (optional)
- 2 medium scallions, thinly sliced (optional)

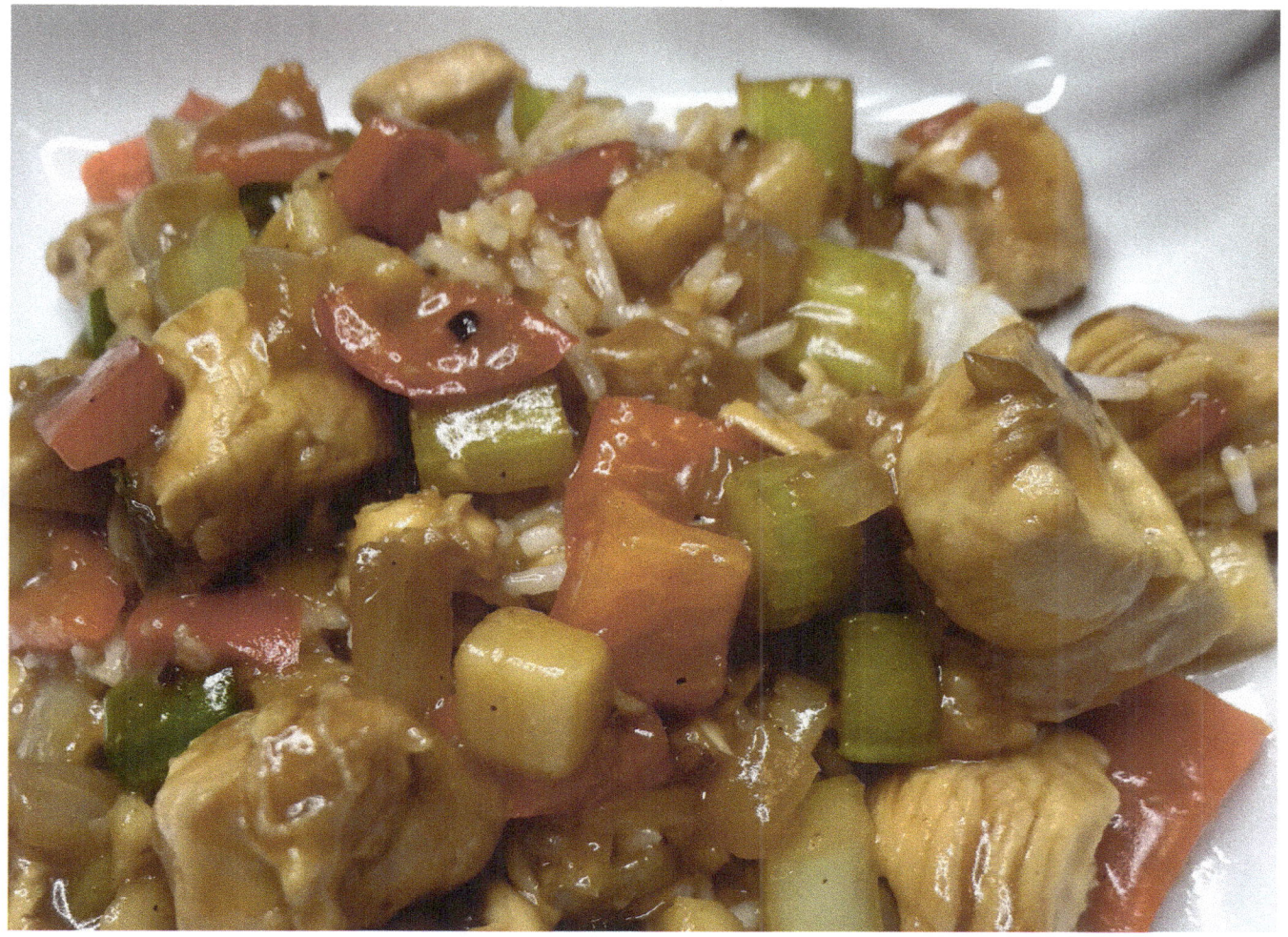

Method

- Place chicken in a medium bowl. Add two - three tablespoons of the marinade over chicken and mix until coated very well. Let sit in refrigerator 30 minutes.
- Add the sauce ingredients to the remaining marinade, set this sauce aside.
- Heat a flat-bottomed wok or large frying pan over medium-high heat until very hot, about 2 minutes. Drizzle in 1 tablespoon of the oil, add the bell peppers, celery, carrot, water chestnuts and stir turning constantly. Add the garlic and ginger and stir-fry until fragrant, about 30 seconds. Transfer to a plate.
- Drizzle the remaining 2 tablespoons oil into the pan. Add the chicken and stir fry until chicken is done. Continually stir and turn the chicken as it cooks.
- Return the vegetables to the pan and heat with the chicken for 1-2 minutes.
- Whisk the reserved sauce to dissolve the cornstarch. Pour into the pan and stir until the sauce thickens, is glossy, and evenly coats everything in the pan. It may take 1-2 minutes. Sprinkle with the scallions, if using, and serve immediately over steamed rice, or noodles..

Spatchcock Grilled Chicken

Ingredients (Serves 4-6)

- 1 whole chicken, thawed.
- Spices or mixes for marinade (BBQ or Mediterranean are always good with this chicken)

Method

- Prepare the grill by laying foil on one side of the grill which will be the side the chicken sits to cook and no heat will be lit underneath.
- Pre-heat the other side of a grill leaving the foil side free from direct heat source.
- Let the grill heat to 300 degrees.
- Prepare the chicken by first removing the backbone from the chicken so the chicken will lay flat on the grill.
- Make a seasoning marinade for the chicken. I typically use Mediterranean spices or BBQ spices for my chickens, but any flavor works.
- Rub the marinade over the chicken, and gently lift the skin to rub spices under the skin. Be sure to get marinade under the legs and all the nooks & crannies of the chicken.
- Make a foil boat that will hold the chicken by taking several sheets of tin foil and lay together flat, making a foil tray with about an inch high side (this holds in the drippings and juices from chicken.
- Place the marinated chicken in the foil tray and place chicken on the grill - the side without direct heat where the foil had been used to cover the grids.
- It is important to check the temperature of the grill often as the 300 degrees F should be maintained.

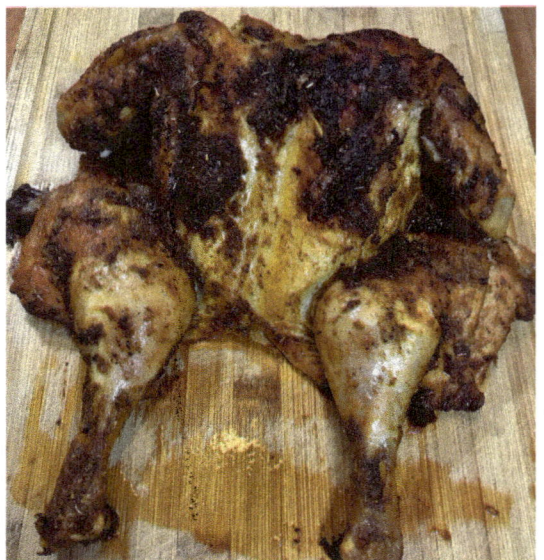

- As chicken cooks, check and brush with the marinade of choice every 30-40 minutes.
- Cook until chicken is done (depending on size of the chicken). Internal temperature at thickest point and through legs should read 165 degrees, and juices run clear.
- Remove chicken to cutting board, cover with tin foil and let rest 30 minutes before slicing.

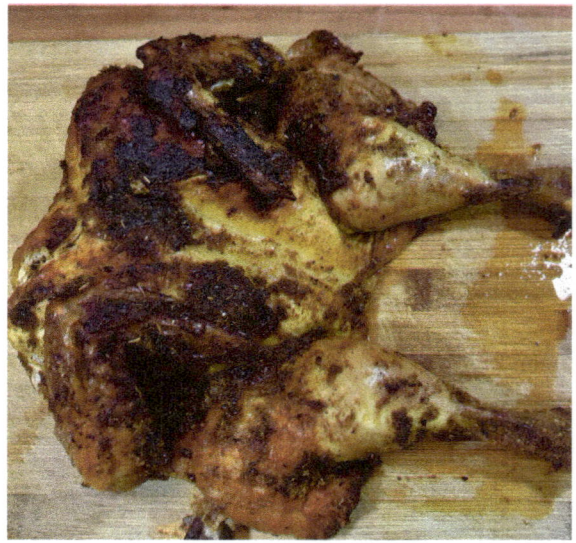

Chinese Chicken & Broccoli Stir Fry

Ingredients (Serves 4)

- 1 large head broccoli, cut into pieces
- 3 tablespoons olive oil
- 2 boneless, skinless chicken breasts, cut into pieces
- 2 cloves garlic, chopped
- 1 small onion, chopped
- 1 teaspoon ginger
- 2 tablespoons hoisin sauce
- 3 tablespoon low sodium soy sauce
- 6 tablespoons honey
- 6 tablespoons hot water

Method

- Steam broccoli slightly. It should be a bit firmer than typically desired.
- Heat a wok on high heat and add one half the oil.
- Add chicken and brown on all sides. Remove chicken and set aside
- Fry garlic, onion, and ginger for 30 seconds in the oil while stirring. This will flavor the oil.
- Add chicken back to the wok. Add soy, hoisin and hot water bringing to a boil.
- Drizzle the honey and cover the wok. Simmer 7-10 minutes.
- While simmering, occasionally add more honey and stir well.
- Add broccoli and stir with sauce until cooked through.

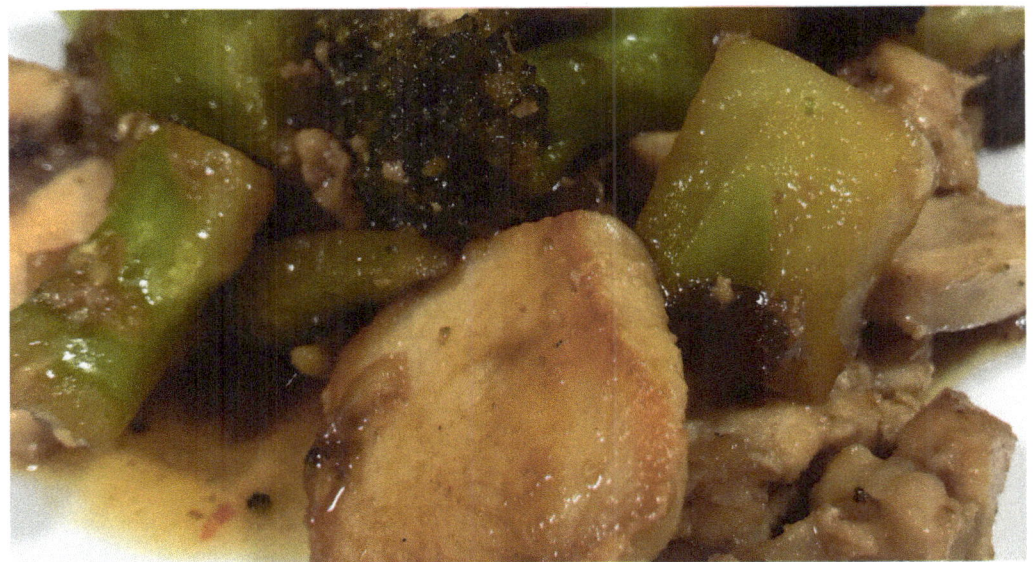

Chinese Chicken Dumplings

Ingredients (Makes 18-24 dumplings)

<u>Dumplings</u>

- 1 package square dumpling wrappers
- 1 pound ground white meat chicken
- 1 medium onion chopped fine
- 1 beaten egg
- 1 tablespoon reduced sodium soy sauce
- 1 teaspoon fresh grated ginger
- ½ teaspoon crushed red pepper
- 1 tablespoon Chinese rice wine vinegar
- ¼ cup non fat Half & Half
- ½ teaspoon salt
- ½ teaspoon black pepper

<u>Dipping Sauce (per person)</u>

- 2 tablespoons soy sauce
- 1 tablespoon rice wine vinegar
- 1 teaspoon sesame oil
- 1-2 chopped scallions
- Dried red pepper to taste, if you like a bit of heat

Method

- Mix the chicken and all spices and sauces together to make the Dumpling mix.
- Add the beaten egg and Half & Half (this gives the chicken moisture it lacks during cooking)
- Lightly flour a bread board
- Fill a small bowl with water (this is used to seal the edges)
- Lay out 6-8 dumpling wrappers
- Place a spoonful of filling in the center of each one
- Fold over in a triangle shape
- Brush a very small amount of water along one edge and pinch to seal.
- Place into one of the bamboo trays for steaming which have been lined with tray paper
- Repeat above and fill the second tray.
- Place the bamboo lid on steamer basket
- Pace the bamboo tray on top of a steaming grid with water boiling slightly. I like using my wok as it fits nicely, but any steamer pan wide enough to accommodate the bamboo works.
- Steam 10-15 minutes.
- Remove from water and serve in baskets.

Cook's note: If you like a crisper dumpling, add a small amount of oil to a skillet and lightly brown dumplings after they have steamed.

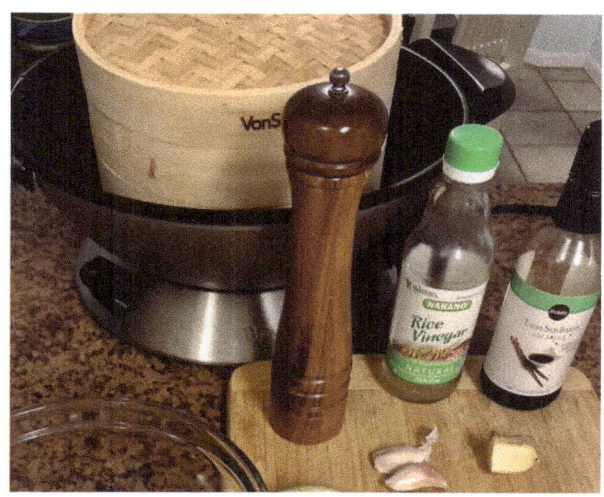
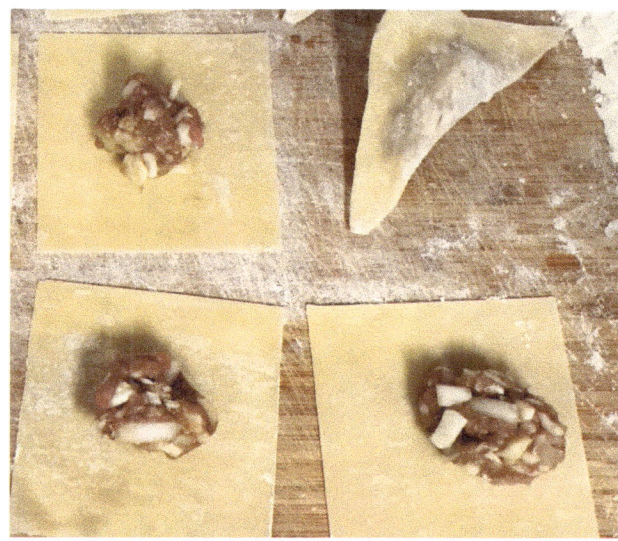
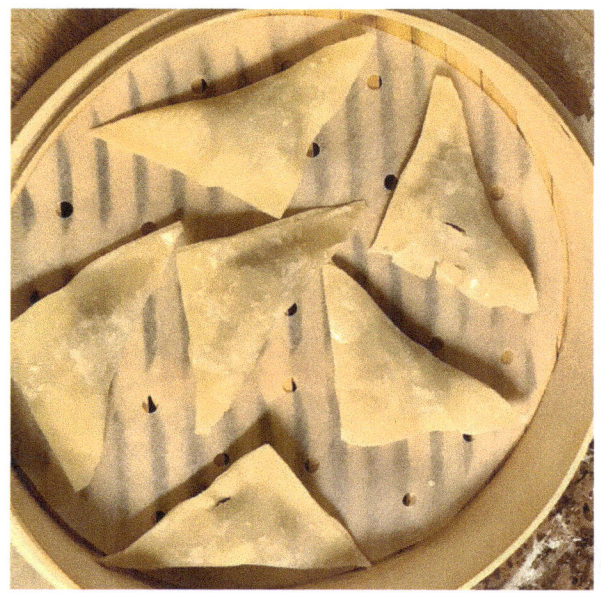
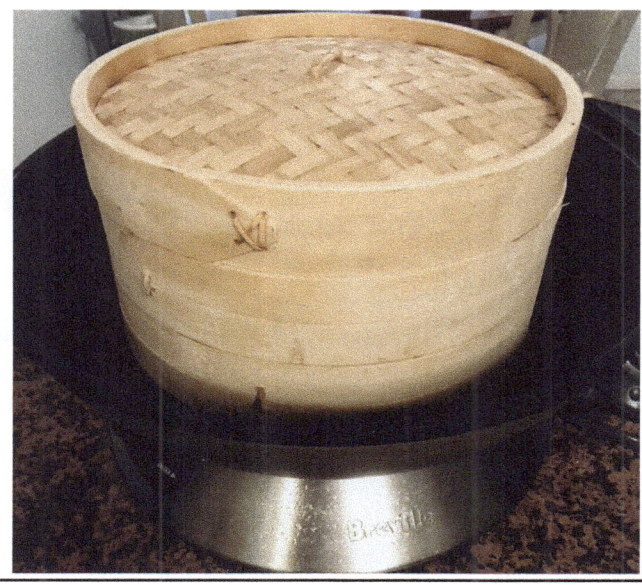

Oh Momma! Where's the Fat?

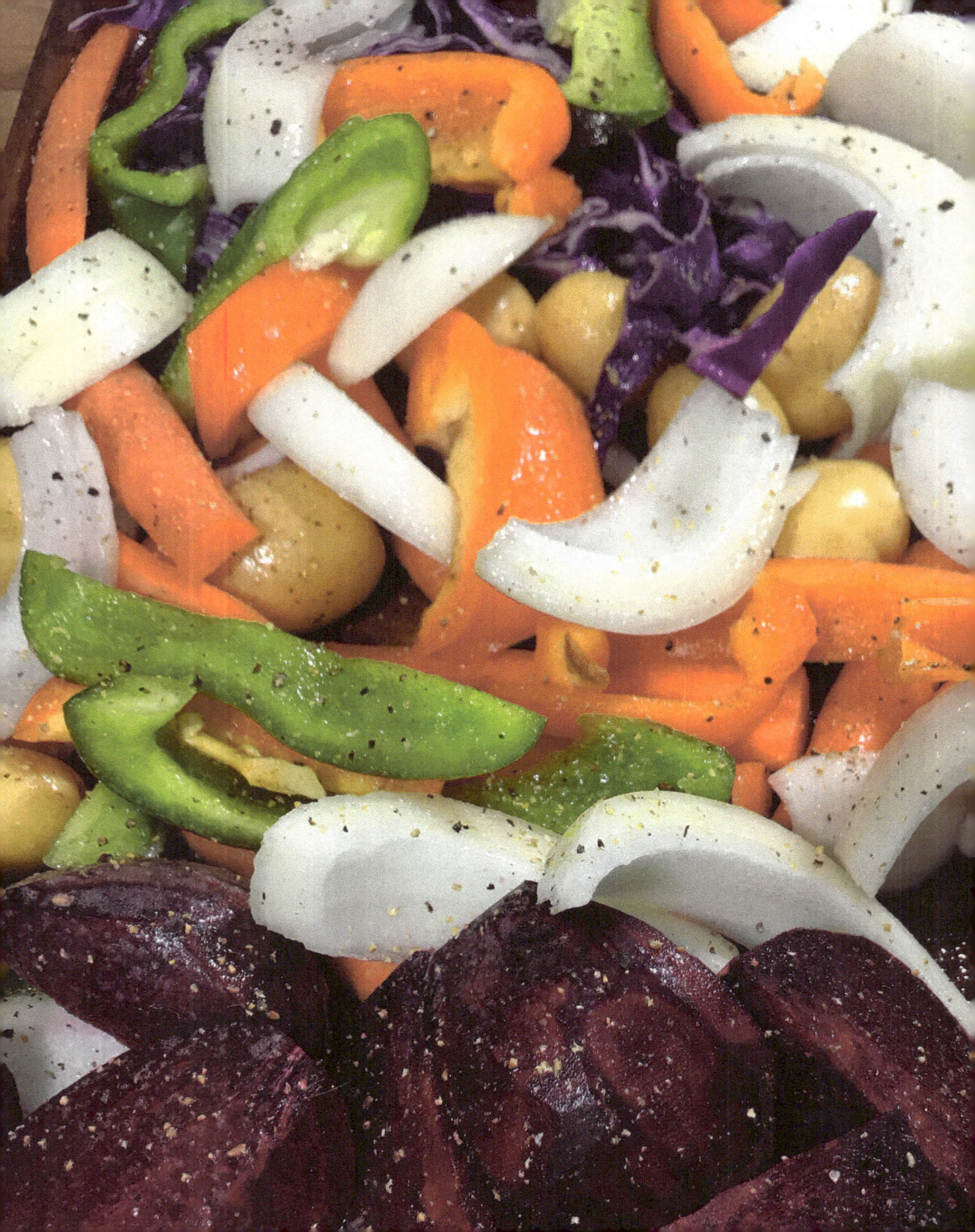

Vegetables

Air Fried Sweet Potatoes 110
Balsamic Grilled Zucchini 111
Mom's Sweet Corn 113
No Crust Cauliflower Quiche 114
Creamy Mashed Potatoes 115
Grilled Corn & Peppers 116
Roasted Sheet Pan Vegetables 117
Mediterranean Cauliflower & Broccoli 118
Spicy Asian Potatoes 119
Honey & Thyme Roasted Carrots 120
Paprika Potatoes 121
Mediterranean Stuffed Peppers 123
Slow Cooked Carrots & Cabbage 124
Cabbage & Carrot Omelette 125
Italian Sausage Stuffed Zucchini 126
Spicy Potatoes & Garbanzos 127
Stuffed Butternut Squash 128

Air Fried Sweet Potatoes

Ingredients (Serves 4)

- 2 large sweet potatoes, sliced
- Olive oil
- Salt and Pepper
- 1 teaspoon Paprika (Use Himalayan Paprika if you want a bit more heat)

Method

- After sweet potatoes have been washed, place on paper towel to drain and dry. Let them dry at least 30-60 minutes.
- Preheat your air fryer per manufacturer's instructions.
- Put 1/4 cup Olive oil in a large bowl.
- Add sweet potatoes.
- Add salt and pepper.
- Add Paprika
- Mix all together with your hands making sure all potatoes are covered in oil.
- When air fryer is finished preheating, remove basket and scoop the oiled and seasoned potatoes into the basket.
- Cook at 400 degrees for 15 to 20 minutes.
- Temporarily stop cooking about half way through and shake pan to mix up the potato layers.
- Continue cooking.
- Potatoes should be done after 20 minutes, but if they need more crispiness, shake them up and let them cook another 10-15 minutes.
- To serve, put on platter and use your favorite dipping sauce.

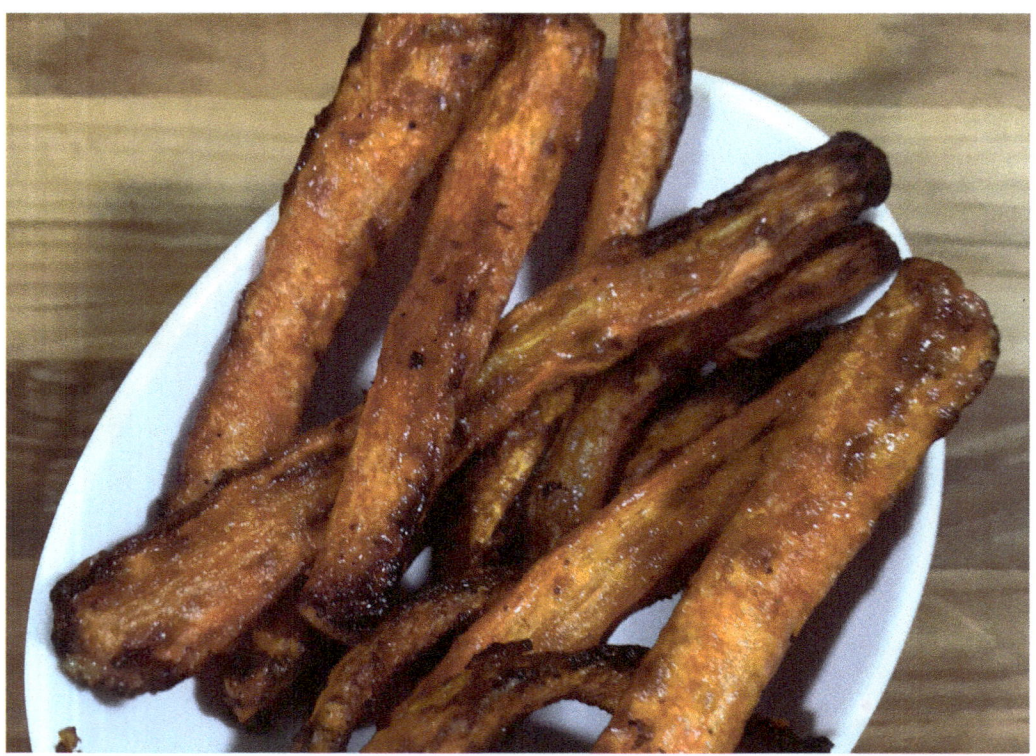

Balsamic Grilled Zucchini

Ingredients (Serves 4)

- 2 zucchinis, cut in quarters lengthwise
- 1 tablespoon olive oil
- 1/2 teaspoon garlic powder
- 1 teaspoon dried Italian seasoning
- 1/2 teaspoon onion powder
- 2 tablespoons white balsamic vinegar

Method

- Preheat the grill, or a grated griddle pan on the stove, on high
- Mix the garlic, onion and dried Italian seasoning together and add Vinegar
- Brush the Zucchini lightly with the olive oil
- Cook on preheated grill for 2-3 minutes per side. The grill marks will show on the sides and be a nice golden brown.
- Remove to serving platter when done.
- Brush with balsamic vinegar mix and serve.

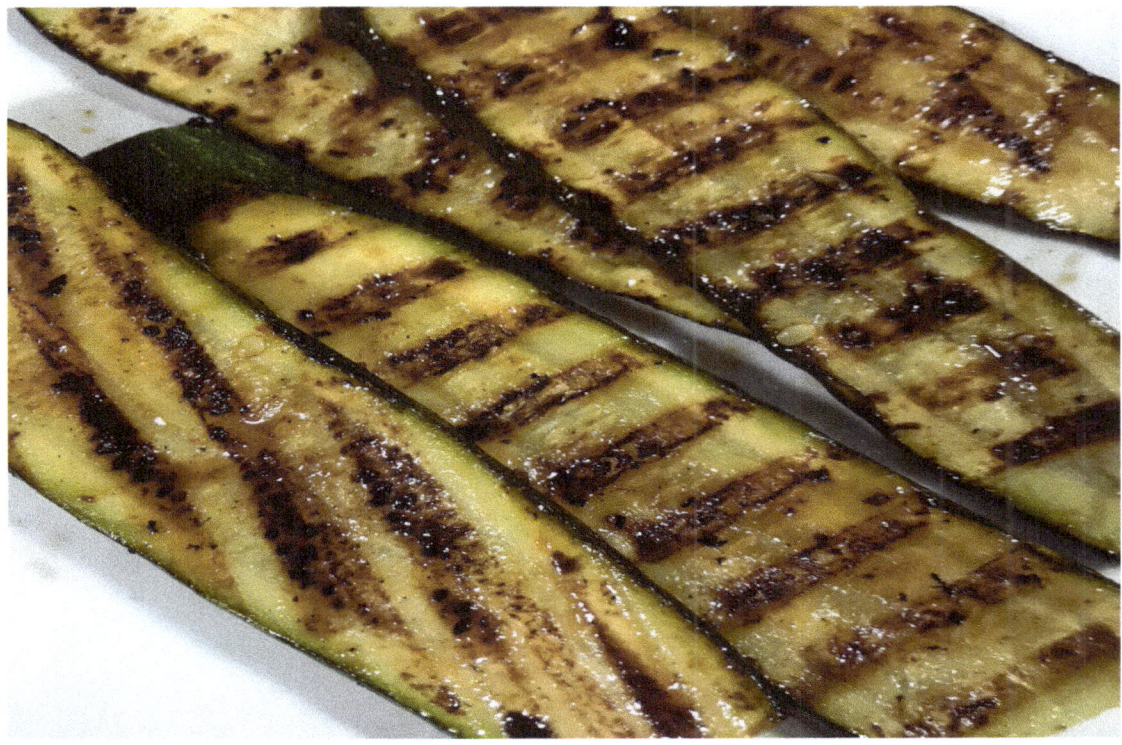

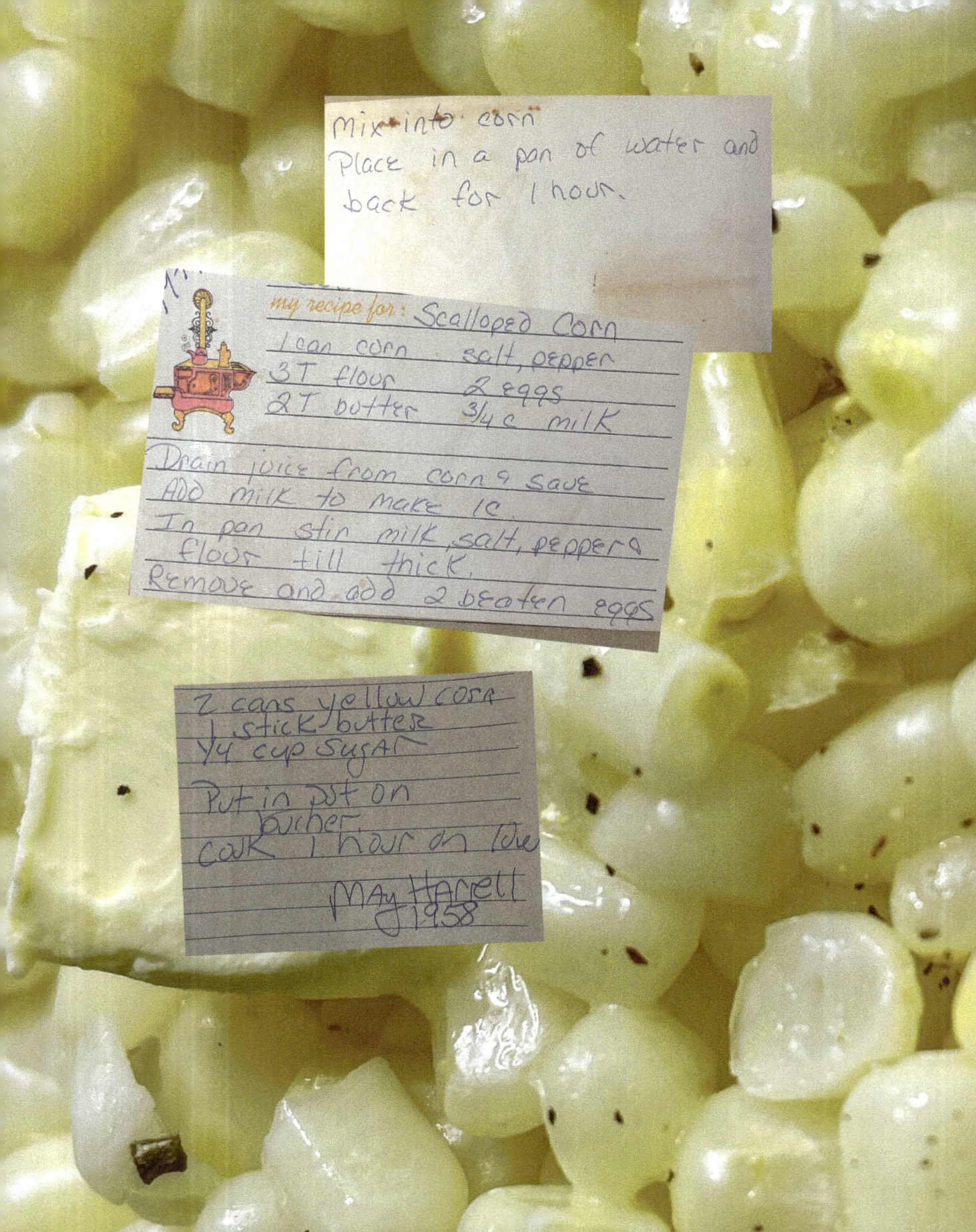

mix into corn
Place in a pan of water and
back for 1 hour.

my recipe for: Scalloped Corn

1 can corn   salt, pepper
3 T flour   2 eggs
2 T butter   3/4 c milk

Drain juice from corn & save
Add milk to make 1c.
In pan stir milk, salt, pepper &
flour till thick.
Remove and add 2 beaten eggs

2 cans yellow corn
1 stick butter
1/4 cup sugar

Put in pot on
burner.
Cook 1 hour on low

May Harrell
1958

Momma's Sweet Corn

There was never a lack of corn living in the middle of Indiana surrounded by cornfields. Corn of many colors, flavors and cooking methods. We ate buttered sweet corn, white corn on the cob, scalloped corn and had corn in all our vegetable soups. But no corn dish was as famous as my mom's sweet corn.

Mom's recipe for corn became well known as a dish in our house and everyone loved it and always wanted her corn when they came for a meal. No matter what the meal, a request for her corn was always forefront. Living close to the Indy 500 race track outside Indianapolis, my mom was known for her cooking and her generosity to those who came from other states that were part of the racing crowd. She knew everyone, and everyone knew her. Indy winners throughout the years, their families, newcomers to the industry, and grandsons of the owner of the Indy 500 track were all frequent dinner guest at our home. I do not recall a night in May during racing season, when a driver, mechanic or owner of a racing team was not at our home having dinner - and always my mom made her special corn. Never was there enough of her corn to satisfy everyone.

As the years passed, Moms reputation grew. She became an icon at the racetrack given special permission to set in the "family section" of the bleacher seats. Mom knew the drivers by their helmet colors and the cars. NBC ask her to be one of the main camera spotters during filming. Her job was to let the camera man know who was approaching. She loved the job and being up on the towers.

After she was diagnosed with melanoma cancer in 1986 and given 3 months to live, she struggled. Everyone who knew her at the racetrack got together and individuals with NBC arranged a special cart to take her around the garages and bleachers at gasoline alley where she could see everyone one more time. There were many greetings and goodbyes that day. Her heart swelled with joy and even a few tears were shed by many. The only thing missing that day was her corn!

Her recipe was simple and is shown in the photograph opposite. She had cooked the corn the same way from 1958 until 1986.

" Open a few cans of sweet corn and put in a pot. Add 1/4 pound of butter, and a few tablespoons of sugar. Heat slow and long to meld the flavors together. "

No Crust Cauliflower Quiche

Ingredients (Serves 6)

- 1 head cauliflower cut into florets
- 2 eggs
- 1/2 cup non fat half and half
- 1/4 cup olive oil
- 2/3 cup nonfat yogurt, plain
- 2 tablespoons flour
- 1 teaspoon paprika
- Salt and Pepper to taste
- 2 tablespoons flour
- 1/2 cup shredded Parmesan cheese

Method

- Preheat Oven to 375 Degrees
- Bring a large pot of water to a boil.
- Boil the cauliflower for 2-3 minutes.
- Mix the eggs with the milk and seasonings
- Add the flour
- Add the yogurt
- Add the cauliflower
- Pour in a pie dish about 8-9 inches.
- Sprinkle the top with the cheese
- Bake at 390 degrees F for 20 minutes (or a bit longer if needed)
- Remove from oven and let cool 5 minutes before serving

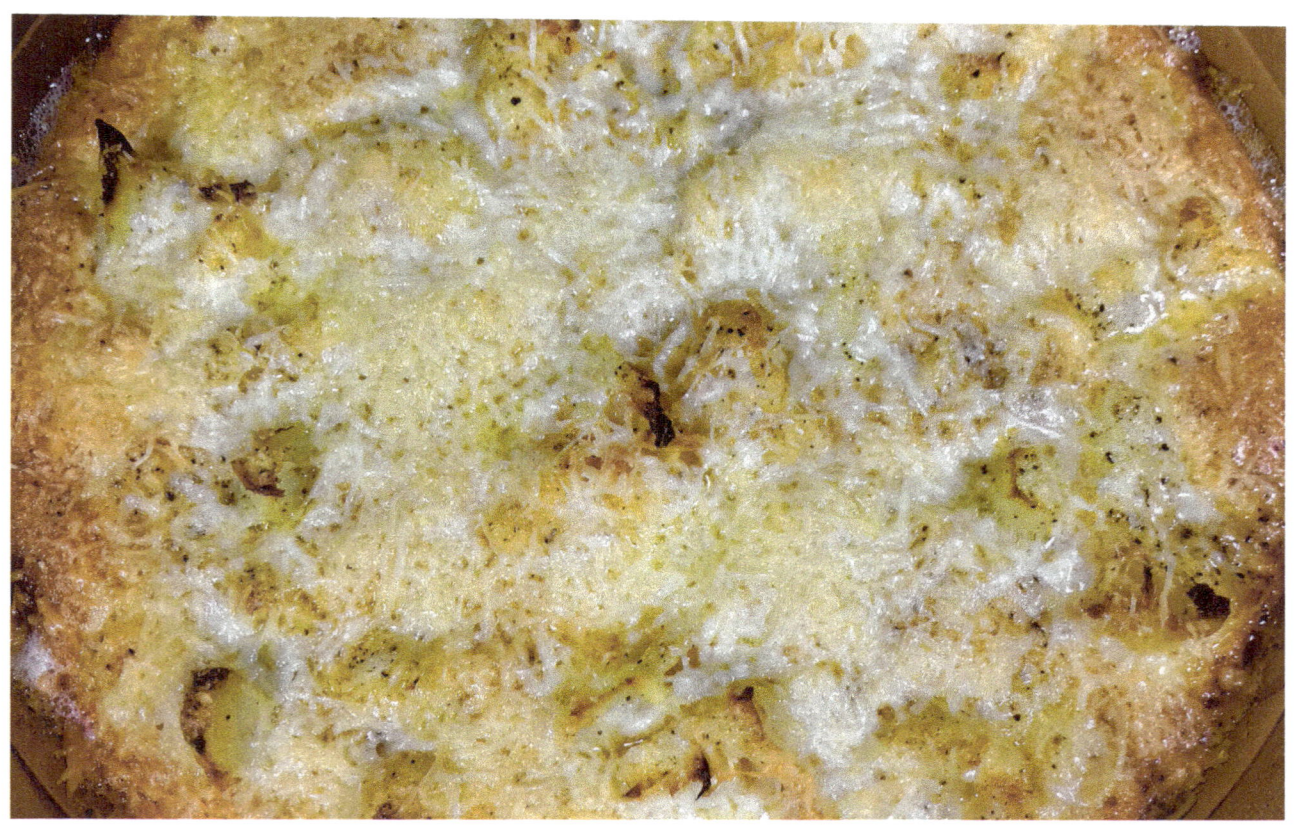

Creamy Mashed Potatoes

These creamy mashed potatoes are used in many of my recipes. This is adapted from my grandmother teaching me when I was 8 years old. You will become a pro in making these quickly, and your guest will rave over them. Today I use non fat half and half and low fat margarine. I have never measured for these potatoes, so start with a little bit of the half and half and chicken broth and add as you mix to get the creamy consistency preferred.

Ingredients

- 8 Golden potatoes (I typically use 2 small to medium per person). This recipe will make enough potatoes for 4 people.
- 1/4 - 1/2 cup Non Fat Half n Half Low Fat Margarine
- 1/4 cup Chicken Broth, Low Sodium
- 2 tablespoons of low fat margarine
- Salt and Milled White Pepper to taste

Method

- Wash potatoes
- Peel or not Peel them. I like the peels left on.
- Quarter potatoes and place in a Dutch oven filled with water and the broth. Cover with lid.
- Cook over medium to high heat until they fork soft.
- Drain the water from the potatoes.
- Place back on the stove top on low heat.
- Add the half n half, broth and margarine.
- Let this mixture heat, but do not boil.
- Turn off the heat from the burner and remove the pan.
- With an electric mixer on low, mix the ingredients together.
- Increase the speed of the mixer and continue mixing until fluffy. If you need to add a bit more half and half to the mixture you can.
- Add Salt and Pepper to taste.
- Serve.

Cook in water until soft and then drain water. Keep on low burner.

Add half and half to potatoes, salt and pepper and margarine. Heat all.

Using electric mixer, start slow speed and increase to high. Mix until smooth.

Grilled Corn & Peppers

Ingredients (2 ears of corn serves 2 people)

- 2 fresh ears of corn, cut from cob
- 1 green bell pepper (or red pepper or poblano), chopped
- 1 small onion, chopped
- 1 tablespoon olive oil
- Salt and Pepper

Method

- Heat a skillet or flat griddle on medium high heat.
- Add Olive oil
- Add corn, pepper and onion
- Stir continuously until peppers and onions appear opaque
- Remove from heat
- Add salt and pepper to taste.

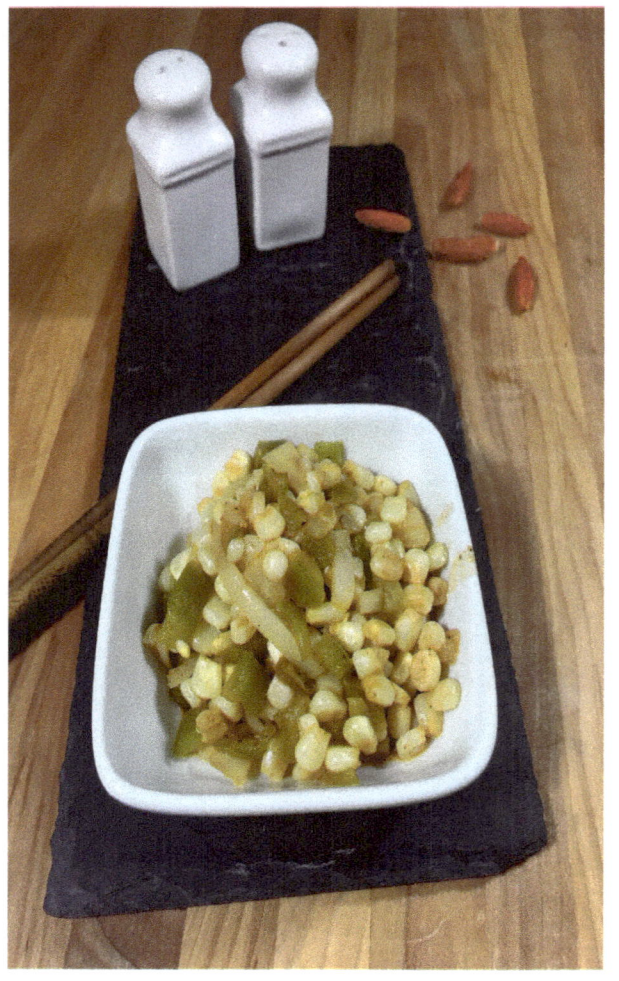

Nothing says summer has arrived like my garden when the peppers are hanging on their vines and ready to pick and eat. As a child, I would walk the garden with my dad, we would pick a green pepper "sampling the fruit as it grows" as my dad would say. I learned to eat green bell and sweet yellow peppers fresh and uncooked, no seasoning. They were never included in the salads at dinner or cooked in any dish, just washed, sliced thin and put on a plate to enjoy their natural flavor. As I got older, I began to include peppers in everything, first experimenting, then in some of my favorite dishes. On a low saturated fat diet, with fats removed, the peppers add a lot of flavor to dishes.

Roasted Sheet Pan Vegetables

Ingredients (Serves 4)

- 2 beet roots, peeled and sliced
- 5 carrots, peeled and sliced
- ½ green pepper, sliced
- ½ orange pepper, sliced
- 1 large onion, peeled and sliced
- ½ bag baby Dutch potatoes (approximately 3-5 per person)
- 4 ½ slices red cabbage
- 1 tablespoon canola oil
- Salt
- White Milled Pepper
- Low Fat Margarine
- White Rice Wine Vinegar

Method

- Peel carrots, wash and slice into stick size.
- Peel beet roots, wash and quarter each.
- Place 1 tablespoon canola oil on a cookie sheet size baking pan. Use a pan that has sides about ½ inch high.
- Place all vegetables on the tray spreading into a single layer.
- Spray lightly with canola oil (1 tsp is plenty)
- Mill ground pepper over top of all vegetables.
- Cover with tin foil and place in preheated 350 degree oven for 20 minutes.
- Remove tin foil, stir vegetables and cook another 10-15 minutes or until beets are soft in middle and moisture from vegetables has evaporated from pan.
- Remove from oven and serve.

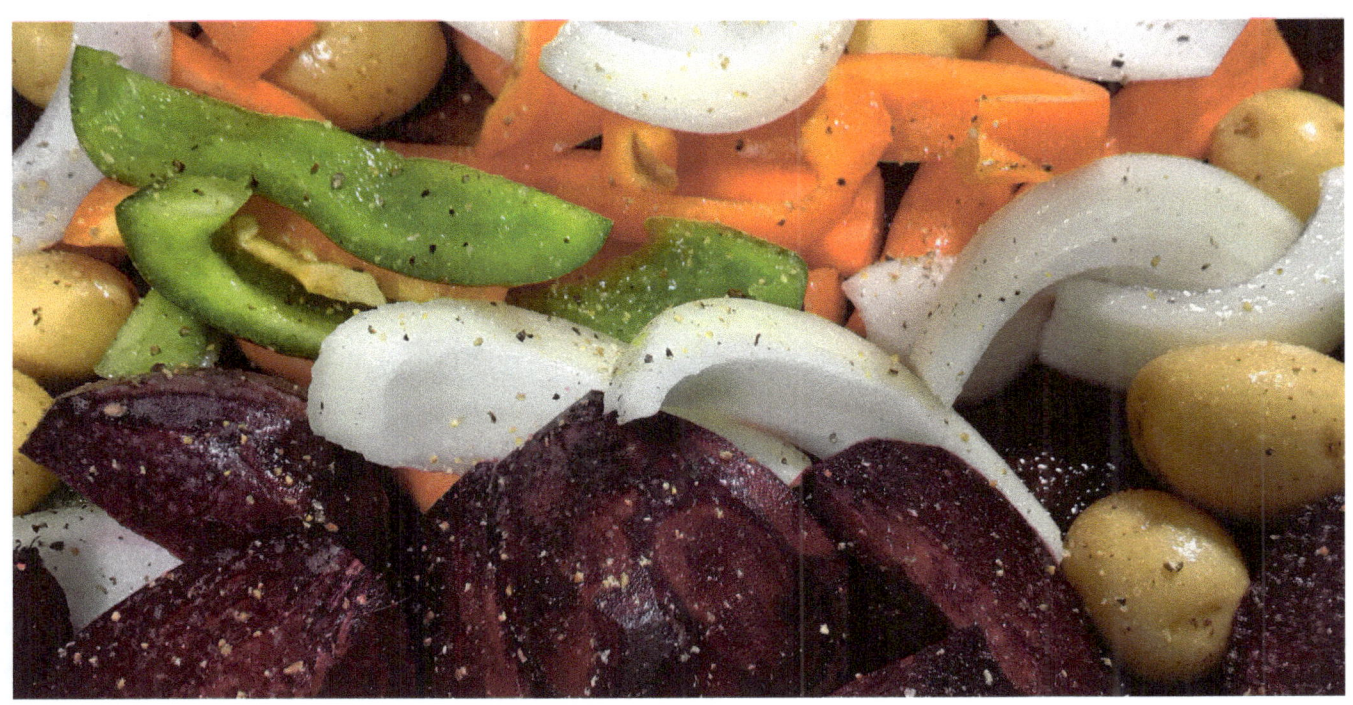

Oh Momma! Where's the Fat?

Mediterranean Cauliflower & Broccoli

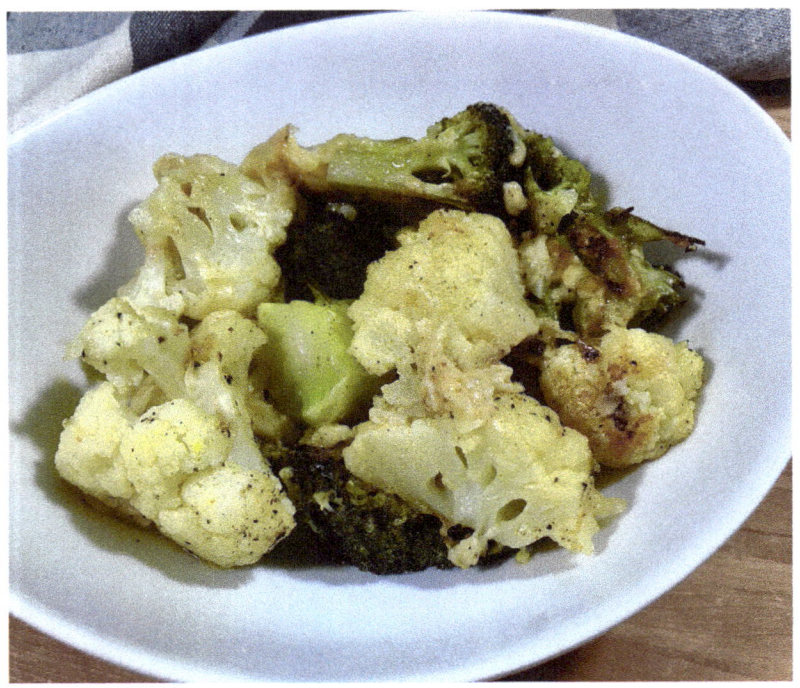

Ingredients (Serves 4)

- 1 small head of broccoli
- 1 small head of cauliflower
- 1/2 cup shredded Parmesan cheese
- 5 cloves of garlic, minced
- 5 tablespoons of olive oil
- 1 teaspoon gold curry powder
- Salt and Pepper to taste

Method

- Preheat oven to 390 degrees
- Chop the broccoli and cauliflower into small florets.
- In a bowl, mix the olive oil, garlic, cheese and curry powder.
- Add the chopped broccoli and cauliflower into the bowl and mix until well blended.
- Using a baking dish approximately 9 x 9, layer the vegetable mixture in the dish.
- Cover with foil.
- Bake for about 20 minutes.
- Uncover and stir very well,
- Cover the pan and bake another 10 minutes or until the vegetables are brown. The vegetables should be firm and not mushy.
- Sprinkle with a bit of salt and couple turns of the pepper grinder before serving.

Spicy Asian Potatoes

Ingredients: (Serves 4)

- 4-5 medium gold potatoes, sliced thin
- 4 tablespoons soy sauce
- 2 tablespoons rice vinegar
- 1 teaspoon sugar
- 1/4 teaspoon red pepper flakes
- 3 tablespoons olive oil
- 4 cloves garlic, minced
- 2 scallions sliced into 1 inch pieces
- 1 Serrano chili pepper, steamed and sliced. You can substitute a Serrano chili pepper with a jalapeno pepper or a mild red pepper.

Instead of a traditional potato salad at your next bar-be-que, try these potatoes. They will not disappoint and are great with burgers, hot dogs, pork chops and chicken.

Method

- Wash, slice and soak the potatoes for 5 minutes. Drain and lay out on paper towel to dry.
- Mix the soy sauce, vinegar, sugar and red pepper flakes with 1 tablespoon of water.
- Heat the oil in a large cast iron skillet over high heat until oil becomes hot (about 5 minutes)
- Add potatoes and fry, turning often. The potatoes should be tender when forked.
- Add the garlic, scallions and pepper, sautéing for about 1 minute. Be careful not to over cook as the garlic will burn.
- Pour the sauce over the potatoes and stir to coat the potatoes. Cook 1-2 minutes until the potatoes have absorbed the sauce.
- Remove from heat and serve

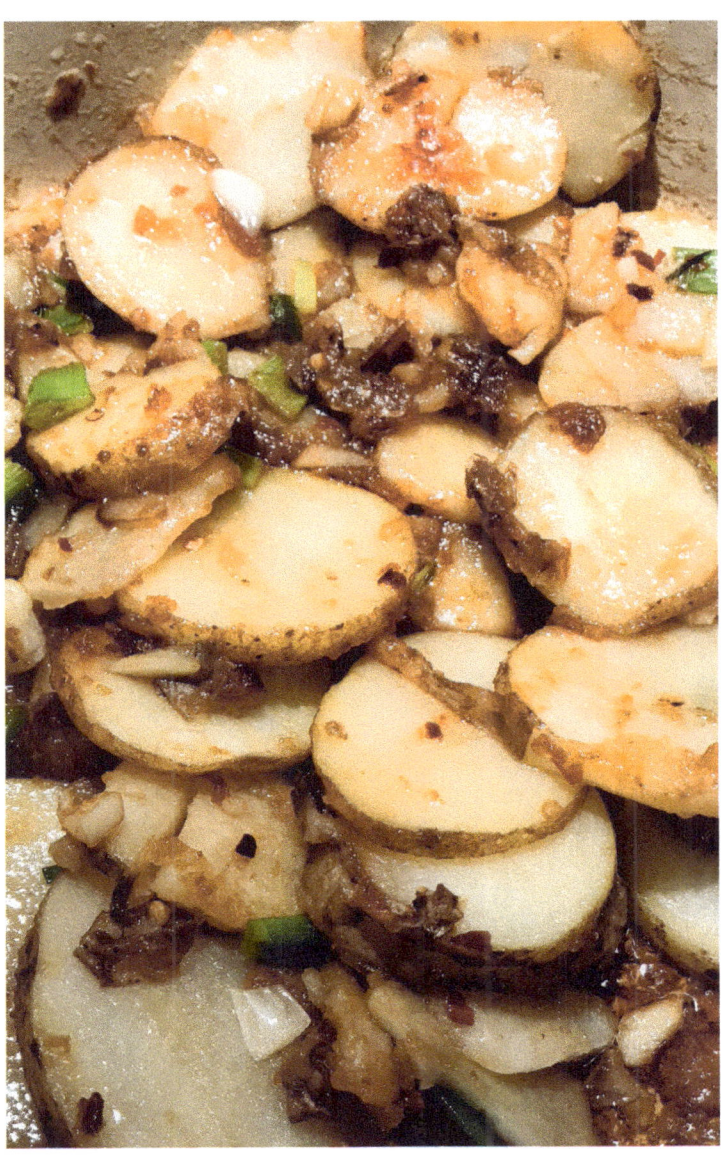

Honey & Thyme Roasted Carrots

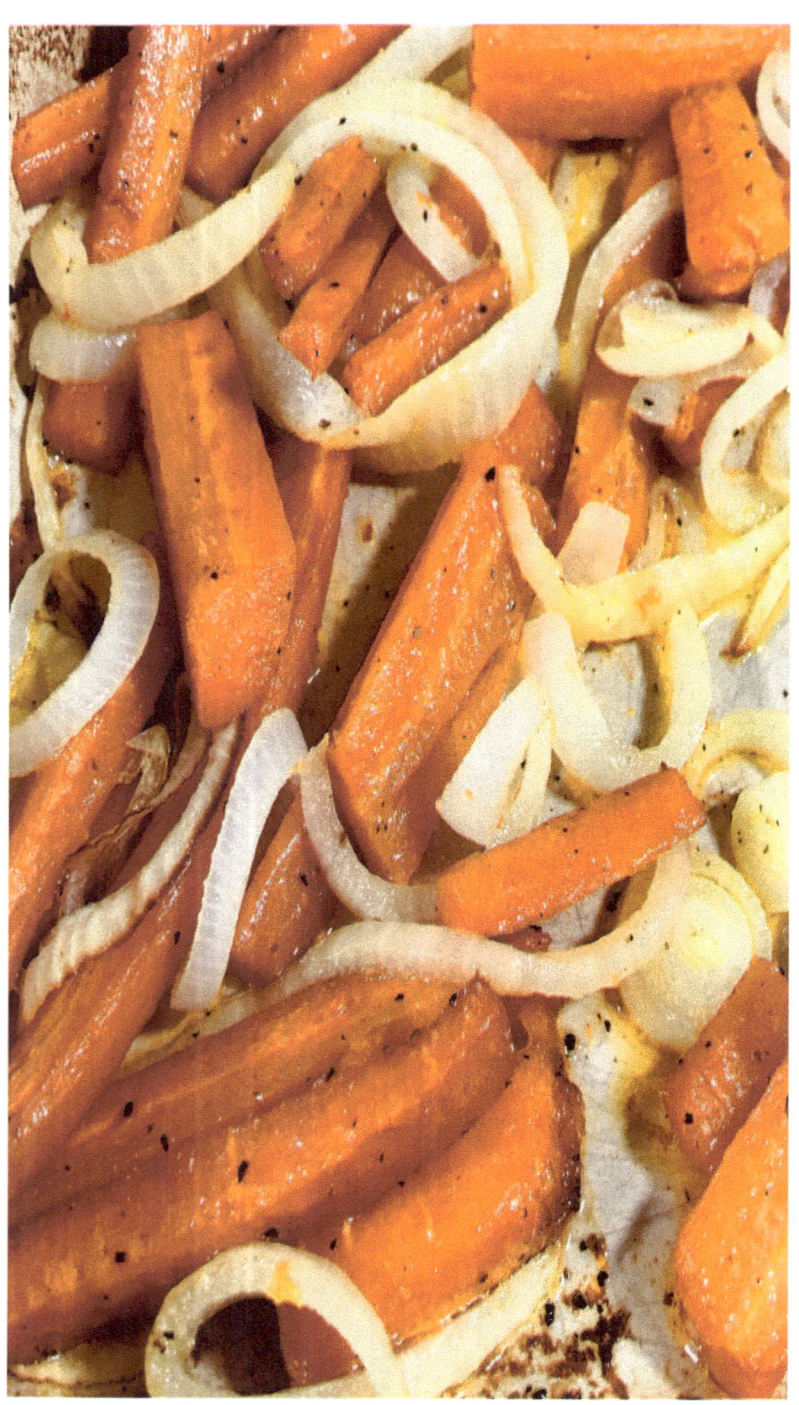

Ingredients (Serves 2-4)

- 6 fresh carrots, peeled and sliced into wedges
- 1 whole onion with rings pulled off (Optional)
- 1 teaspoon dried Thyme
- 2 tablespoons honey
- 2 tablespoons olive oil

Method

- Preheat oven to 375 degrees.
- Mix the honey and olive oil in a bowl
- Add the carrots and mix well to cover carrots.
- Pour mixture into an 8 x 8 baking pan.
- Sprinkle with Thyme
- Cover with foil
- Bake in oven for 15 minutes.
- After 15 minutes, remove foil, add onions and continue baking another 15 minutes.
- When carrots are tender
- Remove from oven and serve.

Paprika Potatoes

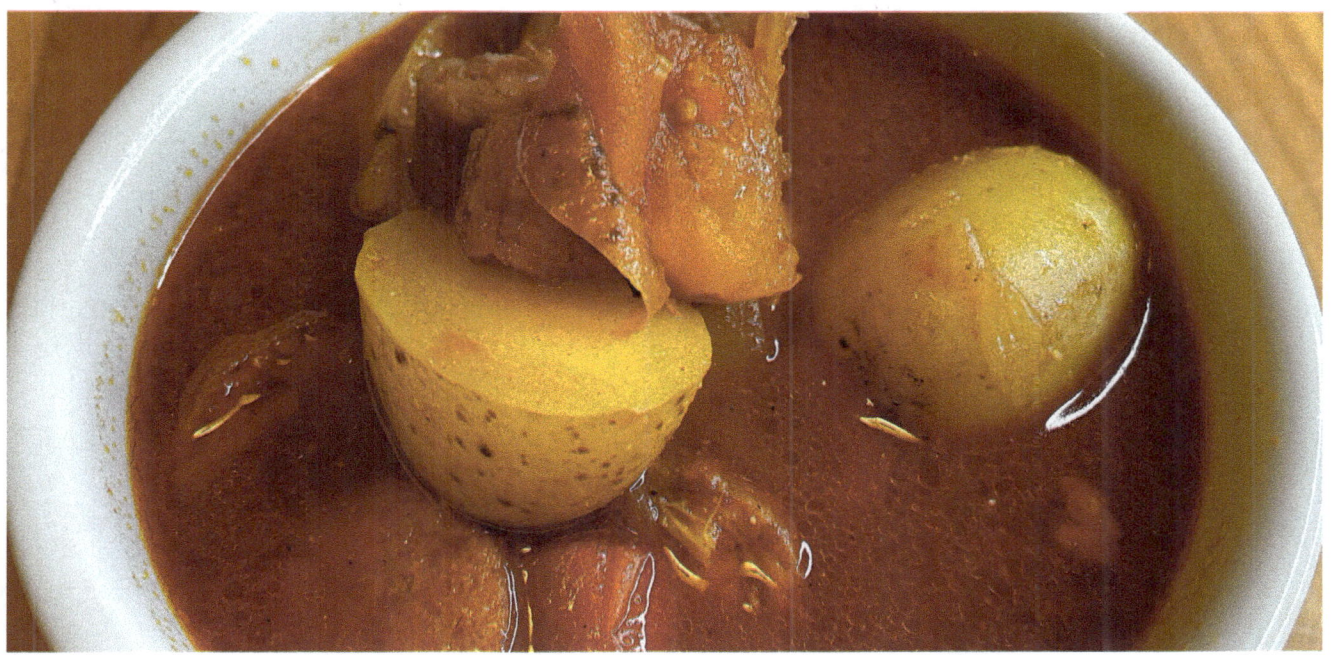

Ingredients (Serves 2-4)

- 4 medium golden potatoes, peeled, cut into medium size cubes
- 1 medium onion, diced
- 1 can chopped spicy tomatoes
- 1 sweet yellow bell pepper, cut into small pieces
- 2 cloves of garlic, minced
- 1 tablespoon Hungarian paprika (add more if needed)
- Olive Oil, approximately 1 tablespoon
- 1/2 teaspoon of caraway seed
- Ground black pepper and Salt to taste
- 1 Cup Water

Method

- In a pot, sauté the onions in olive oil over low heat, stirring frequently, until slightly translucent.
- Add the sweet Hungarian paprika and stir for 30 seconds.
- Add the minced garlic and stir for 30 seconds.
- Add the chopped tomatoes and peppers and stir very well blending all vegetables together.
- Add 1 cup of water and cook for about 10 minutes.
- Add the cubed potatoes, the ground caraway seed and pour in just enough water to cover, salt to taste, sprinkle with ground black pepper.
- Cover, bring it to a boil and slowly simmer until the potatoes are tender.
- Serve warm

If you want to make this a main dish, add 1 pound skinless turkey kielbasa, sliced thin and brown it when cooking the onions.

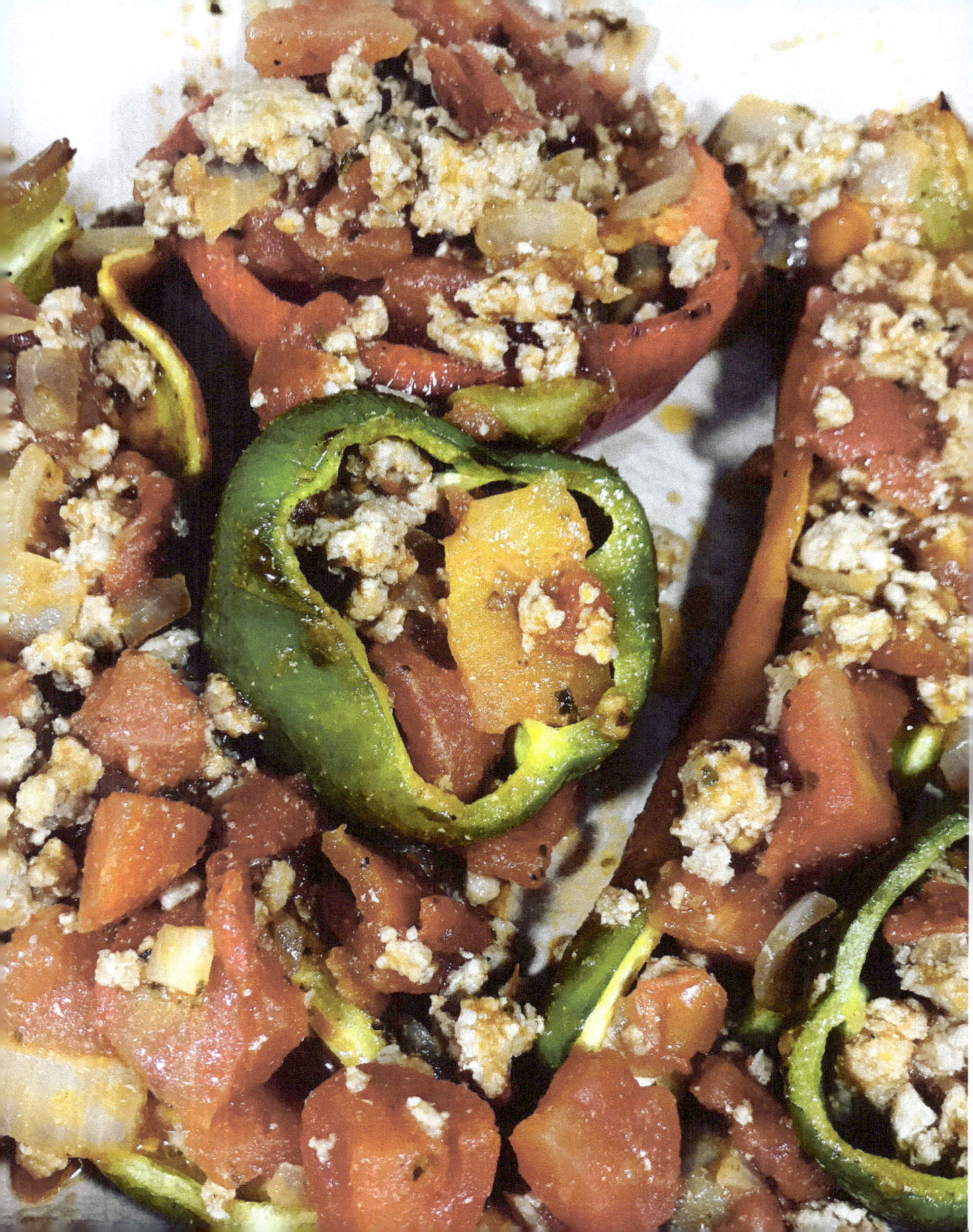

Mediterranean Stuffed Peppers

Ingredients

<u>(Minimum 1 pepper per individual)</u>

- For the Stuffing Mixture (Enough to Stuff 4-6 peppers)
- 1 tablespoon liquid olive oil
- 1/2 pound lean ground turkey breast
- 1 small onion, chopped
- 2 cloves garlic
- 1 teaspoon ground cumin
- 3 portobello mushrooms, cleaned and chopped (optional)
- 1 can chopped tomatoes, Italian flavors
- 1 tablespoon tomato paste
- 1/2 cup fresh oregano, chopped (or 1 tablespoon dry)
- 1/2 cup low sodium chicken broth
- 1/2 cup low fat shredded mozzarella cheese
- Olive oil in a spray can.

Method

- Preheat oven to 350 degrees.
- Wash and cut the peppers in half lengthways and remove the seeds.
- Spray a light coating of olive oil to cover peppers, and place on tray in oven. Let roast 15 minutes.
- Add 1 tablespoon olive oil to a skillet and cook the ground turkey. Add onion and garlic when the meat is just about done.
- Mix in the cumin and mushrooms and heat through.
- Add the chopped tomatoes and tomato paste with the chicken broth.
- Remove peppers from the oven, place in baking dish and fill them with the meat/tomato mixture. Use all the meat mixture even if it overflows and drops into the bottom of the baking dish.
- Sprinkle with 1/2 cup low fat mozzarella, shredded
- Bake in the oven approximately 15 minutes. I like a small brown edge on some of the peppers.
- Remove from oven and let rest 5 minutes prior to serving.

When I make stuffed peppers, I like using a variety of peppers, so even if you do not have a garden, buy a variety of peppers. You can mix and match green bells with red and orange bells, poblano peppers, sweet yellow, spicy red and cubanelle. Pick the peppers you enjoy and have fun making this Mediterranean pepper dish.

Slow Cooked Carrots and Cabbage

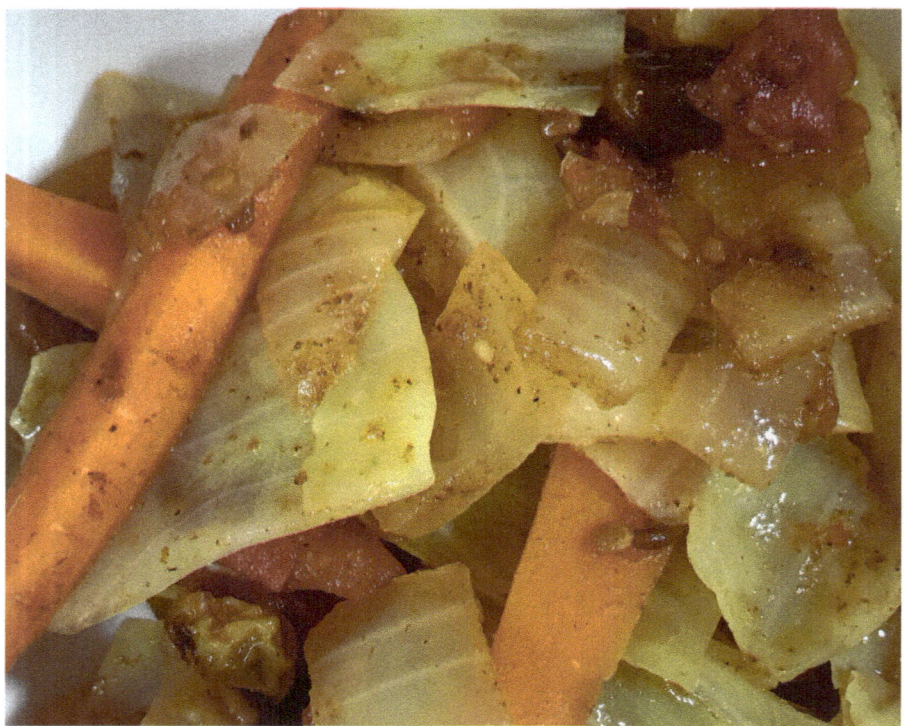

Ingredients (Serves 4)

- 1/2 Small Cabbage, chopped into 1-1.5 inch pieces.
- 6 Carrots, sliced into sticks
- 1 large onion, chopped
- 3-4 Tablespoons of Olive Oil
- 1 tsp Cumin
- 2 tsp Fennel
- 1 teaspoon Fenugreek
- 1/2 teaspoon Turmeric
- 1 teaspoon medium to hot dried Pepper (your choice)
- 1 tsp mustard seeds
- 1/2 cup chopped tomatoes
- Salt and Pepper to taste

Method

- In a heavy pan with lid, add the Olive Oil and heat on medium heat.
- Add the seasonings (cumin, fennel, fenugreek, turmeric and mustard seeds, and stir them constantly for 1 minute.
- Add the chopped onions and cook for 2 minutes or until onions begin to turn opaque.
- Stir in the cabbage and carrots.
- Add tomatoes and hot dried pepper
- Reduce heat to low, put on the lid and steam/cook for 10-15 minutes until carrots are tender.
- Remove pan from heat and plate the carrots and cabbage.

Cabbage and Carrot Omelette

Ingredients (Serves 4)

- 1/2 head green Cabbage, shredded (You can substitute purple cabbage and cook it slower as purple cabbage is more tough)
- 3 medium to large carrots, shredded
- 1 small or 1/2 half medium onion, chopped fine
- 2 large eggs, whisked
- Salt and Pepper to taste
- Salsa or Chutney for serving
- 2 tablespoons of Olive Oil for cooking

Method

- Wash cabbage and carrots after shredding and dry on paper towels
- Once cabbage and carrots have dried, put in a mixing bowl.
- Add the onions.
- Whisk the eggs and pour over the cabbage and carrots
- Add salt and Pepper
- Mix all the ingredients together so cabbage and carrots are very well coated with the egg mixture.
- Heat a shallow skillet (with a lid) on medium heat.
- Add the Olive Oil, enough to cover the bottom of the pan lightly.
- Once heated, pour the cabbage mixture in the skillet.
- Put the lid on the skillet and let cook on medium heat for 5 - 8 minutes or until the bottom begins to brown.
- Using a large spatula or two spatulas, gently flip the mixture over. It should have a nice brown color. Cook another 5-8 minutes or until the vegetables are tender.
- Remove from skillet to serving platter.
- Slice the pieces in wedges and serve.

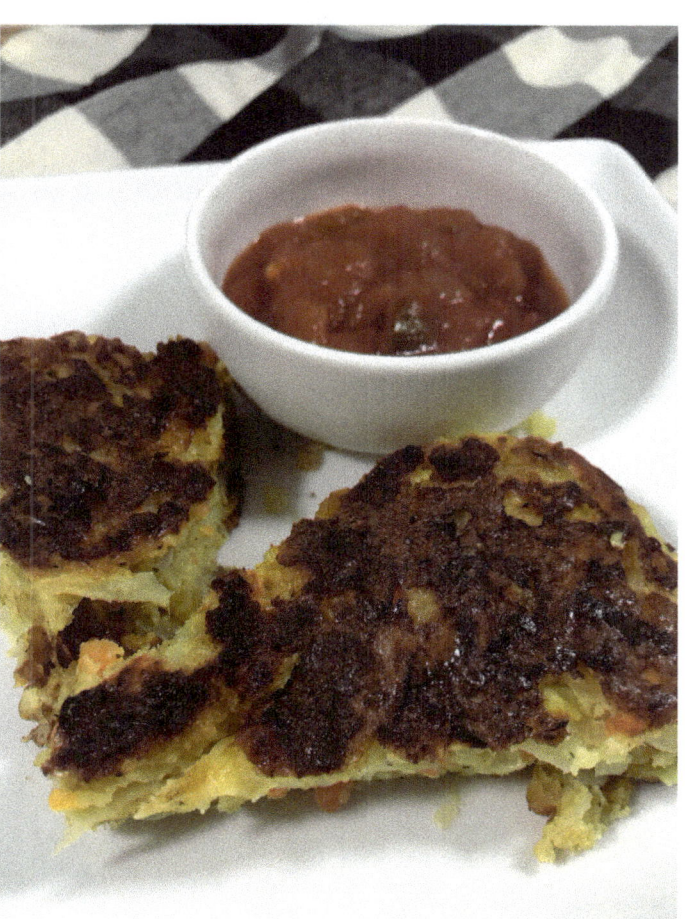

> I like mine a darker brown and crispy, so I cook it longer on each side. I also serve it with my homemade salsa, but a nice chutney or a green salsa is just as tasty.

Oh Momma! Where's the Fat?

Italian Sausage Stuffed Zucchini

Ingredients (Serves 4)

- (You will need one zucchini per person)
- 4 medium zucchini
- 1 pound turkey or chicken Italian sausage links, casings removed
- 1 medium tomatoes, chopped
- 2 cloves garlic, minced
- 1 small onion, chopped
- 1 teaspoon dried oregano
- 1 teaspoon dried basil
- 1/2 - 3/4 cup panko bread crumbs
- 1/4 cup Parmesan grated cheese
- 1/4 cup fresh parsley, chopped
- Salt and Pepper to taste.
- 1/2 cup low fat, shredded mozzarella cheese.

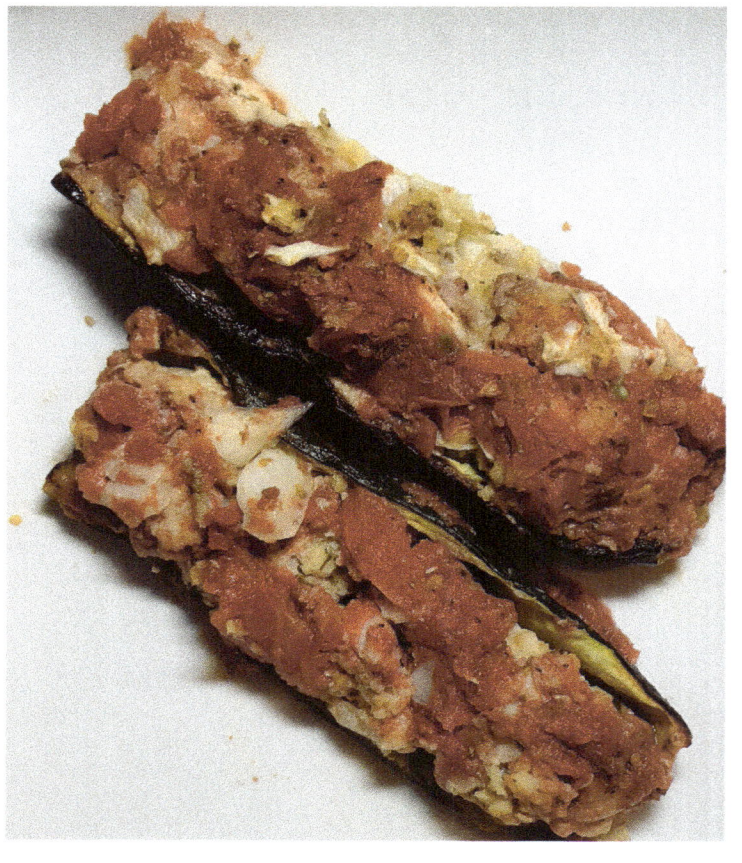

Method

- Preheat oven to 350 degrees.
- Cut each zucchini in half lengthwise. Scoop out the pulp and save it to a bowl.
- Place zucchini shells in a microwave bowl and put in microwave for 2 minutes until they are a bit crisp, yet tender. Remove from microwave and set aside.
- Cook turkey sausage meat and a few scoops of the zucchini pulp in a skillet.
- Add garlic, onions, oregano, basil and tomatoes. Mix well and let cook until tender
- Remove from heat and add the panko crumbs and Parmesan cheese, parsley, salt and pepper. Mix well.
- Select a baking dish that is large enough to hold the zucchini. Place a sheet of parchment paper to cover the pan.
- Seal pan with lid or foil.
- Bake 15-20 minutes or until zucchini is tender.
- Remove the foil and sprinkle with the mozzarella cheese.
- Bake uncovered another 5-8 minutes until cheese is melted.
- Remove from oven and let rest a few minutes before serving.

Spicy Potatoes with Garbanzos

Ingredients (Serves 4)

- 1 pound Dutch potatoes, washed and kept whole. You can also use mini red potatoes.
- 1 onion, diced
- 1 teaspoon ground cumin
- 1/2 teaspoon ground allspice
- 1 can (15 ounce) garbanzo beans, drained. I use dried garbanzo beans and put them in the pressure cooker for 25 minutes. In this way I can control the amount of added salt to the beans. Either method will work for this dish.
- Salt and Pepper to taste
- 1 tablespoon Olive Oil
- 1 cup low sodium vegetable broth.

Method

- Heat oil in skillet over medium high heat.
- Add onions and stir cooking just until soft.
- Reduce pan heat to medium.
- Add the spices and stir well.
- Add potatoes and chickpeas, sat and pepper. Stir well.
- Add the broth and let it come to a boil, then put a lid on the pot and turn heat to medium or medium low. The broth should slow simmer, not heavy boil.
- Cook for 15-20 minutes until potatoes are done and transfer to a serving dish.

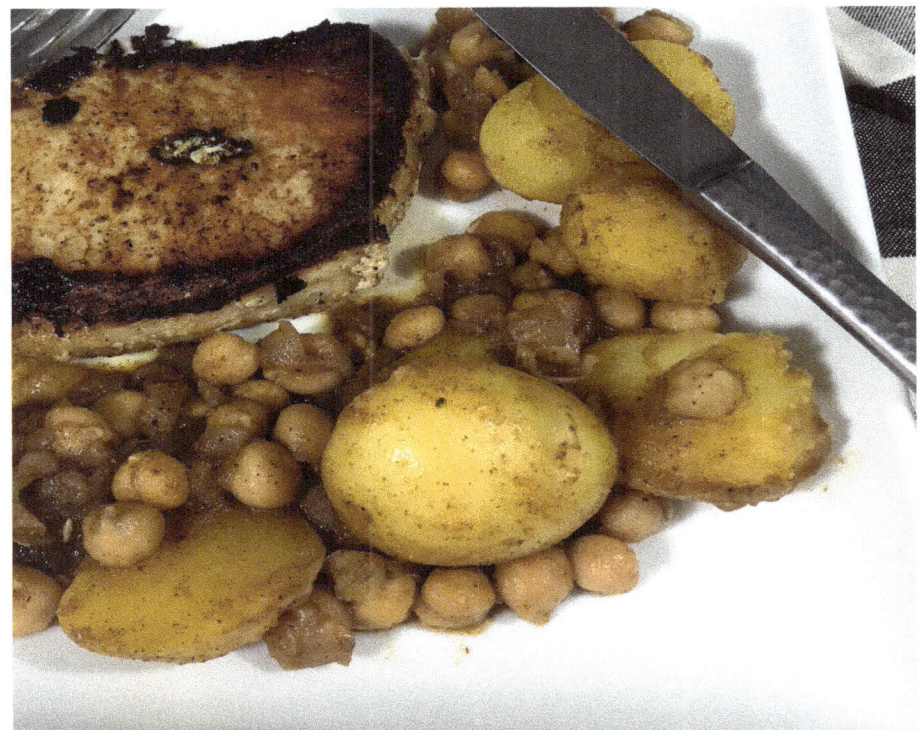

Great side dish with grilled pork chop recipe, "Best Pork Chop Ever"

Oh Momma! Where's the Fat?

Stuffed Butternut Squash

Ingredients (Serves 2-4)

- 2 small butternut squash, halved and seeds removed
- 1 large onion, chopped
- 3 cloves garlic, minced
- 1 pound lean ground turkey meat
- 1 teaspoon cumin
- 1/2 teaspoon chili powder
- 1/2 cup frozen corn (white or yellow)
- 1 can (15.5 ounces) seasoned black beans, drained
- 8 ounces of jarred salsa (I use my homemade salsa)
- Olive oil
- Salt and Pepper
- 1/2 cup shredded Parmesan cheese

Small squash can be replaced with one large squash. It will make enough for 2-4 individual servings when sliced in half after baking.

Method

- Preheat oven to 425 degrees.
- Place squash halves on baking sheet and drizzle with olive oil, season with salt and pepper.
- Roast until almost tender, 25-30 minutes.
- Remove from oven and let cool.
- Scoop out inside of squash, but leave 1/2 inch around edges. This will make the butternut squash boats for the filling. Save the squash in separate bowl.
- Reduce oven heat to 350 degrees.
- In a heavy skillet, add olive oil to cover bottom of pan and heat on medium
- Add the ground turkey meat and when it starts turning brown, add the garlic, onion, cumin, and chili powder.
- Mix very well and stir occasionally until onion begins to become translucent.
- Stir in the corn and black beans, mixing well.
- Add the salsa and the squash that was scooped out, and blend very well. Heat mixture until warm. Add the filing meat to the squash.
- Sprinkle with the Parmesan cheese
- Bake until the cheese melts, about 2-3 minutes. Remove from oven and cool.
- If you made one large squash, let it set a few minutes, then cut in half and serve.

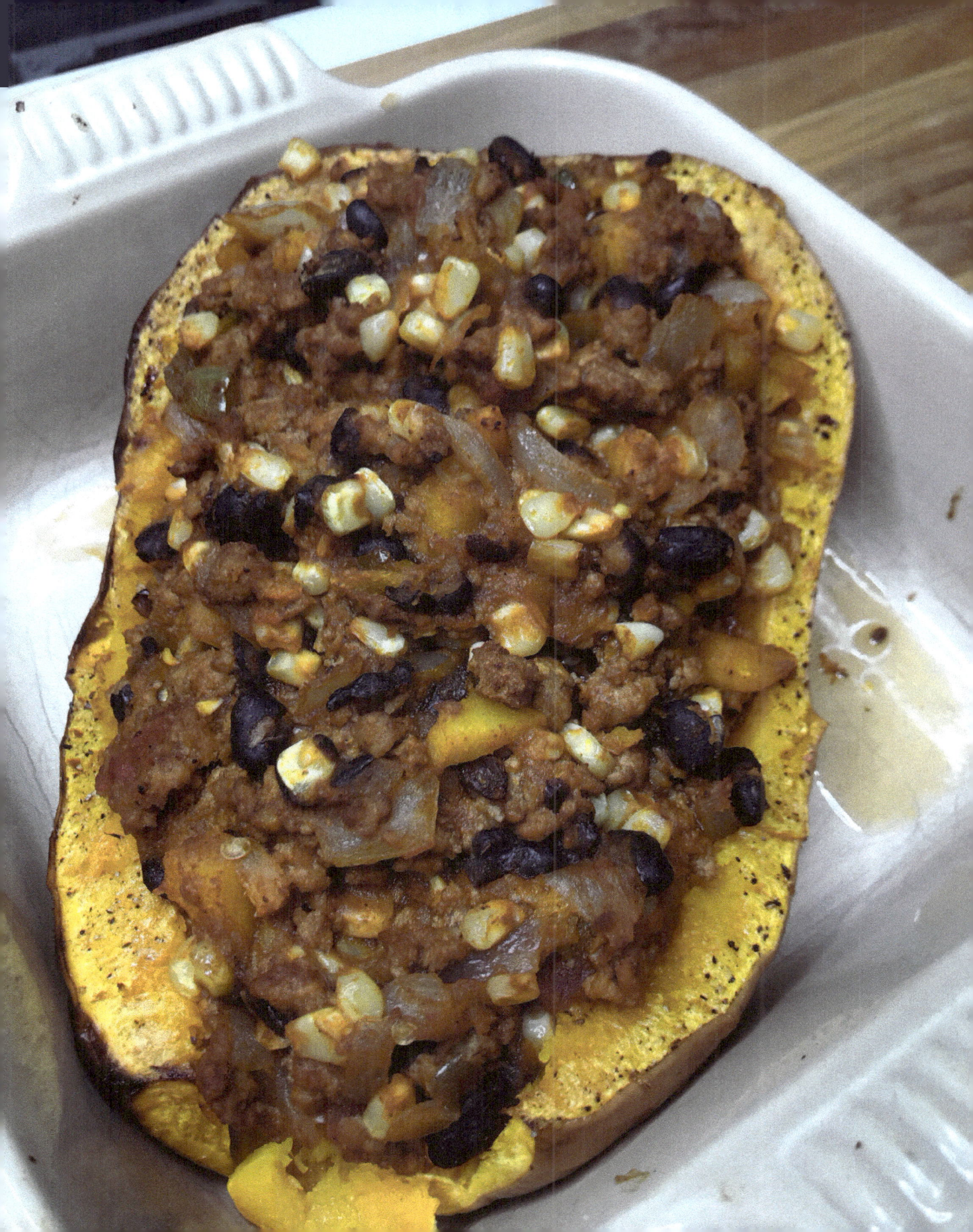

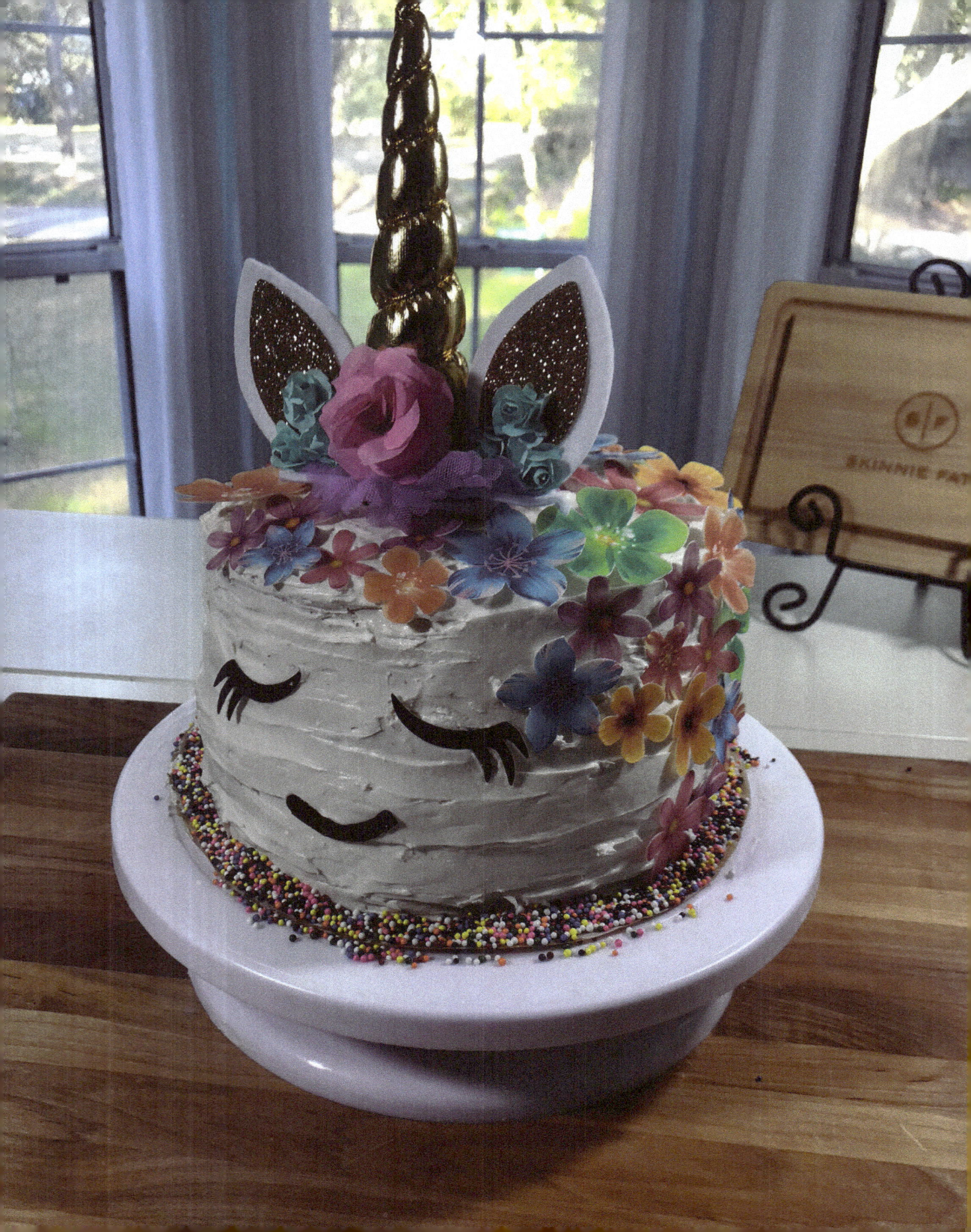

Desserts

Rum Pound Cake 136

Lemon Glaze..138

Lemon Curd 139

Apple Pie Cake 140

Pistachio Pudding Cake 142

Madeleines - Lemon 144

Madeleines - Blueberry 145

Carrot Cake 146

Pineapple Chunk Pie............................147

Red Velvet Cake 148

Fruit Filled Coffee Cake Ring 150

Old Fashioned Apple Pie 152

Do Not Forget the Desserts

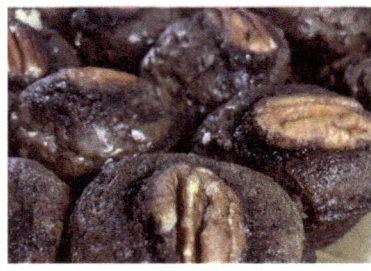 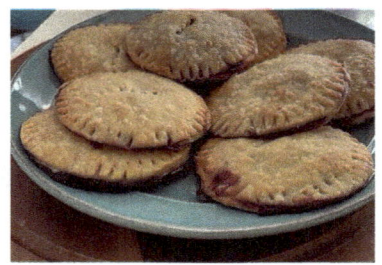 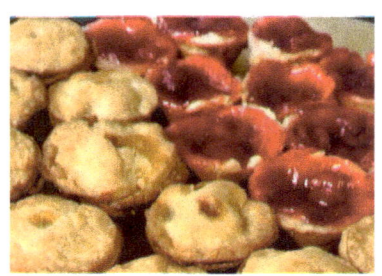

I love desserts. Growing up in the Midwest, dessert was part of the meal. I cannot remember a time no matter what family home we were having dinner, dessert was always served.

Back then no one thought about fats and calories and no one spared the butter, cream, sugar or chocolate. All my family dessert recipes were full of fat and sugar. It has been quite the task to revise them to low saturated recipes, but with a lot of trial and error, I got a few of them right.

One of the first lessons I learned was a little bit of a delicious cake was better than "no delicious cake at all". So when making cakes, I used hard stick margarine instead of butter. Cakes and cookies rise differently when butter is not being used and baking times vary.

In addressing the rise of a baked dessert with lower fat, I found that being creative in the shape and decorative affects of a pan made a difference. With my rum cake, instead of a two layer cake, or a large bundt pan cake, I have a one layer cake made in a decorative Charlotte pan. My carrot cake is made in either a bread loaf pan (long and narrow) or in a smaller decorative bundt pan. Brownies have become "Brownie Bites", smaller versions but just as tasty and less saturated fat in a mini bite.

Breads were easy to convert since most bread is flour, sugar, salt and yeast. Same with bread rolls and sweet doughs that do not call for butter, but margarine or olive oil substitute well.

Pie crusts, on the other hand, have been a challenge for me. I grew up making some of the flakiest pie crusts around. In my cooking class when I was 14, I beat out my teacher (who had been baking many years) on the Lemon pie because my crust was better. I tried all these oils to substitute for the Lard I use to use: olive oil, canola oil, low fat margarine, margarine stick and

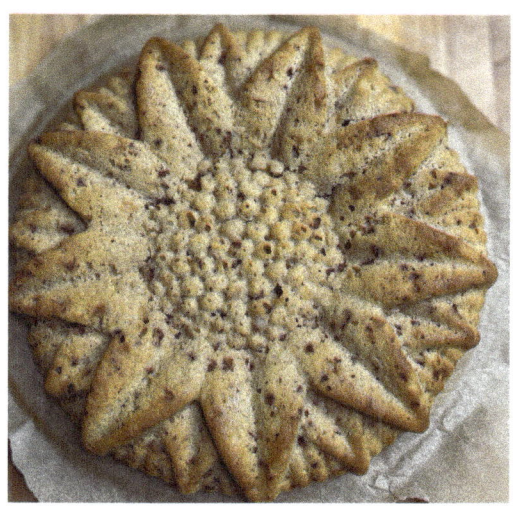

Crisco sticks. They all came out a little disappointing due to lack of great flakiness, but had good flavor. I typically stick with canola oil since olive oil adds flavor I do not want in a pie.

I have found some pre made pie crusts, box cake mixes, and phyllo dough to be very good for many desserts. I use a box brownie mix and box banana nut bread mix. However, read the labels to make sure that per serving, the saturated fat is less than 2 grams. The serving size is important to keep saturated fats lower. When using box mixes, do not be afraid to add more flavors. For example in the banana nut bread mix, reduce the water and add a whole smashed banana and some walnuts or pecans. Always remember, "a little bit of deliciousness is better than none."

For cream cheese flavored icing, use the cream cheese flavored oils; use lemon oils and other flavored oils. The butternut rum oil is wonderful! Be sure to use just a drop at a time since too much artificial flavor can ruin an otherwise great dessert. I also like the no fat cream cheese. It does not bake as well, but it works great as fillings in brownie cups, mixed with icing for cakes, and even as toppings when whipped with non fat whipping cream.

For puddings, I always use non fat Half & Half. No whole milk or cream, just the Half & Half whenever it calls for milk or cream. To make buttermilk, I added vinegar to the non fat Half & Half.

I am perfecting homemade, no fat and no added sugar ice cream, which has been quite a hit with the kids who have no clue it is non fat. A few strawberries and non fat whipping cream on top makes it even more delicious.

So, "Do Not Forget the Desserts." They are part of the meal, part of the 15 grams of fat per day, and a great way to wrap up the evening.

# Mom's Rum Cake
(Just for fun)

When I found this rum cake recipe, I had to laugh out loud and read it often. I didn't know my mother had such a great sense of humor and found this in my dad's safe-box after his death in 2001. My papaw, her father, always loved a good joke and a great laugh. The apple didn't fall far from the tree with my mom.

RUM CAKE

Before you start, sample the rum, and check for quality. Good, isn't it?

Select a large mixing bowl, measuring cup, etc. Check the rum again for quality. It <u>must</u> <u>be</u> just right. Try it again.

With an electric mixer, beat 1 cup butter in a large fluffy bowl. Add 1 teaspoon sugar and beat again. Meanwhile make certain that the rum is of the finest quality. Add 2 large eggs and 2 cups fried fruit and beat until very high. If the fruit gets stuck in the beaters, just pry it loose with a screwdriver. Sample the rum again for consistency.

Next, sift in 3 cups baking powder and a pinch of rum, 1 seaspoon toda, and 1 cup pepper or salt. Anyway, don't fret. Just sample the rum again.

Next sift in ½ pint lemon juice, fold in chopped buttermilk, and the strained nuts. Sample the rum again. Not in 1 tablespoon sprown sugar, or whatever color is around. Mix well. Grease oven and turn on cake pan to 350°. Now pour the whole mess into the oven and, Oops, where did I put the mop?

Maybe I'd be better to forget the oven and the cake. Just check the rum again and go to bed. It's been a long day.

Wonda May Harrell

Mom & Dad Wedding 1948

Rum Pound Cake

My mammy taught me to make pound cake with one pound of butter, one pound of flour and one pound of sugar plus 6 eggs. The butter in that recipe is 224 grams of saturated fat which is about 28 grams of saturated fat per serving (without any icing). So I came up with this alternative, and it is wonderfully delicious.

Ingredients (Makes 24 Slices in Charlotte Pan)

- 1 cup Low Fat margarine. I have found that Blue Bonnet stick margarine works quite well for baking cakes and is lowest in fat.
- 1 + 3/4 cups granulated sugar
- 3 whole large eggs
- 3 large egg yolks (save the whites in freezer for other recipes)
- 1 + 1/2 Tablespoons vanilla extract
- 1/2 teaspoon salt
- 1 + 3/4 cups all purpose flour
- RUM, optional but highly recommended (I use 2 Tablespoons, but add to your own taste).

Note: if you are out of rum, you can substitute rum/butter extract, but use carefully as it is quite powerful.

Method

- Preheat oven to 350F and spray pan very well with no fat canola oil spray,
- Put margarine in a mixing bowl (I use stand mixer, or you can use hand mixer) and mix until margarine is creamy.
- Scrape the sides down and add the sugar. Mix 1-2 minutes until well blended.
- In a separate bowl, combine eggs and the egg yolks, vanilla, salt.
- Lightly beat the egg mixture with fork until all eggs are blended.
- Slowly add egg mixture (about 1/3 of it at a time) to butter and sugar while mixer is at low speed, and mix thoroughly to blend.
- Once all egg mixture is incorporated, scrape sides of bowl into batter and mix at medium to high speed for 2 minutes.
- Reduce mixer speed to low and gradually add in the flour, about 1/4 cup at a time, until all is added.
- Add RUM to taste but remember too much alcohol will cause cake to rise less.
- Scrape the sides and bottom of bowl to be sure all flour has incorporated, then mix on medium speed until very well blended (but not longer than another minute).

- Pour batter into prepared pan (see note below) and bake for about hour or so in center of oven. Every oven is variable, and you will want to check on the cake after 30 minutes.
- To test for doneness, skewer the center with a toothpick, or cake tester, and when it comes out clean with just a very slight moisture on the stick, take out of oven. Over-baking will dry out cake.
- Let cake cool for 20 minutes before removing from pan.
- To remove from pan, run knife carefully along edge, then invert the cake pan onto a cooling rack.
- Once cake is completely cooled, pour the lemon glaze over top and drip down the sides. Serving size is based on the width of each piece shaped by the pan which serves 24. Saturated fats in a serving of this size is approximately 3 grams.

Note: This recipe makes a one layer pound cake baked in a Charlotte pan. If you do not have a Charlotte cake pan, you can use a 9 inch by 2.25 round heavy duty cake pan. I have adapted our family old fashioned homemade pound cake to use low fat margarine and bake in a shallow pan. I use a shallow cake pan instead of loaf pan as low saturated fat margarines do not make the cake rise as much as real butter and a loaf pan will not bake thoroughly and stay moist.

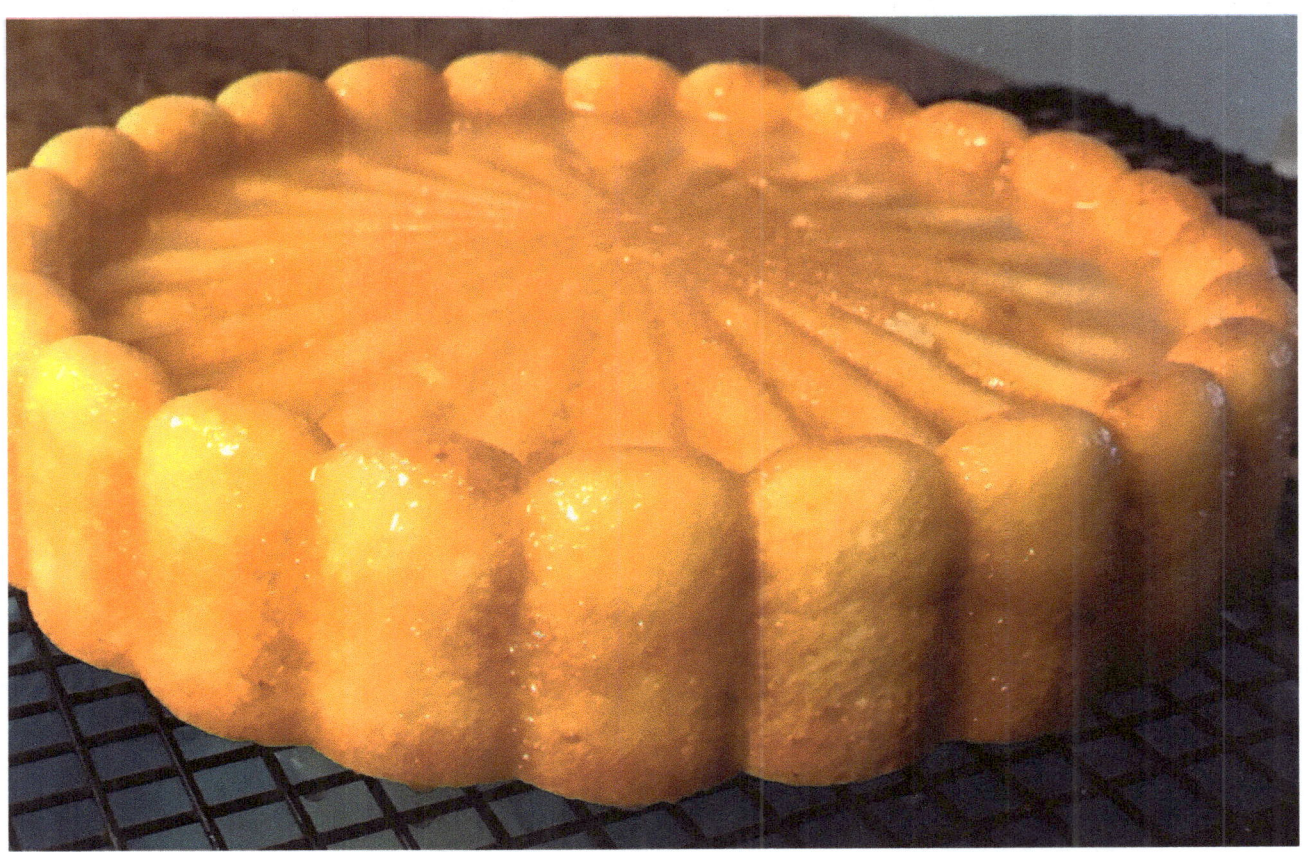

Lemon Glaze for Pound Cake

Ingredients (Enough for a Pound Cake or Rum Cake)

- 6 tablespoons of low fat margarine
- 3 cups powdered sugar
- 1/4 cup lemon juice (I squeeze my own lemons for juice, but you can use the concentrate from the market)

Method

- Mix all ingredients using a whisk to be sure all clumps are removed.
- Keep at room temperature until the cake has cooled.
- Pour on cake and let it drizzle down the sides.

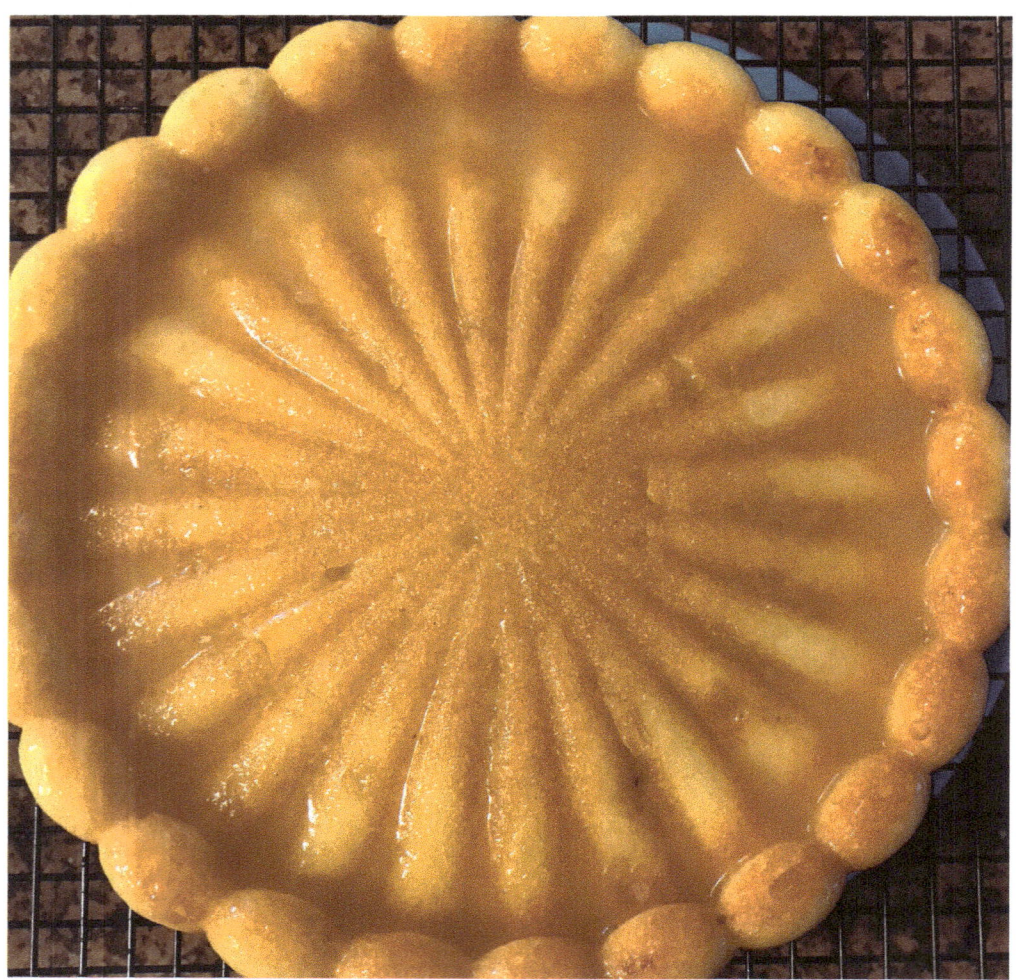

Lemon Curd

Ingredients (Serves 2-4)

- 3 fresh lemons, washed and cut in half
- 1 1/2 cups sugar
- 4 Tablespoons of low fat stick margarine
- 4 extra large eggs
- 1/2 cup lemon juice from lemons
- 1/8 teaspoon salt

Method

- Using a fine grater/zester remove the zest from the 3 lemons. It is important that the white pith is avoided.
- Put the zest in a food processor, add the sugar and pulse until the zest is minced into the sugar.
- Cream the margarine on low speed and beat in the sugar and lemon zest. Add the eggs, one at a time, then add the lemon juice and salt.
- Mix the ingredients until well combined.
- Pour the mixture into a 2 quart saucepan and cook over low heat until mixture thickens. It is important that the mixture is stirred constantly to avoid sticking to the pan or creating lumps in the mixture.
- The mixture should begin to thicken within 10 minutes.
- Remove the thickened mixture from the heat and cool on counter, or in refrigerator.

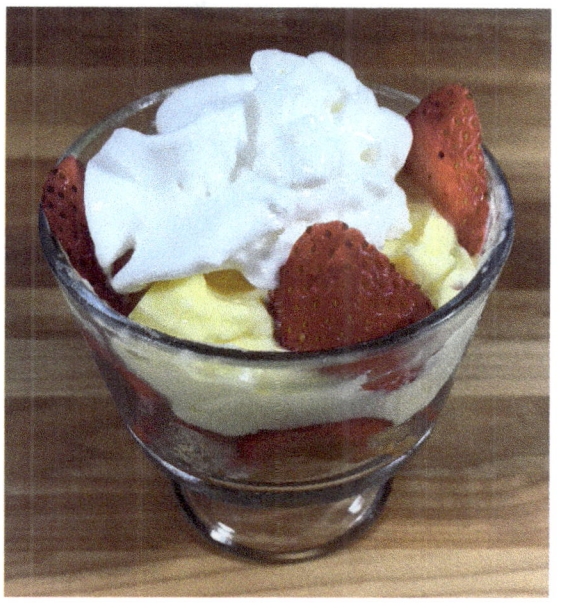

Uses for the Lemon Curd

- The filling between cake layers.
- Filling for pocket brownies
- A layer in a fruit and sponge Trifle
- A drizzle over a bowl of fresh fruit
- Or just a bowl of curd by itself.

Apple Pie Cake

Ingredients (Serves 12)

- 4 Honey Crisp Apples (You can substitute for Gala or any firm crisp apple)
- 2 teaspoons lemon zest
- 2 small lemons juiced
- 13 tablespoons of low fat margarine stick (1 stick plus 5 tablespoons)
- 1/4 cup brown sugar
- 1 teaspoon ground Vietnamese cinnamon
- 1 cup fine ground sugar
- 1 teaspoon vanilla extract
- 2 eggs
- 1 1/4 cup all purpose flour
- 1/2 teaspoon baking powder
- 1/4 cup non fat half and half
- 1/4 cup powdered sugar
- 2 tablespoons butter

Method

- Peel and thinly slice the apples, placing in bowl
- Drizzle lemon juice over apples and mix thoroughly
- In a small sauce pan, mix 4 tablespoons butter, the brown sugar and cinnamon over low to medium heat until butter is melted and sugar is dissolved. Set this aside

<u>For the cake</u>
- Separate the egg whites from the yolks.
- Beat the egg whites until stiff.

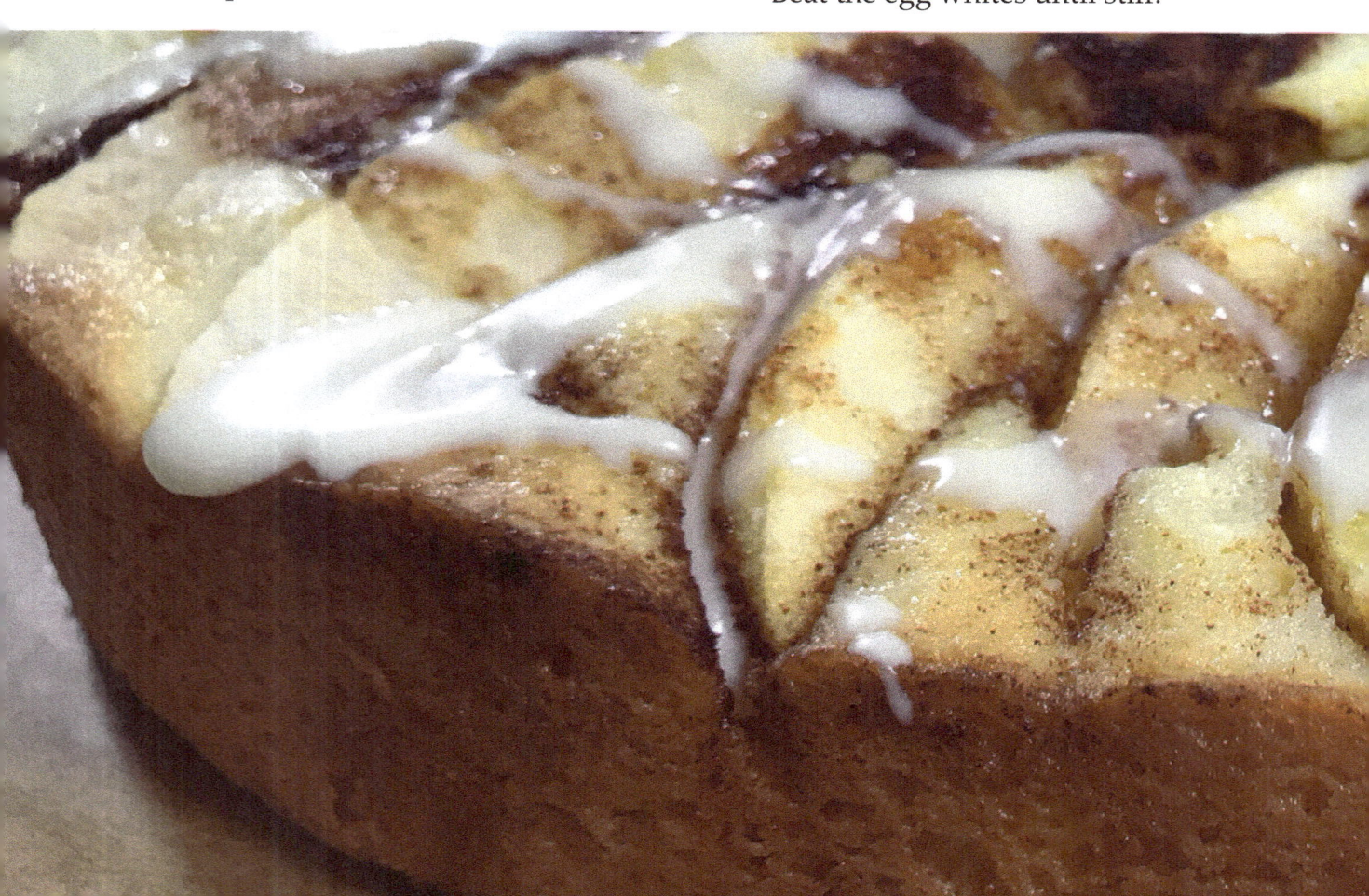

- In separate bowl, mix the flour and baking powder.
- In a stand mixer bowl, beat 9 tablespoons of the low fat margarine with the sugar, lemon zest and vanilla until smooth and color changes to lighter shade.
- Add the egg yolks one by one while the mixture continues to beat at medium speed.
- Add the flour mixture and then slowly add the non fat half and half. Mix well.
- Remove bowl from mixing stand and fold in egg whites until completely mixed in.
- Preheat oven to 320 degrees
- Prepare a 10-inch, deep round cake pan with a piece of parchment paper on bottom and lightly spray sides with canola oil.
- Pour cake batter into the pan.
- Drain apples from the lemon juice
- Place the apples on the dough in a circular pattern.
- Pour the melted butter/brown sugar mixture over the apples.
- Bake for approximately 45 minutes until cake tester shows no signs of batter sticking to it.
- Remove from oven and drizzle with powdered sugar icing

Powdered Sugar Icing (Mix all together)
- 1/2 cup powdered sugar, 1/2 teaspoon vanilla,
- 1 tablespoon low fat margarine
- 1 tablespoon non fat half and half
- If mixture is thick, add a bit more half & half.

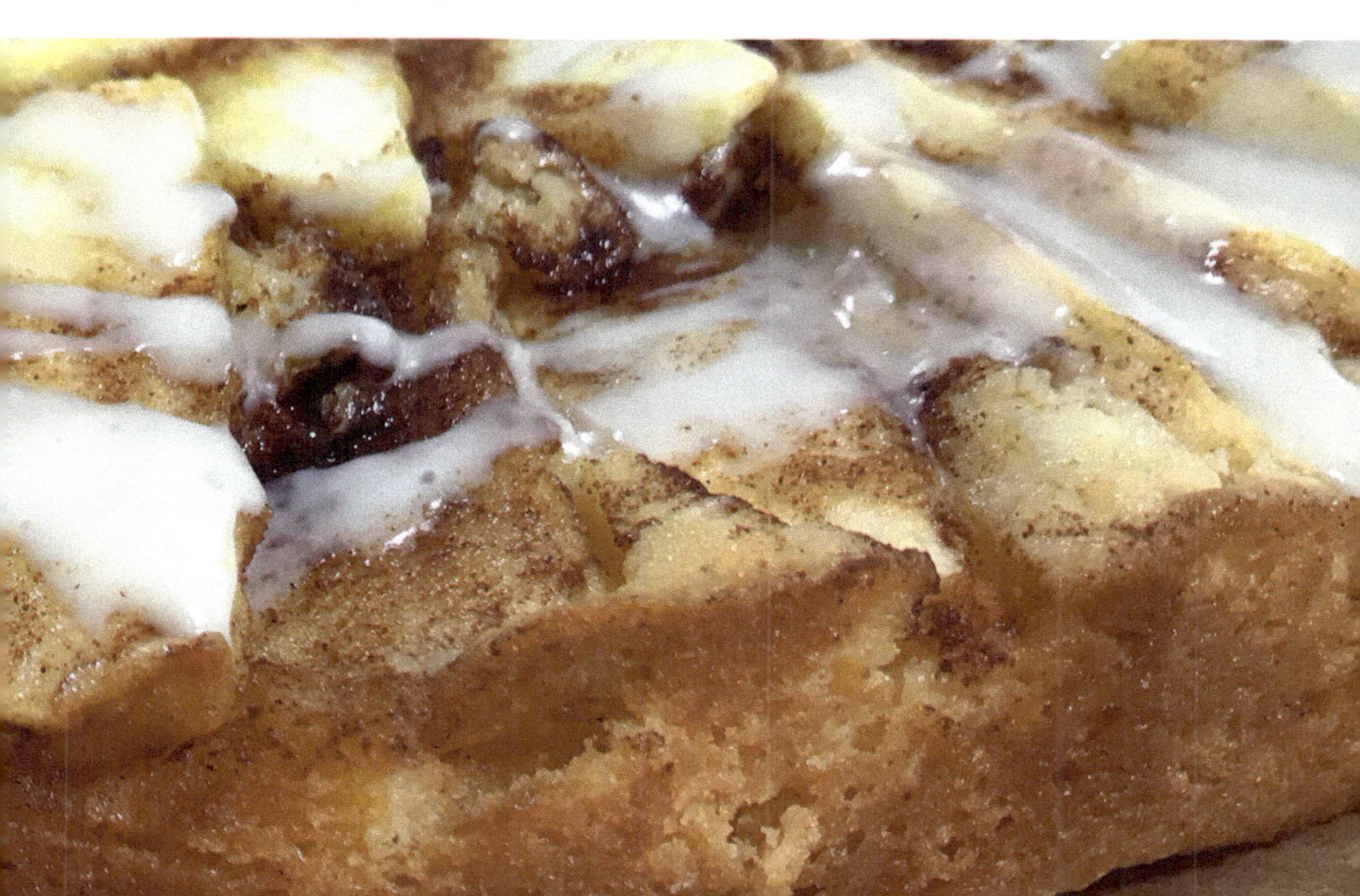

Pistachio Pudding Sponge Cake

Ingredients (Serves 12)

- 1 box pistachio instant pudding mixture
- 1/2 cup pistachio chopped nuts
- 2 eggs
- 1/2 cup fine sugar
- 1/2 cup ail purpose flour
- 1/2 teaspoon baking powder
- 1.5 tablespoons melted low fat stick margarine
- 1 tablespoon water
- 1/2 tablespoon vanilla extract

Method

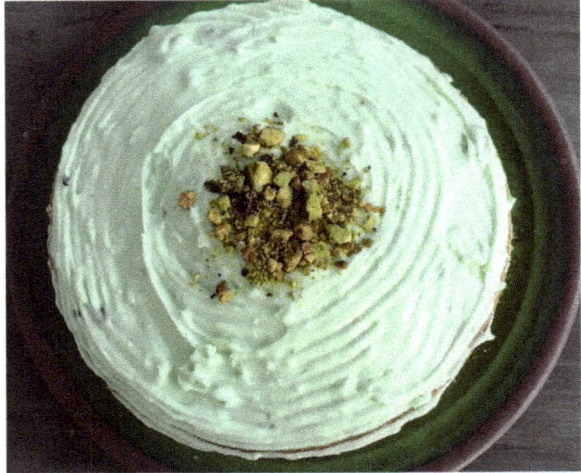

Pudding

- Follow Method on the pistachio instant pudding mixture but use non fat half and half as the liquid. Mix well and store covered in refrigerator until cake is ready to ice.

Cake

- Preheat oven to 350 F and place the rack in the middle of the oven.
- Line an 8 inch pan with parchment paper and sprayed with nonstick canola oil.
- Whip the eggs in a stand mixture on high speed for 1 minute, then add the sugar in thirds while continuing to whip. The eggs and sugar need to whip for 15-20 minutes or until the batter falls off the whisk and stays on it for at least 2-3 seconds.
- Shift the flower and baking powder together.
- Combine melted margarine with water and mix together
- To the egg mixture, add the vanilla
- Add the flower into the whipped eggs in halves and carefully fold with a spatula. Do not over fold the flour or the rise will be lost with the whipped eggs.
- Add the melted butter mixture and fold carefully.
- Pour batter into the prepared cake pan.
- Bake for about 30 minutes in the preheated oven. Use a skewer or toothpick to check cake by inserting into the middle.
- When done, remove to a cooling rack and let set undisturbed 5-10 minutes. Once it has set, invert pan on the cooling rack and remove pan from cake.
- Once cake is cool, carefully cut the layer into two equal pieces. Make sure cake is completely cooled.
- Place pudding on the bottom piece and spread across and sprinkle a few pistachios on top.
- Add top piece and add more pudding. Do not spread on the sides.
- Top with the chopped pistachios.
- Refrigerate prior to and after serving.

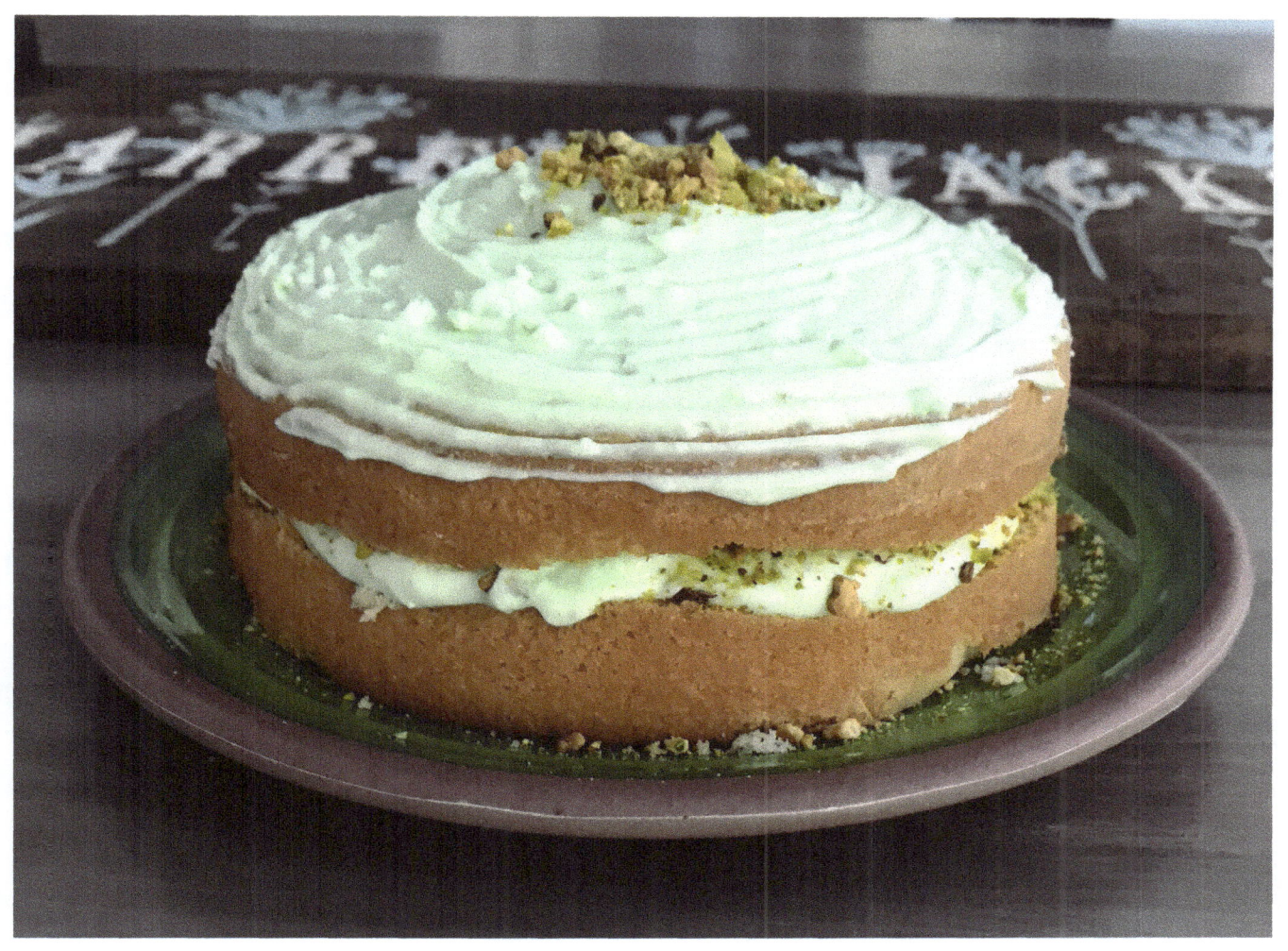

I first made this cake while in college, and it was always a hit with guests or at work for special occasions. It can be made in a long cake pan as one layer for entertaining. If you are not a fan of baking from scratch, pick up a low saturated fat boxed yellow cake mix, and follow the instructions skipping the homemade cake. The cake will still be a "hit".

Madeleines (Lemon and Blueberry)

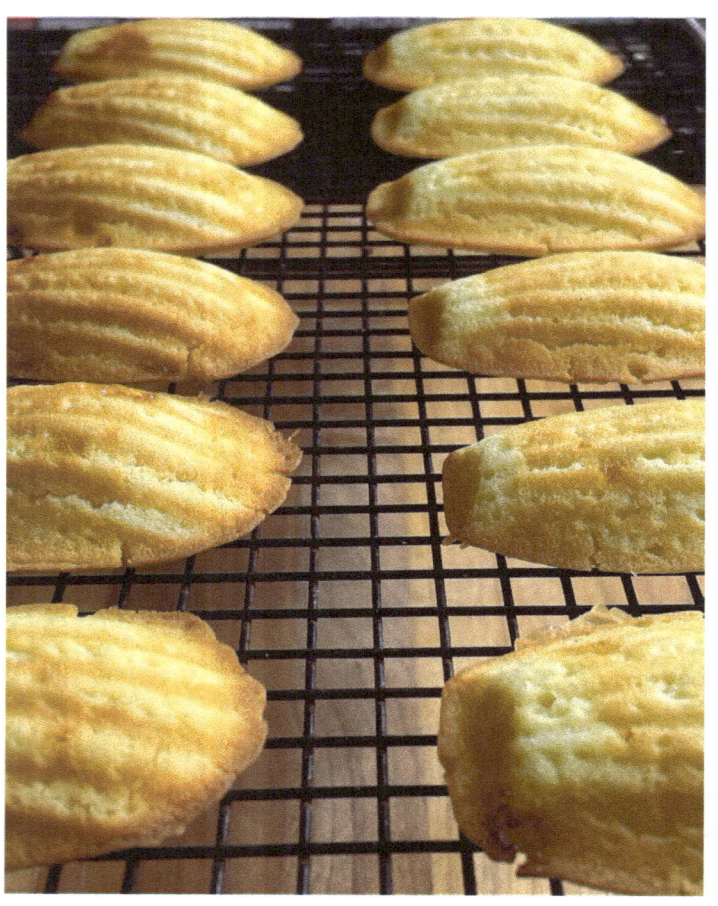

Ingredients (Makes 12-18)

- 2 eggs
- 1/2 white sugar
- 5 tablespoons low fat stick margarine
- 3/4 cups all purpose flour
- 1 teaspoon baking powder
- 1/4 teaspoon vanilla extract
- 1/2 lemon, juiced and zested
- 1/3 cup confectioner's sugar for decoration

Madeleine pans are available on line at many merchants. The key for the madeleines to release easily from pan is to use oil generously. I like using spray Canola Oil.

Method

- In a large bowl blend eggs, sugar and then add the butter. Mix well on low speed then blend in the flour, baking powder, lemon, vanilla.
- Once mixed, cover bowl with towel and let sit for one hour.
- Preheat oven to 375 degrees F.
- Spray Madeleine mold pan with non fat canola oil
- Whisk batter and then pour into the Madeleine molds.
- Bake 10 minutes (check the doneness) and remove from oven. Let cool 5-7 minutes, then gently turn pan over onto cooling rack to release Madeleines.

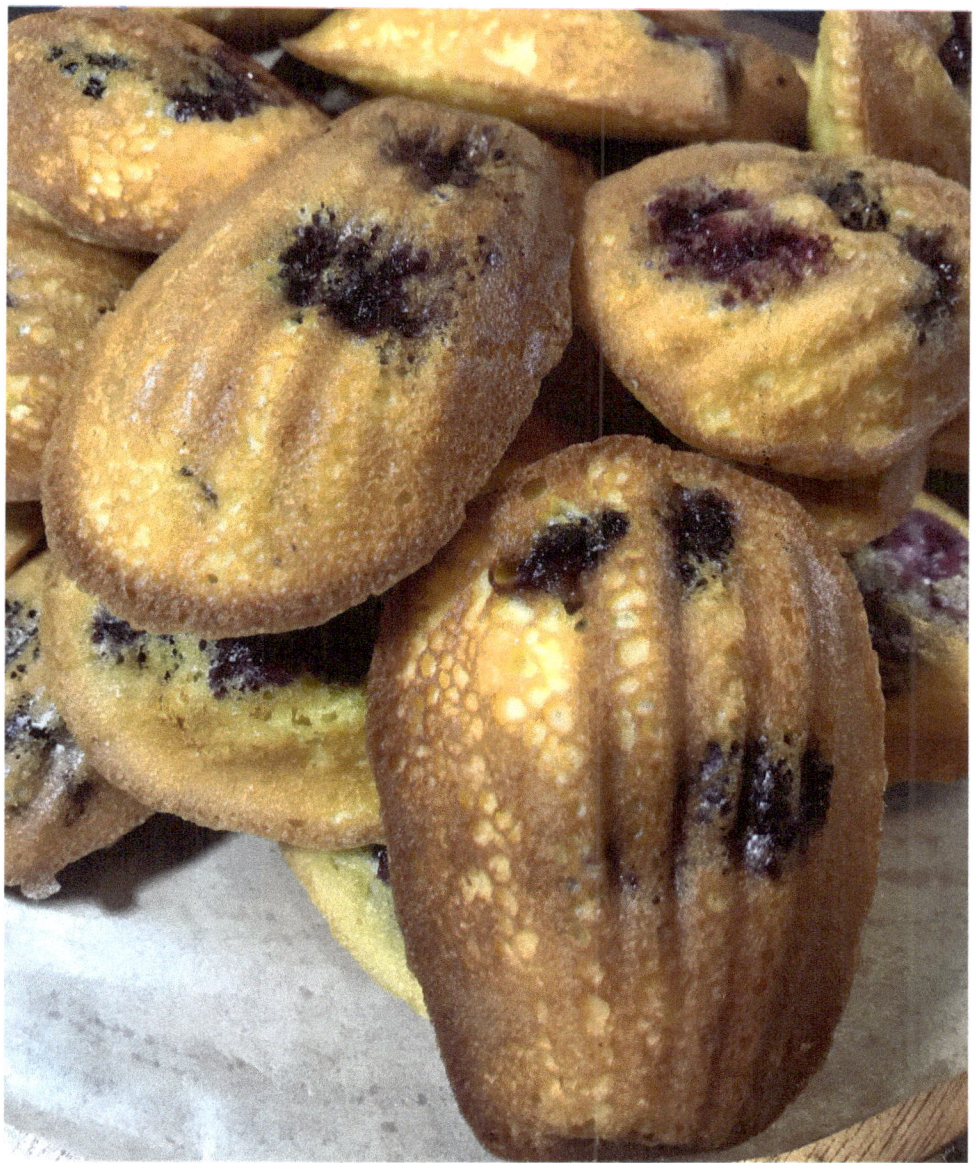

Blueberry Madeleines

Follow the recipe for the Lemon Madeleines, except leave out lemon juice and zest.

- Add 1/2 cup blueberries to the batter after it has set for the one hour.
- Spoon the batter into the molds and be sure to get 3-4 blueberries in each mold.
- Bake and cool as in instructions for the Lemon Madeleines.

Carrot Cake

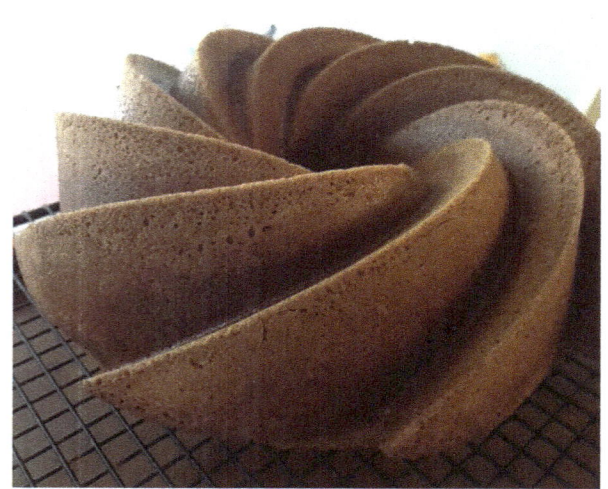
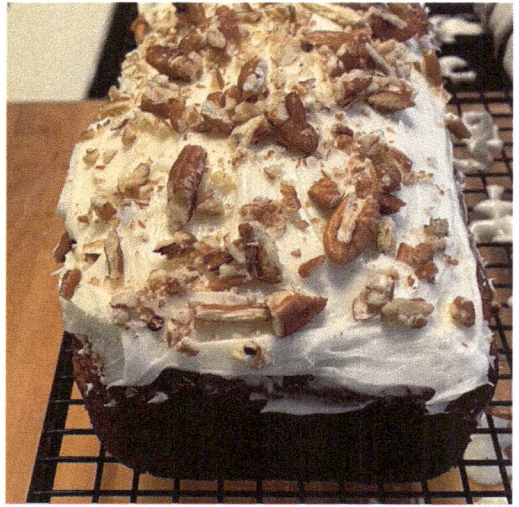

Ingredients (Serves 16)

For the Cake
- Spray canola or olive oil for the pan
- 2 cups all purpose flour.
- 2 cups sugar
- 2 teaspoons baking soda
- 2 teaspoons ground Vietnamese cinnamon
- 1 teaspoon salt
- 4 eggs, slightly mixed
- 1 and 1/2 cup olive oil or canola oil
- 3 cups grated carrots (you can use 2 cups grated carrots and 1 cup grated zucchini if desired; but be sure to squeeze the water out of the zucchini before adding to cake)
- 2 1/2 cups chopped pecans or walnuts

For the Cream Cheese Icing (mix all the items together and blend well):

- 1 - 8 ounce pack of non fat cream cheese
- 1/2 stick low fat margarine
- 8 ounces box powdered sugar
- 1 1/2 teaspoon vanilla
- 1/4 cup chopped pecans or walnuts

Method

- Preheat oven to 350 degrees.
- Spray with the canola oil or olive oil the inside of a cake pan, quite generously. If using a rectangular pan, line it with parchment paper to make it easy to release after cooling. I personally like experimenting with various pans.
- Combine flour, sugar, baking soda, cinnamon and salt. Add the eggs and canola oil. Mix well until all is combined.
- Add carrots and nuts, and mix again just until blended.
- Pour in cake pan and bake 40 minutes, or until a toothpick or skewer in center of pan comes out clean.
- Cool 5 minutes; remove cake from pan.
- Once cake has cooled completely, spread the icing on top.

Pineapple Chunk Pie

Ingredients For Filling (Serves 8)

- 16 ounce can chunk pineapple, drained
- 1 jar apricot preserves
- 1 package instant French vanilla pudding mixed with non fat half & half
- 1 cup non fat sour cream
- Non fat whipped topping
- Ingredients For Graham Cracker Crust
-   1 1/2 cups crushed graham crackers
-   2 tablespoons sugar
-   ½ cup melted stick margarine

Method

- For the Pie Crust - Mix all items for Graham cracker crust together and place in bottom of 9 inch pie dish. Press crumbs on bottom and up the sides of the pie dish
- Spread the non fat sour cream on the top of the prepared pie crust
- Pour the pudding on top
- Let it set until chilled very well.
- Add the pineapple to the top of the pudding mixture after it has chilled.
- Spread the apricot preserves on top
- Spread or pipe the dream whip on top.
- Chill 4 hours or overnight.

Serve with a spoonful of whipped topping or non fat ice cream scooped on top.

My mammy made this cake with full fat whipping cream and used real butter in the crust. It is such a great summer dessert that I worked a few times on the recipe to get it as tasty and low saturated fat.

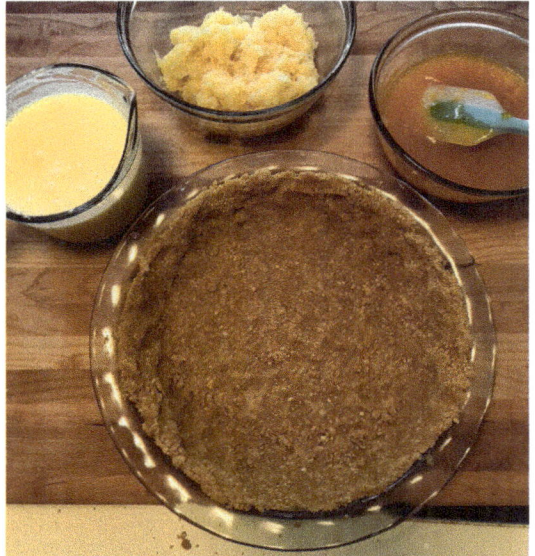
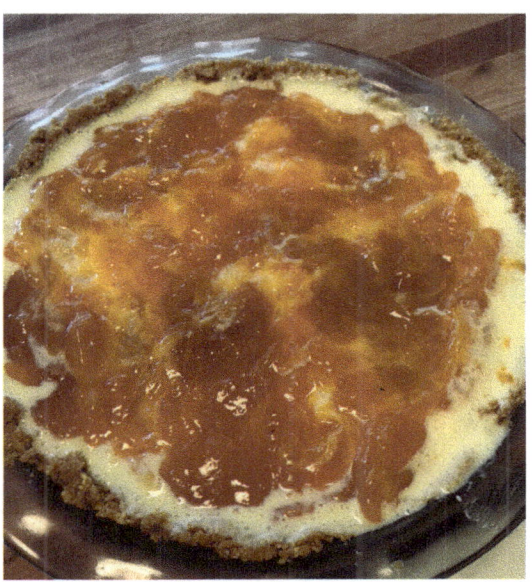

Red Velvet Cake

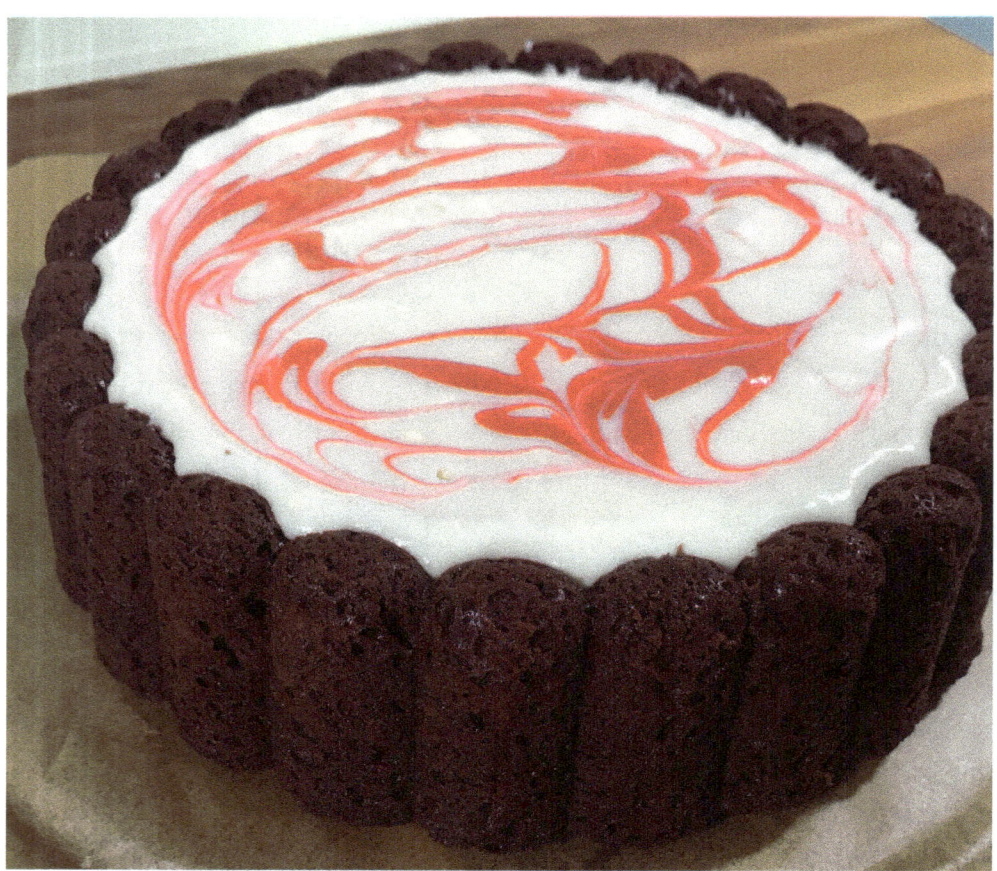

Ingredients (Serves 24)

For the Cake
- 2 - 2/3 cups cake flour
- 1/4 cup cocoa powder
- 1 teaspoon baking soda
- 1/2 teaspoon salt
- 1/2 cup low fat margarine
- 1 3/4 cups fine sugar
- 2 large eggs
- 1/2 canola oil
- 1 tube red food coloring
- 2 teaspoons pure vanilla extract (I use my homemade vodka vanilla)
- 1 teaspoon white vinegar
- 1 1/3 cups butter milk (make this using 1 - 1/3 cups fat free half and half plus 2 tablespoons white vinegar, mix and let set about 5-7 minutes)

For the cream cheese frosting:
- 6 ounces fat free cream cheese
- 1/4 cup low fat butter
- 1.5 cups powdered sugar
- 1 teaspoon pure vanilla extract
- 1 teaspoon cream cheese extract flavoring

Method for Cake

- Preheat oven to 350 degrees
- Spray the Charlotte pan with canola oil spray
- Whisk the cake flour, cocoa powder, baking soda and salt together in a bowl. If there are lumps in the mix, sift it.
- Cream the margarine and sugar on medium speed in a mixing bowl (stand mixer or hand mixer)
- Add the eggs, then mix in the oil and red food dye, vanilla and vinegar. Be sure to scrape the sides of the bowl as it mixes. Mix 4-5 minutes.
- Alternately add the dry ingredients and buttermilk to the creamed butter mixture. Mix thoroughly after each addition. However, do not over mix the batter.
- Pour the cake batter into the prepared Charlotte or round, deep cake pan.

<u>Baking</u>

- Bake at 350 for 30 minutes or so. Each oven is a bit different, so be sure to test the center of the cake with a cake probe to make sure it comes out clean. Do not over bake.
- Remove cake from oven and place on wire rack to cool.
- When cake has cooled, turn cake out onto a wire rack, then flip it over to a serving platter.

<u>Method for Icing</u>

- Combine all ingredients and mix well.
- If batter is too thin, add more sugar; if batter is too thick, add non fat half and half. Be careful not to add too much of either - just a teaspoon at a time.
- When the cake has cooled, and icing is ready, pour all but a couple tablespoons of icing into the center of the cake. Add red food color gel to the tablespoons of icing in the reserved icing and mix well. Drop a few of the red color icing on top of the cake in little polka dots. Use a toothpick and drag through the dots of red to create a swirl.

This cake was baked in a Charlotte pan and creates a stunning display for dessert. Each serving is noted by the knobs around the cake. One serving is approximately 2 grams of saturated fat.

Fruit Filled Coffee Cake Ring

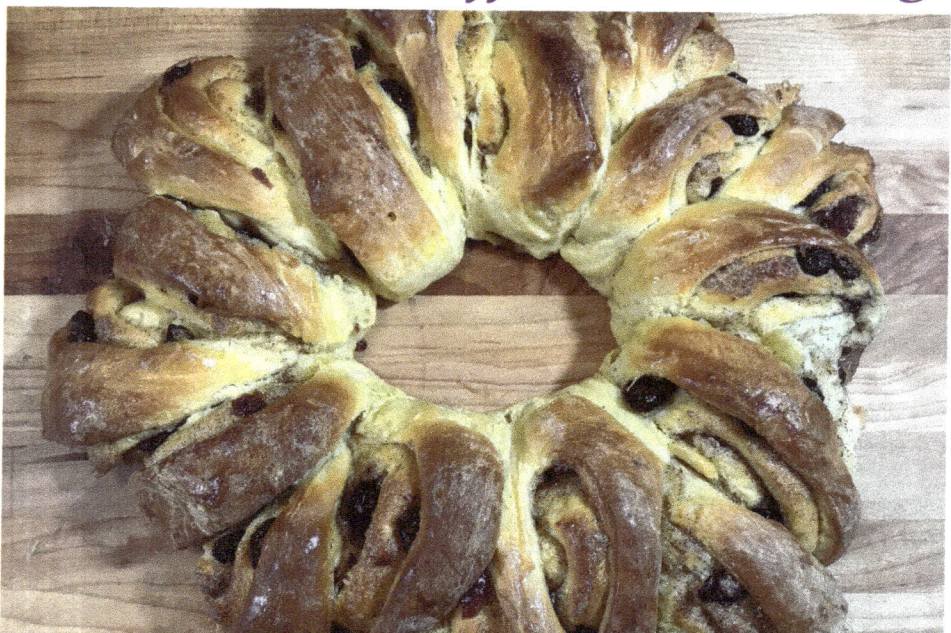

Ingredients (Serves 12)

- Bread
- 1 cup non fat Half and Half
- 1/2 cup (100g) white sugar
- 1/2 cup (4 oz) stick margarine
- 2-pkg active yeast dissolved in 1/4 cup warm water
- About 4 cups (560g) all-purpose flour
- 1 large egg
- 1/2 teaspoon salt

Filling
- 2 tablespoons melted stick margarine
- 1/4 cup (54g) brown sugar, packed
- 1 tablespoon white sugar
- 3 teaspoons Vietnamese cinnamon
- 1 bag of dried mixed fruit (raisins, cranberries, mango, chopped - and chopped pecans, walnuts or almonds if desired)

- Egg glaze
- 2 egg yolks
- Sugar glaze
- 1 - 1/4 cups powdered sugar
- 1 tablespoon non fat half and half
- 1 teaspoon vanilla

Method - Dough

- Put milk into a small saucepan and heat on medium heat until steamy (but not boiling). Remove from heat.

- Stir in the butter and sugar until the butter has melted and the sugar dissolved. Pour into a mixing bowl. Mix in yeast mixture and egg.

- Mix in salt. Slowly add in 2 cups of the flour. After the first two cups of flour gradually add more flour until a soft dough starts to form a ball and pull away from the sides of the bowl.

- Turn out onto a floured surface and knead

dough for 7 to 10 minutes until smooth, OR use a dough hook in a stand-up mixer and knead the dough that way for 7 to 10 minutes, adding more flour as needed to keep the dough from being too sticky.

- Note that the dough should remain soft, so take care not to add too much flour.
- Place the dough in an oiled bowl, covered with a clean tea-towel or with plastic wrap. Let rise for an hour or until the dough has doubled in size.

Make the Wreath Form

- Press the dough down to deflate. Divide the dough into 2 equal parts. Take one part (saving the other for a second wreath) and shape the dough 8-inch by 16-inch rectangle on a lightly floured surface.
- Brush the dough with melted butter, leaving at least a half inch border on the edges so the dough will stick together when rolled. Mix together the brown and white sugar and the cinnamon and sprinkle the dough with half of the mixture
- Sprinkle on the fruit fillings leaving 1/2 inch around edges.
- Carefully roll the dough up lengthwise, with the seam on the bottom.
- Transfer to a greased baking sheet.
- Form a circle with the dough on the baking sheet, connecting the ends together.
- Using scissors, cut most of the way through the dough, cutting on a slant. Work your way around the dough circle.
- After each cut, pull out the dough segment either to the right or to the left, alternating as you go around the circle. The dough circle will look like a wreath when you are done.
- Cover lightly with plastic wrap and set in a warm area for a second rise. Let rise for about 40 minutes to an hour; the dough should again puff up in size.
- While the dough is rising, preheat oven to 350 F
- Whisk together the egg yolks. Use a pastry brush to brush over the dough.

Bake in the oven for 25-30 minutes.

- After the first 15 minutes of baking, if the top is getting too browned, tent with some aluminum foil.
- Remove from oven and let cool completely.
- Drizzle the glaze in a back and forth motion over the pastry.

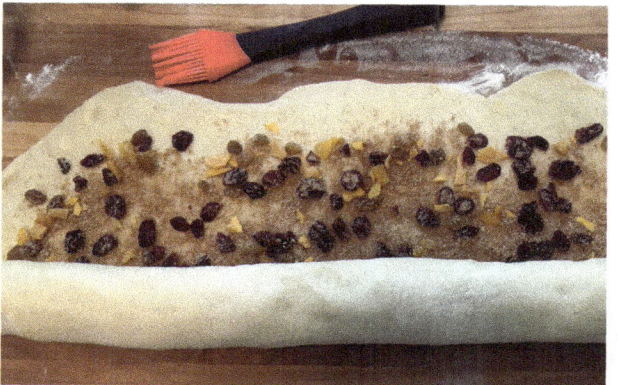
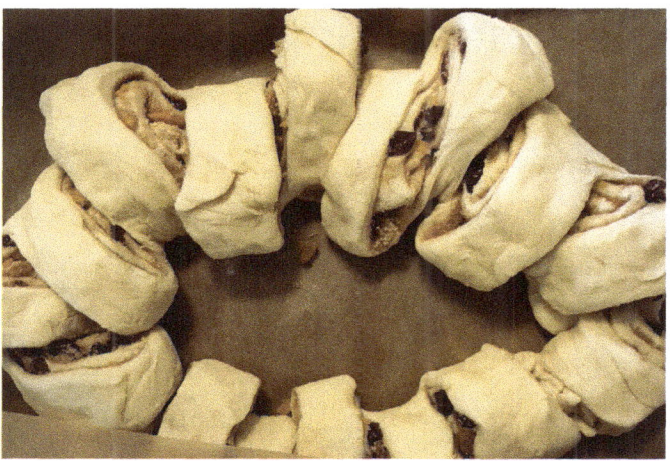

Oh Momma! Where's the Fat?

Old Fashioned Apple Pie

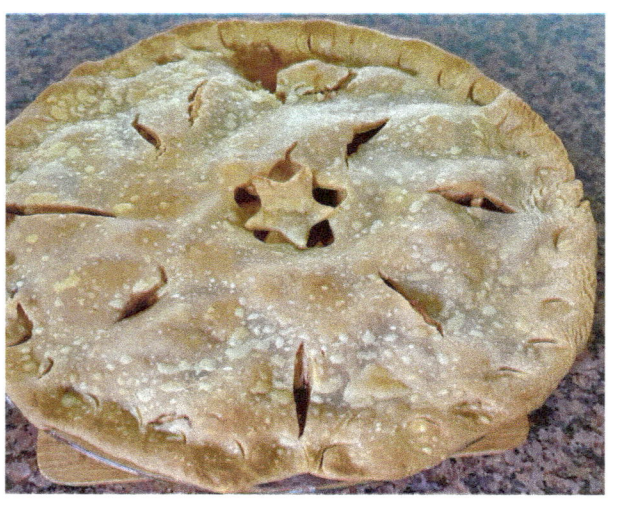

When I was little, I lived in Indiana where apples grew everywhere. We would buy bushel baskets full of apples from Orchards around my grandparent's small farm. This apple pie recipe is one I created when I was 9-10 years of age. I use to make my own crust full of butter or lard. However, I have found a nice pie crust I can use that has less fat and is quite fresh and has a flaky feel.

Ingredients for Pie (Serves 8)

- Store bought pie dough crusts (from dairy department - not frozen), 2 in a box
- All purpose flour for rolling out dough
- Corn Starch
- 7 medium Gala Apples or other Tart Applies
- Brown sugar
- White fine sugar
- Cinnamon
- Low fat Margarine Stick
- 1/2 Lemon
- 9 inch regular pie plate
- Small decorative cookie cutter
- Paring knife
- Bread board, floured

Method

- Peel and core apple pieces, and then cut into slices
- Put apple pieces in bowl and squeeze juice from 1/2 lemon over apples. This keeps the apples from oxidizing.
- Mix well.
- Add 1/2 cup brown sugar to apples
- Add 1/2 cup white sugar to apples
- Add 1 teaspoon cinnamon to apples
- Add 2 tablespoons melted margarine to apples
- Add 1 tablespoon of Corn Starch to apples
- Mix all these well and set aside.
- Unfold one of the pie crusts on a very well flowered board.
- Fold the crust in half and in half again.

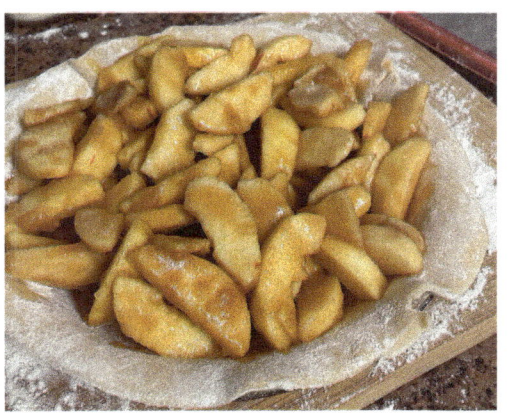

How to Serve Apple Pie

While warm, or reheated lightly, place some sprinkles of non fat cheddar cheese on top

Add a scoop of non fat ice cream and sprinkle with sugar ginger bites.

Add a spoonful or two of non fat whipped cream; or put pie in bowl and pour non fat cream over pie.

- Take a 9 inch pie dish and unfold the pie dough carefully and press gently down into the bottom of the pie dish. The crust will be a bit bigger than the pie dish but that is okay.
- Pour the apple mixture in the pie dish
- Unroll the next dough piece
- Using a small decorative cookie cutter, cut a hole in the center. Save the piece that was cut out.
- Carefully fold the dough in half and lift on top of the pie placing it on top of the apple filling. Unfold the other half carefully so you do not tear the cookie cutout.
- Take the cookie cut out and lightly dab water on the back side. Put at an angle over the hole in the crust so it leaves just a little bit of the area open. This allows steam to flow from the pie's center.
- Using a sharp knife, cut some slits in the pie crust. This allows the steam to escape along the sides and the pie crust not to explode in the oven.
- The crust should overlap the plate. Take the top edges and fold down and under the bottom crust.
- Once all the crust dough is folded, use your thumb to make an indent all around the edge of the pie.
- Preheat oven to 375 degrees and place the oven rack on the second from bottom.
- Make a tin foil boat to place the pie dish into so if it boils over or drips, it will not burn in the oven bottom.
- Place pie in the oven, uncovered, for 45 minutes. Check pie to see if it is bubbling. Also, if crust looks like it is getting too brown on top, place a sheet of aluminum paper on top the crust.
- Cook another 10-15 minutes or until pie is bubbly and crust is brown.
- Remove from oven and let pie cool on rack or insulated pot holder for 3-4 hours before eating.
- Store pie in refrigerator after serving. Pie pieces can be heated on a microwaveable plate in the microwave for a few seconds, if needed.

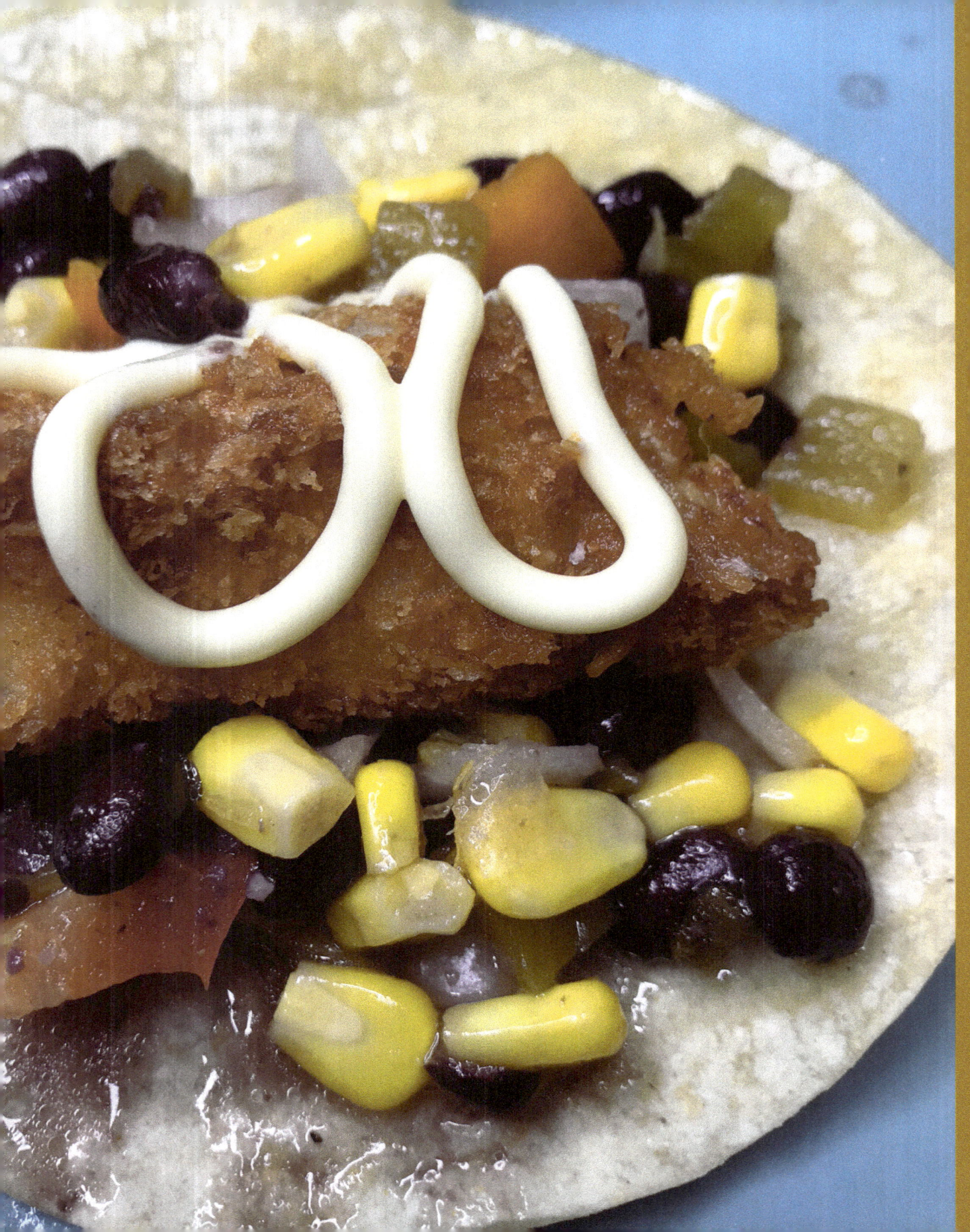

Fish

Stuffed Tilapia......................................157
Blackened Tilapia 158
Fried Cod Tacos..................................159
Mediterranean Tuna Salad 160
English Fish & Chips........................161
Grilled Fish Fajitas 162

A Fish Tale to Believe

I did not eat fish growing up. On Friday's the school cafeteria would have a fish dish for those who could not eat meat on Friday, and I just ate the vegetables. My mom and mammy never cooked fish. My other grandmother, Gammy liked to go fishing, but she didn't eat it either. So my experience in eating fish was lacking much education and flavor and fish variety.

I stayed away from fish for a long time during my school years. In college I would buy a can of Salmon and mix it up like meatloaf and fry it in a pan. I would pour ketchup over it and eat it. Sometimes, I would buy a can a tuna and add mayo and pickles to it. It was cheap and easy. However, I remember the first fish sandwich I ordered came from MacDonald's. I asked for extra tarter sauce. The fish was lightly flavored and with cheese and tarter sauce, I thought it was pretty good. I made it a favorite when I would order, not knowing the cheese and sauce made it more unhealthy than healthy.

It wasn't until I left college and moved to California that I started experiencing real fish cooked properly. Not those square patties on a burger, but real fish. I was working in the electronic consumer business in Los Angeles and then San Francisco, so when we had vendors or sales reps come to town, we would take them out to dinner. Most wanted fresh fish. One night when my sales group learned I had not tried most items on the menu, they ordered a bit of everything, including my meal and the night became a delightful array of flavors and new tastes, and my introduction into the seafood.

One of my French students in my group I tutored introduced me to swordfish. He use to leave for a weekend fishing with friends (not sure if off California or Mexico) but would come back with one in his truck packed in ice, and then he would fillet it for grilling. Instead of paying me to tutor him, he would cook me fresh swordfish.

I never took to shell fish and still do not eat it. Tilapia and Swordfish became some of my favorites, along with fried Calamari. While in England, I was introduced to "fish and chips" made with Cod. I believe the fresh Cod in England is some of the best fish I have eaten. It is much different than what I can buy here. I have tried fish pies in England and fish stews and these recipes are in the works for altering to low fat cooking.

Stuffed Tilapia

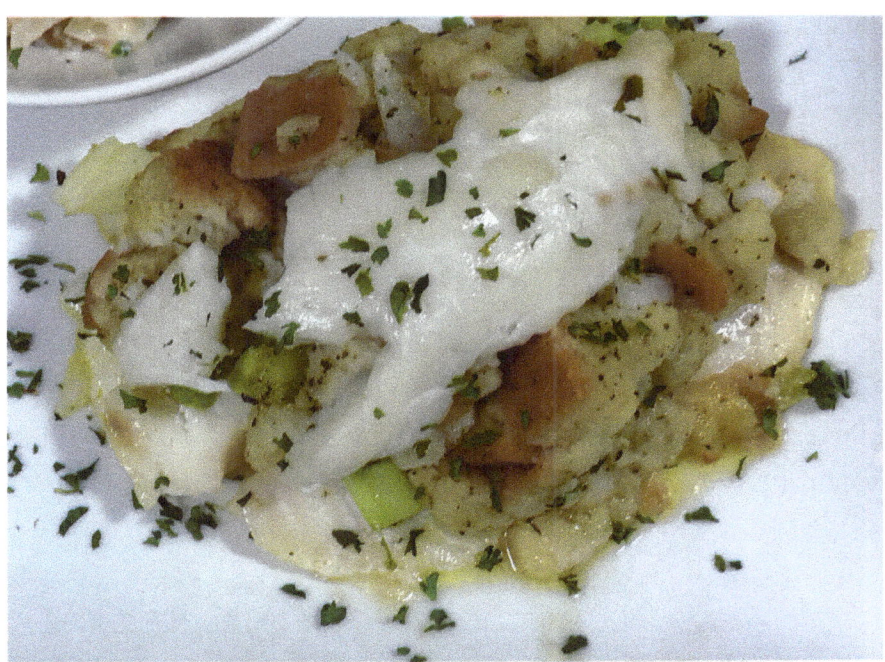

Ingredients: (Serves 2-4)

- 2-4 Tilapia fillets
- Olive Oil
- 1/2 small onion, chopped
- 1/2 cup celery, finely chopped
- Salt and Pepper
- 1 teaspoon dry sage
- 1/2 cup vegetable stock
- 2-3 cups dried bread crumbs
- Parsley for Garnish

Method

- Preheat oven to 350 degrees.
- In a small skillet, saute the onion and celery in a teaspoon of olive oil until tender.
- Add the vegetable stock, sage, salt and pepper to the onion and celery mix.
- Add the dried bread crumbs one cup at a time and mix after each cup until well blended and moist but not soupy.
- Slice the fillets down the middle to make a pocket being careful not to cut in half.
- Place a spoonful or two of the mix into the fillets.
- Place the fillets in an oiled roasting pan. If there is extra dressing, spoon it around the pieces of fish.
- Lightly brush Olive Oil on top of each fillet.
- Bake in preheated oven for 30 minutes or until fish flakes and is white throughout.
- Serve with a garnish of parsley.

Blackened Tilapia

Ingredients (Serves 4)

- 4 Tilapia Fillets
- 1 tablespoon canola oil
- Blackened Seasoning (Pre-mix or Homemade)
- Pineapple or Mango Salsa (shown on plate with Tilapia)

Method

- Rub the Tilapia fillets with the Blackened seasoning on one side only.
- On a seasoned cast iron flat griddle pan, pour 1.5 teaspoons of canola oil and heat pan.
- Put Tilapia, seasoning down, on hot griddle and cook 5 minutes.
- Flip the Tilapia and cook another 5 minutes.
- Serve Tilapia on a warm plate with your favorite fruit salsa or chutney

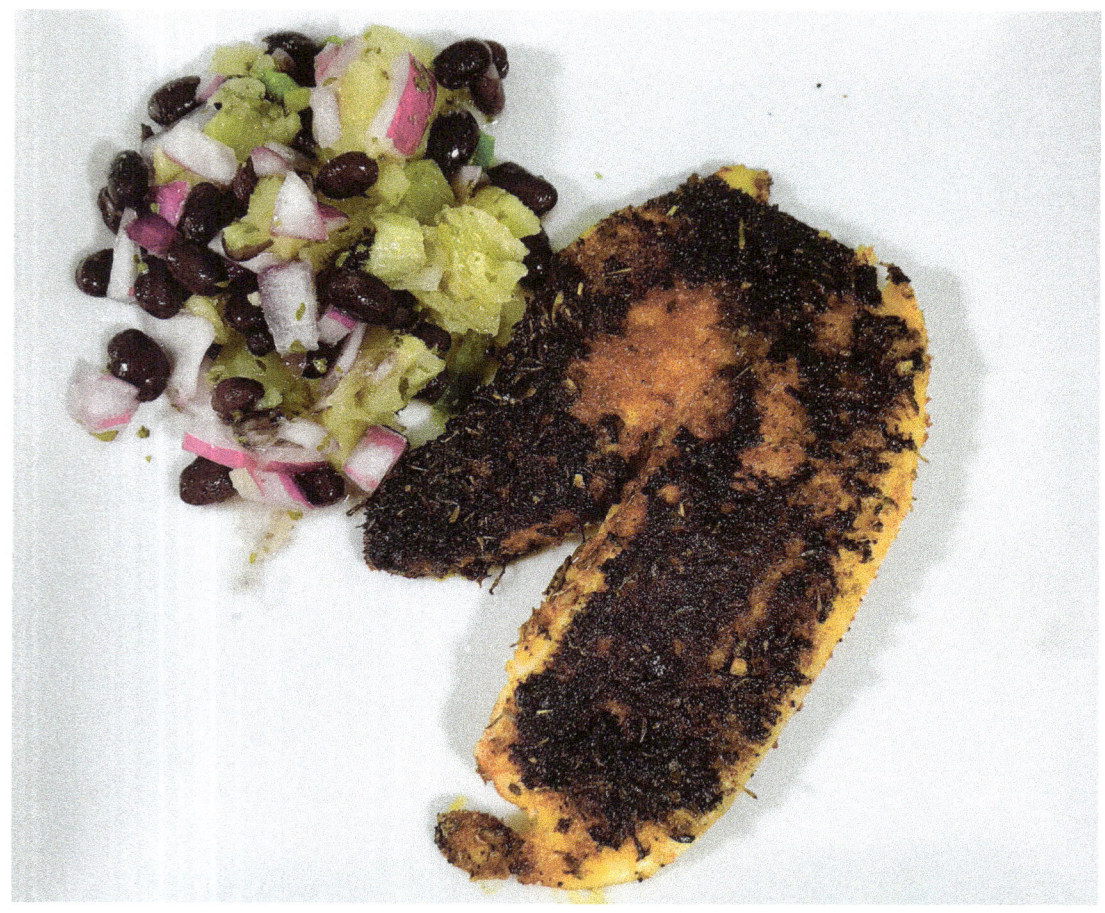

Fried Cod Tacos

Ingredients (Serves 2)

- 1 pound thick cod fillet, cut into 4 pieces
- 4 flour or corn tortillas
- 1/2 cup flour
- 1/2 cup Panko crumbs
- 2 eggs whisked in a bowl
- Sometimes I add a bit of smoky paprika to the flour for a slight flavoring of heat.
- Favorite Taco toppings (corn salsa, red or green salsa, onions, hot sauces)

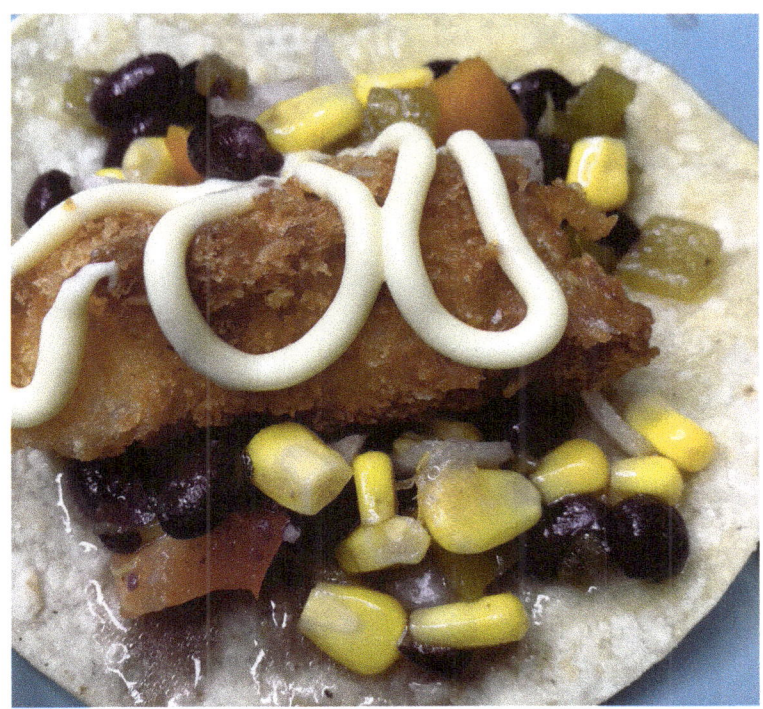

Method

- Preheat air fryer following manufacturer's guidelines. If you do not have an air fryer, you can bake the cod in the oven at 375 degrees.
- Put the flour on a small plate
- Put the Panko crumbs on a small plate
- Whisk the eggs in a low flat bowl
- Take a piece of the cod and lay it on the flour turning it over so the piece is covered.
- Dip the cod into the egg, covering all areas of the cod.
- Lay the egg dipped cod on the Panko crumbs and flip over so the piece is covered. Slightly press on the crumbs so they adhere to the egg.
- Sit the cod on a large plate
- Repeat this procedure for the other 3 pieces of cod.
- Once all pieces are breaded, spray the bottom of the air fryer basket with oil and lay each piece of cod in the basket.
- If you are using the oven, spray the bottom of a baking dish and lay the cod on the bottom of the baking dish.
- Air Fry the cod for 5 minutes then flip over, spray lightly with oil again and cook for another 5 minutes
- If baking, then Bake the cod in the oven for 5-7 minutes and flip over for the same.
- Cod is done when it is flaky white in the middle.
- Remove the cod to a serving tray along with the tortillas
- Place a piece of cod on a heated tortilla, and add your favorite toppings.

Mediterranean Tuna Salad

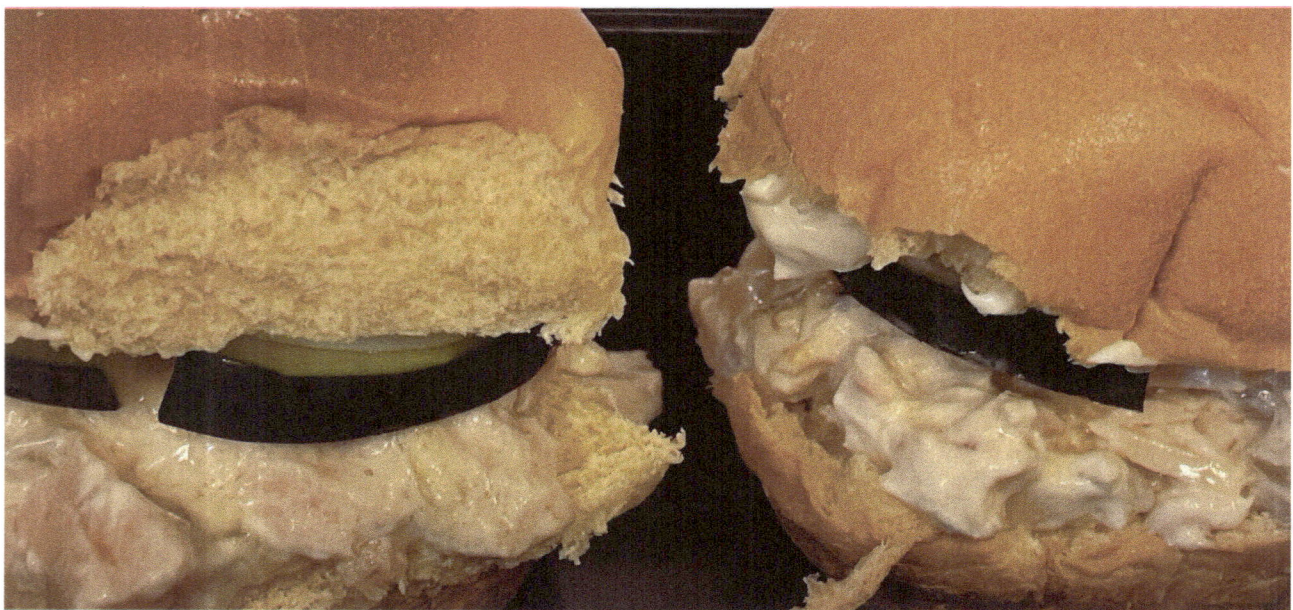

Ingredients

- 1 can light tuna in olive oil. The light tuna has less mercury, especially in Slip Jack Tuna. The olive oil adds the "good fats" to the dish.
- 1 tablespoons (more if desired) low fat, olive oil mayonnaise
- 7-9 chopped Kalamata olives
- 1 rib celery, washed chopped
- 1/2 teaspoon Dijon mustard
- Bread of choice (I like pitas, homemade buns, olive bread)
- 1 thin sliced cucumber
- 1 hard boiled egg sliced (optional)

Method

- Mix all the above ingredients, except the cucumber, together in bowl.
- Put one scoop of tuna salad on a piece of bread or bun of your choice.
- Top with a slice of cucumber and hard boiled egg (optional)
- Top with other half of bread

As a young adult and living away from home, I had to make one can of tuna last several days and multiple sandwiches. I ate it for lunch and dinner. So I would add vegetables to it like cabbage, carrots, pickles and dash of mustard for tartness. This Mediterranean Tuna Salad I make now reminds me of those days.

English Fish and Chips

Ingredients

- One cod fillet per person
- 2 eggs, in bowl and beaten slightly
- 1 cup flour, in a bowl
- Salt and Pepper

Tarter Sauce
- 1/2 cup olive oil mayonnaise
- 1 small onion diced
- 2 cloves garlic diced
- 1/4 cup pickle relish (I use dill)
- Juice from 1/2 lemon

Method

- Preheat air fryer per manufacturer's instructions

Tarter Sauce
- Make the tarter sauce by mixing all ingredients
- Refrigerate until ready to eat

Fillets
- Take each fillet and dip in flour, dip in egg again and back in flour
- Lay the fillets gently in the basket of the air fryer
- Set air fryer to 400 degrees for 10 minutes. After the first 5 minutes, turn the fillets over and continue frying.
- Fish is done when centers are white.
- Serve with tarter sauce and your choice of a side. I like cole slaw and hand cut French fries in the air fryer. Sometimes I make mushy peas (baby peas cooked and mashed).

Tilapia (or Cod) Flat Top Fajitas

Ingredients (Serves 1 person per Tilapia)

- 1 piece of Tilapia for each person
- Blacken Seasoning
- 1 -2 Onions, peeled and chopped in large pieces. One onion will be for topping each fajita and one onion will be used in the corn.
- 1 Green Pepper, sliced in sizes to match onion
- 1 Red or Orange Pepper, sliced in sizes to match onion
- 1 can Seasoned Black Beans
- 2 cups Frozen White Corn
- 1 Large or 2 Medium Poblano Peppers
- 1 Tomato, sliced in small piece. 1/2 will be to top tacos and 1/2 to warm in corn.
- 1 Cup Non-Fat Cheddar Cheese
- Your favorite Salsa
- Shredded lettuce
- Hot sauces
- Pickled Jalapenos
- Salt and Pepper
- Flour and/or Corn Tortillas – 2 per piece of tilapia
- Oil for cooking

Prepare a Serving Tray - keep warm at 150 degrees

Method Black Beans

- Open the can of Black Beans and put in a stove top or microwave pan.
- Put two cups Frozen White corn in bowl and add the chopped Poblano peppers and onions.
- Place Tilapia on plate and rub one side with the Blacken Seasoning mix. Let set a few minutes

Method Fried Corn & Vegetables

- Place 1 tablespoon cooking oil in skillet and heat.
- Cooke onions, green and red peppers until slightly soft. Remove to serving tray and keep warm.
- Place 1 tablespoon cooking oil in a skillet and heat.
- Slightly brown the Poblano pepper and then add the corn and corn seasoning.
- Cook until corn is soft.
- Add tomatoes to the corn and stir until heated.
- Remove the corn to the serving tray and keep warm

Method - Tilapia

- Put 1 – 2 tablespoons of oil in a skillet and heat.
- Take the seasoned Tilapia and place on a prepared skillet with seasoning side down.
- Cook for 2 minutes or until you see the edges starting to crisp.
- Flip the Tilapia and continue cooking until white and flaky throughout.
- Remove to warming tray.

Method - Tortillas & Black Beans

- Lightly spray a skillet with non-fat oil and heat.
- Place tortillas on skillet and brown on each side.
- Heat the black beans to a boil.
- Remove the Tilapia to the warming plate and cut each piece in half.
- Add the cooked pepper and onion mixture to the plate
- Remove the Heated and Browned tortillas to the heated serving tray.
- Add the fried corn to the plate along with a bowl of the black beans
- Serve with toppings of cheese, salsa, hot sauces, jalapenos, lettuce and any other favorite ingredients. If you like sour cream, be sure to buy non fat sour cream.

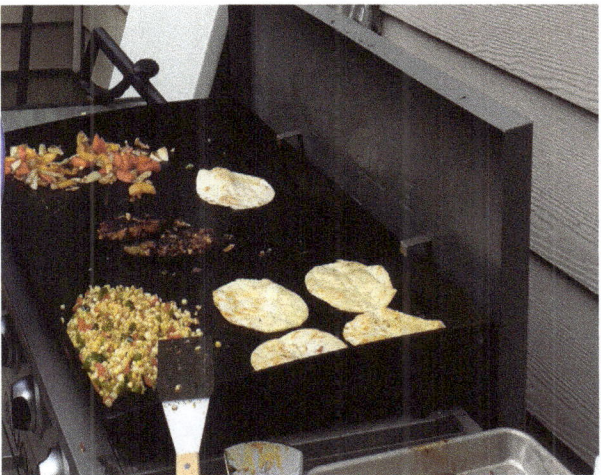

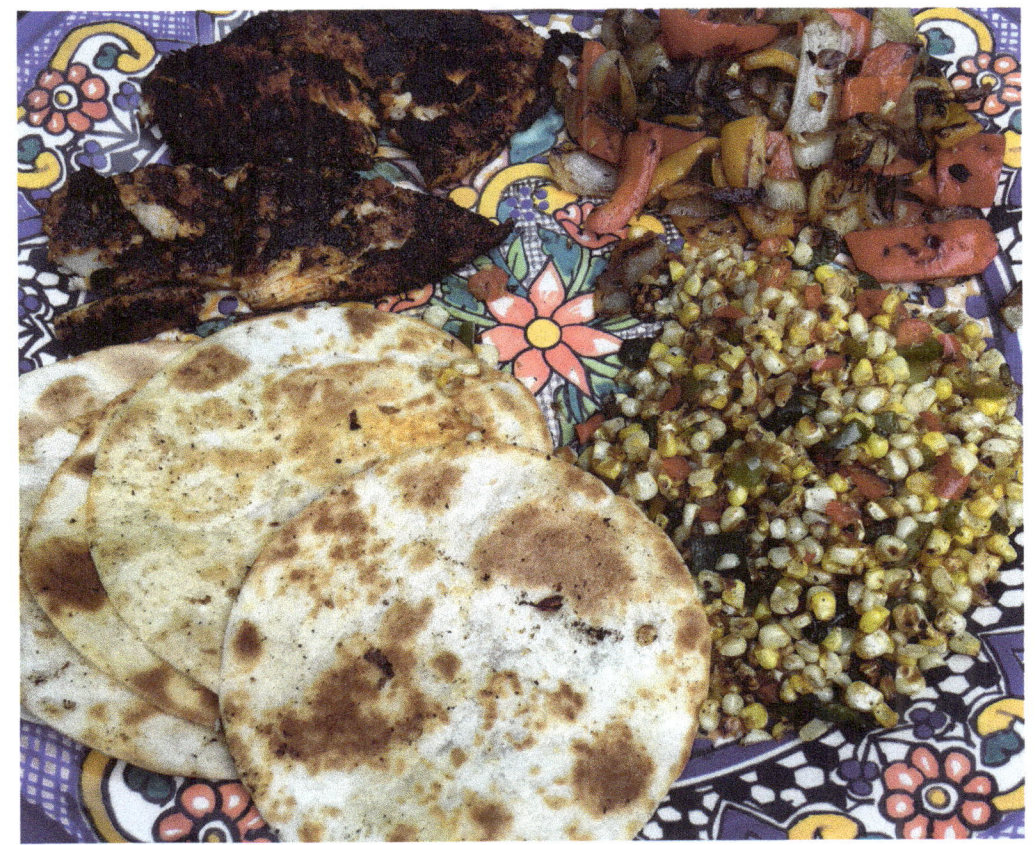

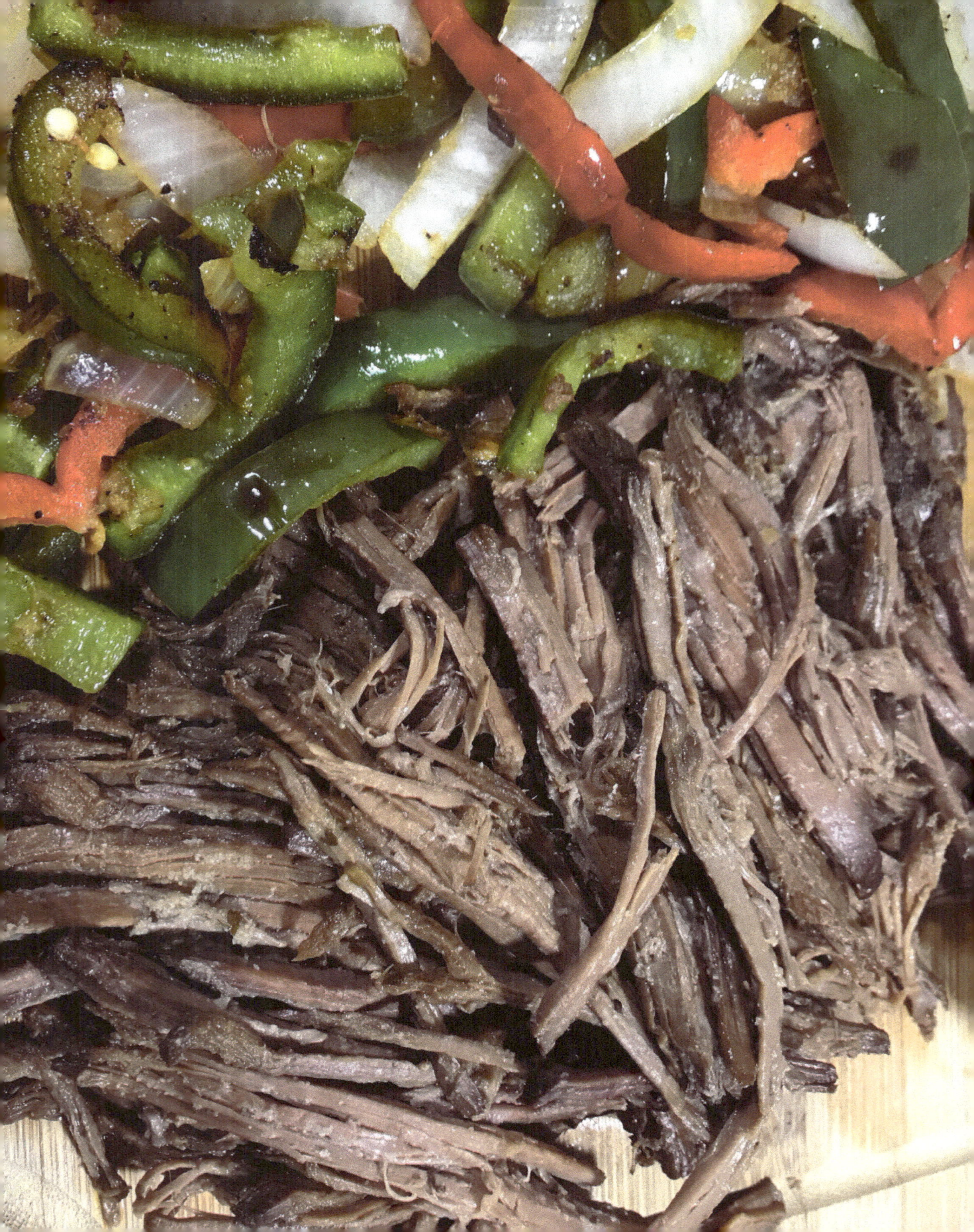

Beef

Old Fashioned Beef Stew 167

Thai Fry 168

Beef Stroganoff 170

Italian Roast Beef 173

Italian Roast Beef Sandwich 173

Borscht 174

It's Not the Other White Meat - It's Beef

I honestly think people fail with this and that diets because it is not easy to go "cold turkey" with habits and things we love. While I do not promote low saturated fat eating as a diet plan, reducing saturated fats in the diet will assist anyone with weight loss. This is regular food, cooked a bit different and some ingredients substituted, but these recipes are "Happy Eating".

You can still enjoy Burger Night, celebrate birthdays and enjoy holiday meals and vacation dining. It's called SPLURGE NIGHT. We celebrate it at least once every 6 weeks or so.

This is a day where we have a meal we want without regard to saturated fats. Sometimes it's a regular pizza at our favorite joint. Other times, it is a steak or some onion rings or even a piece of real cheese cake. But we make it a day or a meal in the day and repeat the SPLURGE DAY every 6 to 8 weeks.

Typically, a day with beef is a Splurge Day. Beef contains trans fats which are bad fats for the heart. So in consideration of healthier beef meals, a lot of thought has gone in to the cut of meat. I grew up eating pot roast at least once each week. We at meatloaf with fatty hamburger meat. We ate steaks grilled and cube steaks deep fried. Hamburgers were generous, fatty and juicy.

Today, I cook beef a couple times each month, if we have a craving. To be honest, I do not miss it as much as I thought I would since I have found other meats and seasonings to take the place. But I am not denying myself of its flavor, and I make dishes where a small amount of beef can go a long way.

So enjoy beef, but do so in moderation and with the right cuts of meat. Balance a beef meal with the other meals in the day and the 15 grams of saturated fat per day can still be achieved.

Beef Choices for Lower Saturated Fat

Top Loin Roast (per 3.5 oz serving is 3.7 g saturated fat*)
Bottom Round (per 3.4 oz serving is 3.1 g saturated fat*)
Eye of Round (per 3.0 oz serving is 3.1 g saturated fat*)

*Nutritional values provided by USDA

Old Fashioned Beef Stew

Ingredients (Serves 4-6)

- 3 pounds Sirloin Tip roast, cut into bite size chunks
- 1/4 cup white flour
- 8 Dutch potatoes
- 2 onions, peeled and cut into pieces
- 3 carrots, cut into bite size pieces
- 2 celery stalks, cut into bite size pieces
- 6 ounces sliced mushrooms (any type)
- Beef broth from a box 32 ounces
- Olive oil for browning meat (1-2 tablespoons)
- Salt and Pepper to Taste

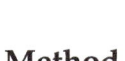

Method

Brown and flour meat then add broth.

- Use a heavy Dutch oven and pour in the oil to preheat on medium high
- Add the cut up meat, dash of salt and pepper.
- Turn the meat continuously as it browns and keep cooking until the water has evaporated.
- Sprinkle the meat with the flour and continue stirring to incorporate all the flour.
- Add the 3 cups beef broth

Add vegetables to meat and broth.

- Add the potatoes, onions, carrots and mushrooms.
- Mix very well.
- Cook with cover on, medium heat until boiling, then low heat for 2 hours.
- Check it often to make sure there is still plenty of liquid that creates the thick gravy. You can add 1/2 - 1 cup of water or more broth if necessary.

Cook until meat is tender. Then enjoy with a slice of bread.

- When meat and vegetables are done, the gravy can be thickened if desired. Measure out a couple tablespoons of flour and then add about 1/4 cup of the stew gravy. Mix it very well, then add it back to the pot of stew. Stir for a few minutes and the gravy will thicken.

Oh Momma! Where's the Fat?

Beef Thai Fry

Ingredients (Serves 2-4)

For the Stir Fry

- 3/4 pound Sirloin Tip, fat trimmed and sliced in thin strips
- 1 red bell pepper, sliced in thin strips
- 1 medium onion, chopped
- 1 large carrot, chopped in small pieces
- 2 celery stalks sliced down middle and chopped
- 1 small can chopped water chestnuts, drained.
- 4 cloves of garlic, minced
- 1 1/2 tablespoons of Sesame Oil (for frying)

For the beef Marinade

- 1 teaspoon water
- 1 teaspoon cornstarch
- 1 teaspoon low sodium soy sauce
- 1 teaspoon Mirin

For the Sauce

- 2 tablespoons low sodium soy sauce
- 1 tablespoon Chinkiang Vinegar
- 1 tablespoon fish sauce
- 1 tablespoon oyster sauce
- 1 tablespoon hoisin sauce
- 1 teaspoon Chili Garlic sauce
- 1/4 cup water
- 2 tablespoons light brown sugar

For the Noodles

- 2 packages cooked ramen or Homemade Thin Noodles.

Method

- In a small bowl, mix the Marinade ingredients until the cornstarch is well blended and smooth..
- Add the sliced Sirloin tip to the marinade and mix well. Cover and set in refrigerator to marinate for 30 minutes (or longer).
- Whisk the Sauce ingredients together and set aside.
- Boil the Noodle Water
- Heat the oil in a large skillet over high heat (or you can use your Wok which is what I prefer)
- Remove the meat from the marinade and sear the beef until it is brown on all sides. This should take 3 minutes. Remove the meat from the pan to a plate and set aside.
- To the hot skillet or Wok, add the vegetables, except garlic and water chestnuts. Cook approximately 3 minutes, turning them constantly in the pan for even cooking. Add the garlic and water chestnuts at the last minute.
- Add the Raman noodles and the packet of beef flavor to the boiling noodle water.
- Add the beef back to the pan of vegetables, stir well and then add the sauce. Continue stirring the mixture until it thickens, typically 2-3 minutes.
- Ladle a scoop of noodles into a bowl.
- Top with a scoop of the meat and vegetables mixture. Serve.

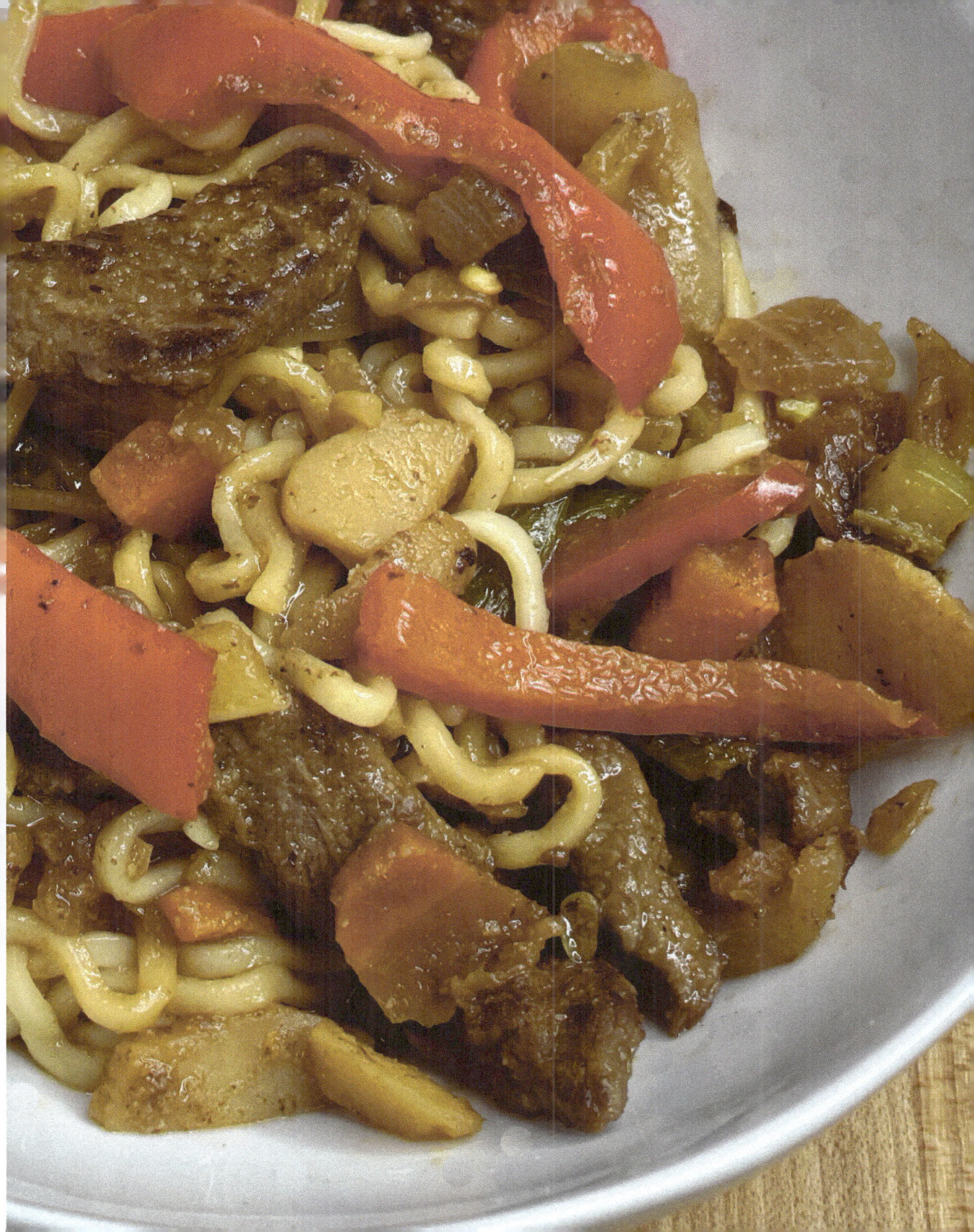

Beef Stroganoff

Ingredients (Serves 4)

- Cooking spray - Olive Oil
- 1 pounds top boneless sirloin, fat trimmed and cut into 1 1/2-inch pieces
- 4 pieces turkey bacon cut into small pieces
- 1/4 cup all-purpose flour
- 1 - 1/4 teaspoons kosher salt
- 1 teaspoon freshly ground black pepper
- 8 ounces shiitake mushrooms, sliced 1/4-inch thick
- 1 medium yellow onion, diced (about 1 cup)
- 2 cloves garlic, minced
- 1 1/4 cups low-sodium beef broth
- 2 tablespoons Worcestershire sauce
- 8 ounces dried egg noodles
- 1 tablespoons olive oil
- 1 cup non fat sour cream
- 2 tablespoons chopped Italian parsley leaves (optional)

Method

- Coat a 5-quart or larger Dutch oven with cooking spray and set heat to medium.
- Place the beef, flour, salt, and pepper in a large bowl and toss until the beef is evenly coated.
- Transfer the beef and any flour left in the bowl to the Dutch oven. Brown meat for 3 minutes, turning occasionally.
- Add the mushrooms, onion, garlic, beef broth, and Worcestershire sauce, and stir to combine. Cover and cook until the beef is tender. If cooking in a Dutch oven on top of the stove, turn burner to low and cook slow for 3-4 hours. If placing pot in oven, set heat to 325 and bake 3 hours. Be sure to check the meat half way into baking. Every stove and oven cooks differently. If the meat needs more liquid, add a bit more beef broth.
- 15 minutes before you are ready to eat, cook egg noodles according to package Method. Drain, toss with a teaspoon of olive oil, and set aside.
- Gradually and slowly stir the sour cream into the stroganoff. Serve over noodles and sprinkle with the parsley if desired.

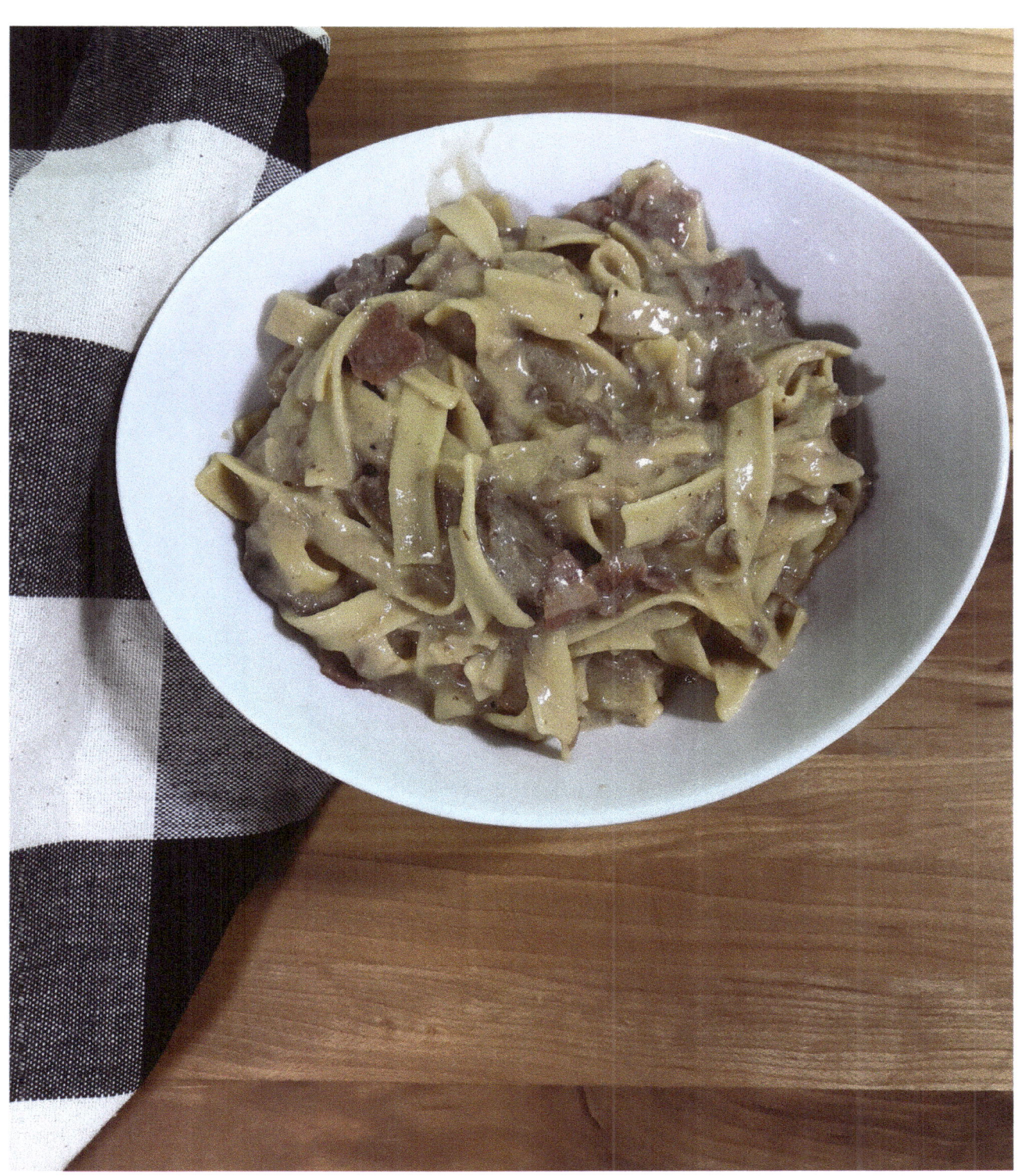

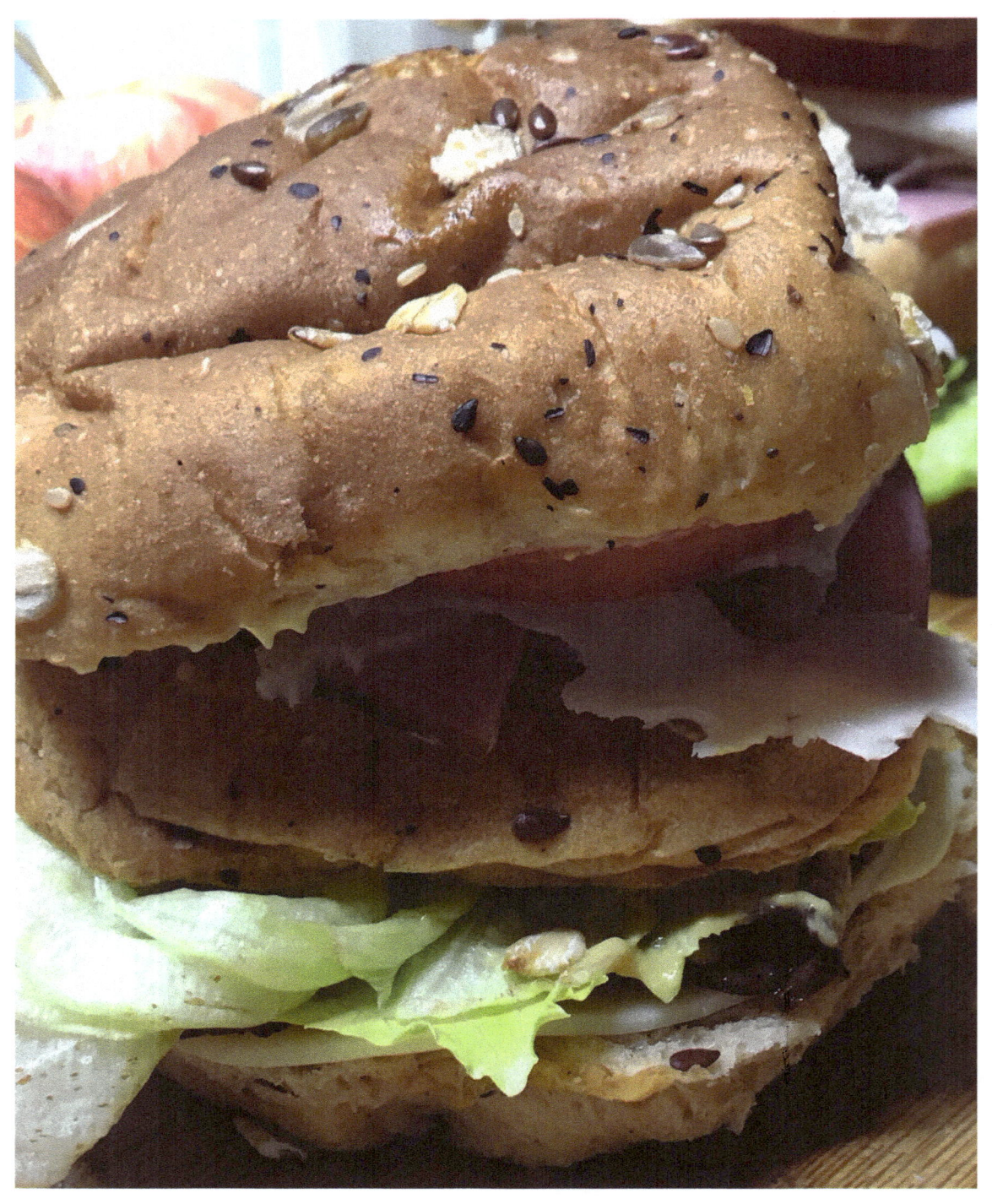

Triple Decker Italian Roast Beef Sandwich

Italian Roast Beef Sandwiches

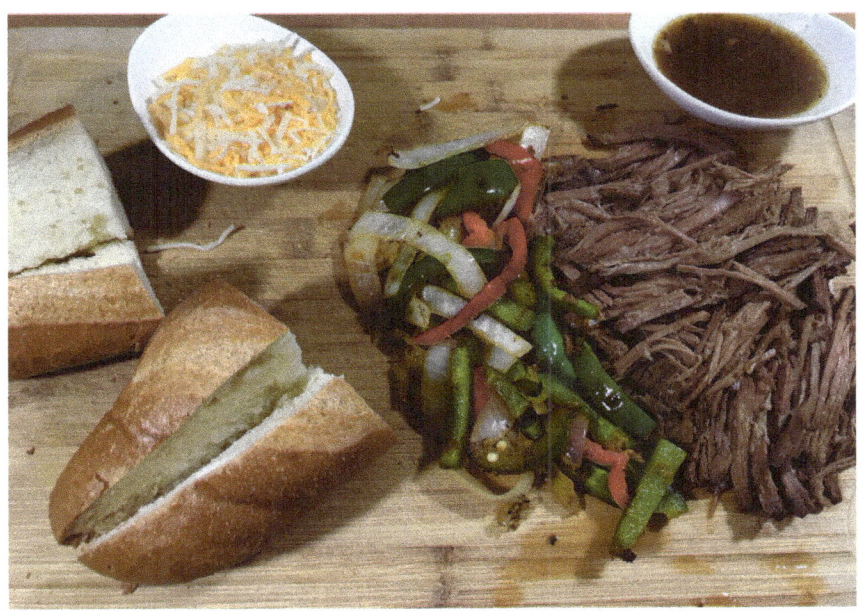

Ingredients (Makes 4-6 Sandwiches)

- 3 pound beef roast

 (Select either Sirloin Tip, Top Loin or Bottom Round for lowest saturated fat content)
- 1 package Dry Italian salad dressing mix, or 1/4 cup Fat Free Italian bottled salad dressing.
- 1 cup beef broth
- 1/2 jar Pepperoncini Peppers; add more if you like,.

<u>Toppings</u>
- Non fat shredded cheddar and mozzarella,, tomato slices, black olives, stir fried peppers and onions, pepperoncini peppers, mustards and olive oil mayonnaise.

Method

- Preheat oven to 300 degrees.
- Place the roast in a Dutch oven that has a tight fitting lid, or a heavy pot that can be covered with aluminum paper.
- Pour in the beef broth
- Add the Italian salad dressing
- Cook in a 300 degree oven on the center rack for 2 hours.
- Check the roast for tenderness after 2 hours. Add the Pepperoncini and 1/2 of the juices from the jar and cook another 1 hour.
- Meat should shred easily when it is done.
- Serve on buns with stir fried peppers and onions, mustard or pickled onions.

Borscht

Ingredients (Serves 6-8)

- Beef Sirloin Tip Roast, 1-1.5 pounds, trimmed and cut into 1 inch pieces.
- Olive oil
- 1 large yellow or white onion, peeled and chopped
- 32 oz beef broth (canned or boxed, but lower sodium option)
- 3-4 medium to large fresh beets, peeled and cut into 1/2 inch cubes
- 4 large carrots, peeled and cut into 1/2 inch pieces
- 1 large or 2 medium russet potatoes, peeled and cut into 1/2 inch cubes
- 2 cups thinly sliced red cabbage,
- 3 tablespoons Red Wine Vinegar
- 1 cup nonfat sour cream (optional)
- Salt
- Pepper
- Garlic Powder
- 3/4 cup Fresh Rosemary, chopped
-

Method

- Season the cut up beef with salt, pepper and garlic powder over each piece.
- Let sit for 10 minutes.
- Take a large Dutch oven and pour in 2-3 tablespoons of olive oil, heat until hot.
- Place meat in pot and brown on all sides at a medium heat.
- When the beef is brown all over and the juices have formed in the pan, add the onions.
- Stir the onions and meat at medium heat until the onions begin to become translucent.
- Add the 4 cups of beef broth. Stir, turn heat to medium low, place lid on pan and let simmer slowly for 1-2 hours.
- While meat is cooking, prepare the beets, carrots and cabbage.
- Preheat the oven to 400 degrees.
- During the last 45 minutes of the beef simmering, place the beets and carrots in a bowl and drizzle with olive oil - just a small amount - and mix to cover vegetables.
- Place the vegetables in an even layer on a sheet pan.
- Pace in oven on middle shelf and cook 15 minutes.
- While beets and carrots are cooking, take potatoes and put in a bowl and drizzle with olive oil - again, just a small amount.
- At the end of the 15 minutes bake for beets and carrots, add potatoes to the pan, spreading out in single layer. Bake an additional 15 minutes.
- Take the sheet pan of vegetables and add them to the stock pot of beef and onions.
- Add the sliced cabbage.
- Add 3/4 cup chopped fresh Rosemary.
- Cook until cabbage is tender.
- Add the red wine vinegar. I like a bit more vinegar, so add it to your taste, whether a bit more or less.
- Serve in deep bowls with rolls or bread on the side.

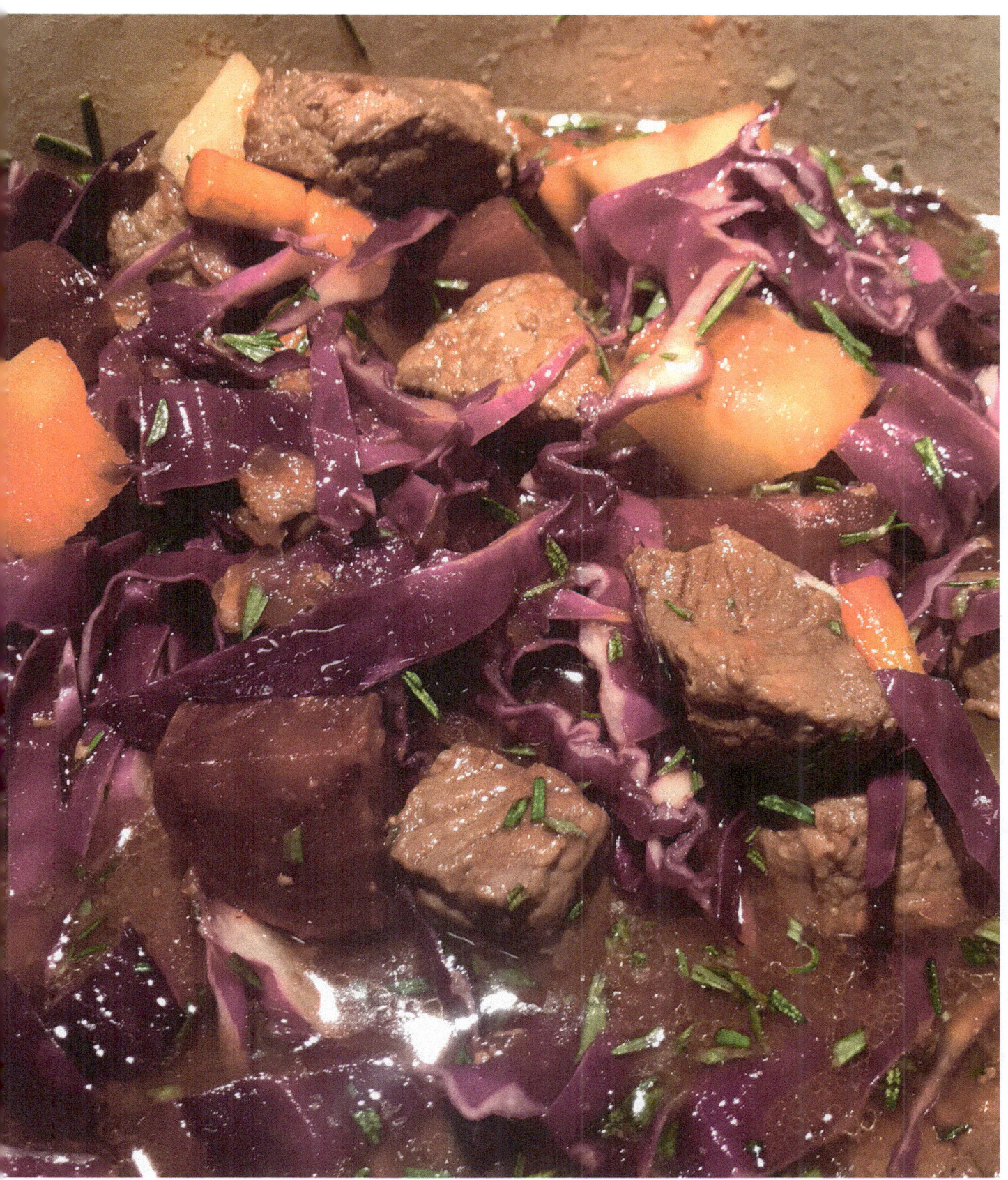

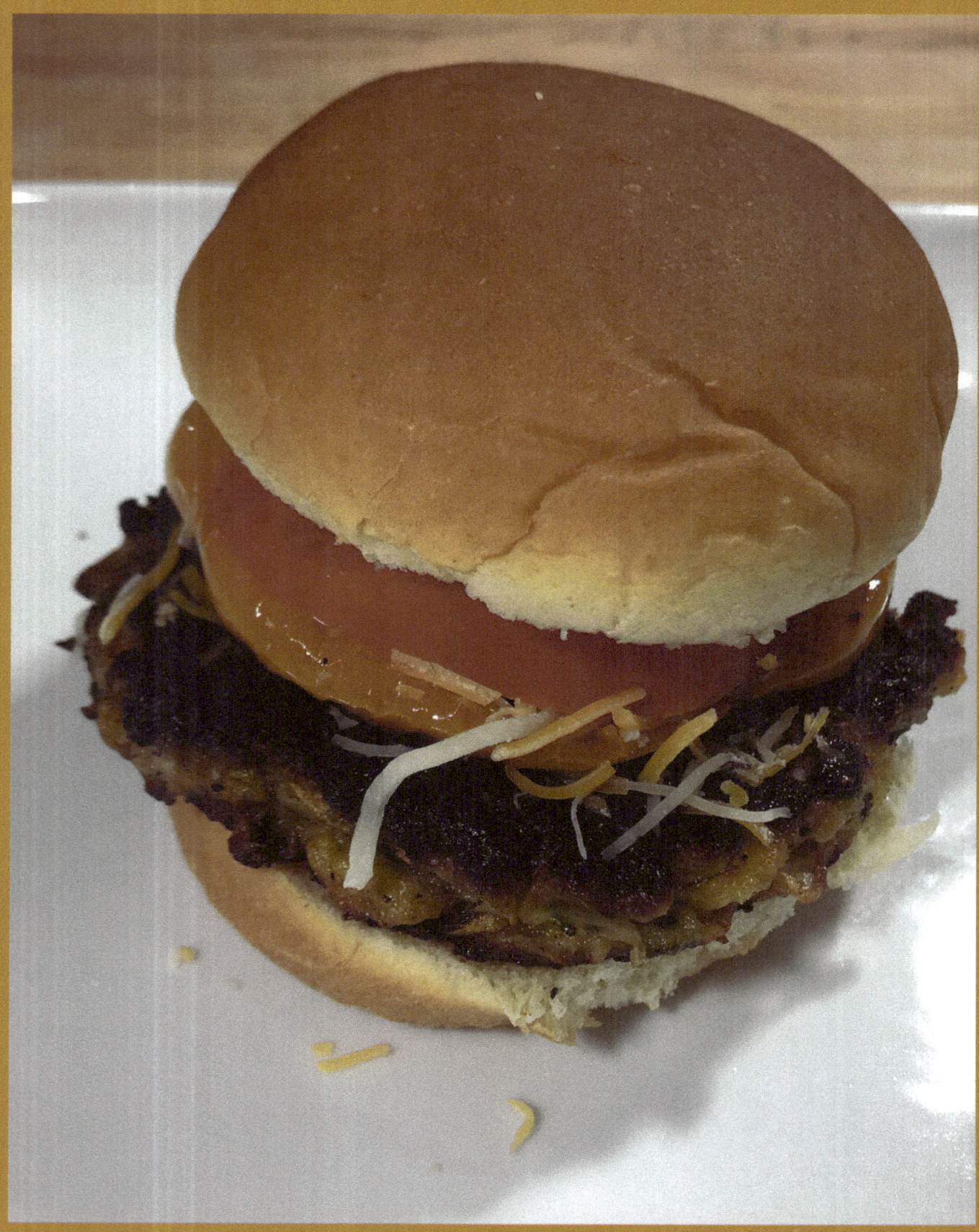

Burgers

Turkey Burgers 179
Zucchini Burgers 180
Portobello Burgers 181
Eggplant Burgers 182
Salmon Burgers 183

Hamburgers - The Best Meal Ever

Around the age of 8 or so, I would only eat hamburgers, and made it my choice of food for any meal. The time of day to eat a hamburger never mattered. I would eat one at breakfast or lunch or dinner, maybe even all meals. A hamburger on a white bun with only a spread of ketchup was my choice but later years it became mayonnaise and onion. Sometimes a few chips thrown on the plate or a side of baked beans would be added, but that was it. The best meal ever.

Once when my family was traveling to the northern part of our state to visit my aunt, we stopped for breakfast in a little diner. Never being the egg and toast type, I asked the waitress if I could have a hamburger on a white bun with ketchup. I still remember the look on her face as if she were going to get sick. Then I saw her lean in to my father and talk quietly, but I do remember hearing his answer. 'My daughter would very much like the hamburger, and if you can make one for her, it will be very much appreciated.' And sure enough, a hamburger was served. I do not know if it was my dad's flirtatious behavior or if it was just the kindness of our waitress, but I certainly enjoyed my hamburger.

My dad and mom almost lost me when I was in second grade. I fell on the school playground during group play and fractured my skull. At the hospital, my parents were told that I may not wake up the next day, and there wasn't anything they could do but wait. The fracture was severe. However, surprising everyone, I woke up and was alert and responsive the next day. I was hungry and wanted a hamburger, but it was not allowed. My mom was with me during the days and my dad came every evening. He couldn't bring me my coveted hamburger (he said the smell would give it away), but he did sneak in chocolate bars for me to hide under my pillow and eat after everyone went to sleep. I made it home to recover a few more weeks, and life returned to normal except I could tell my dad had changed. He seemed to keep a watchful eye on me and spent more time with me than he had before.

So while we were ordering breakfast in the small cafe that morning, me asking for a hamburger for breakfast was his way to know I would be okay from there on out.

Today, my burgers are all very different. First, I don't eat ketchup on them anymore. The main ingredients of the patty vary and can be anything from pork, chicken, turkey, salmon, tuna, eggplant, mushroom and zucchini. Toppings are as varied as the ingredient, but always delicious. At breakfast while traveling, I make sure to go to a restaurant that has long hours and still serves burgers in the morning even at 6:00 a.m.

Marinated Ground Turkey Burgers

Ingredients (Makes 4 - 4 ounce burgers, 1 per serving)

- 1 pound of lean turkey meat (pork or chicken)
- 2 cloves garlic minced
- ¼ cup Worcestershire sauce
- Salt
- Milled Black Pepper

This recipe is for a basic burger made with ground turkey. Substitute chicken or pork if you want. From this basic burger recipe, make it your own with your favorite ingredients added. Sometimes, I add mushrooms, peppers, onions, BBQ sauce, Italian spices, curry spices, rubs and hot sauces.

I like to serve these burgers on slider buns which have been toasted and spread with homemade non-fat Sriracha mayonnaise or Black pepper mayonnaise. Dijon mustard is always good, too.

Chicken meat expands when it is cooked, so make patties smaller and thinner for burgers.

Method

- Mix the turkey meat and spices in a bowl.
- Shape the burgers into four equal pieces.
- Place on a prepared flat griddle or cast iron pan that has been preheated with 1-2 tablespoons olive oil.
- On medium high heat, brown the first side about 5 minutes.
- Flip burgers
- Pour the Worcestershire Sauce over each of the buggers and let cook another 5 minutes until done.
- While cooking the second side, add the sliced Jalapenos to the skillet and brown well on both sides (about 2 minutes while burgers finish cooking)
- Burgers are done when juices run clear or 164 degrees.

Oh Momma! Where's the Fat?

Zucchini Burger Sliders

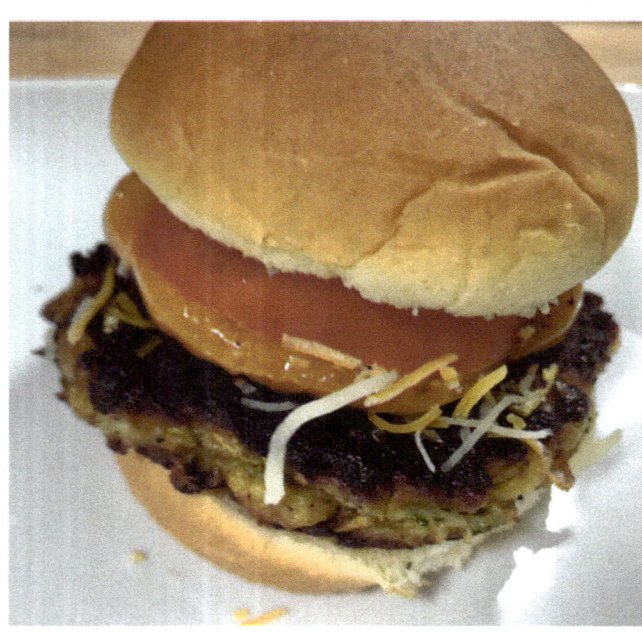

Ingredients (makes 4 sliders)

- 1 cup grated zucchini (1-2 zucchini depending on the size)
- 1/4 cup Parmesan grated cheese
- 1/4 cup breadcrumbs
- 1/8 cup flour
- 1 small onion, finely chopped
- 1 teaspoon dill, chopped
- 1 egg, beaten
- Dash of salt (optional)
- Dash of pepper
- Olive oil for frying (or olive spray)

Toppings

- Sliced Tomato
- Non Fat Cheese Mixture Sprinkled on top
- Sriracha Low Fat Olive Oil Mayonnaise

I like the flavor of Cheddar Cheese, but no fat cheddar does not melt well. So, after the burger is on the bun, sprinkle the non fat cheddar on the bun. Or, if melted cheese is desired, use a lower fat cheese like Parmesan.

Method

- Grate the zucchini into a colander.
- Rinse well and let drain. Once water has drained, put the zucchini on several sheets of paper towel and squeeze the remaining water from them. Lay the zucchini on a piece of parchment paper and let it dry. Typically this takes about 10-15 minutes.
- Mix the grated zucchini with the Parmesan cheese, breadcrumbs, flour, onion, dill, eggs, salt and pepper. Mix very well. If the mixture seems a bit too moist, add more flour.
- In a skillet or flat griddle pan, heat a tablespoon of Olive oil or enough to cover the bottom of the pan.
- Shape the zucchini patties into round slider size patties and place on hot oil.
- Do not cover the pan as it will create too much moisture.
- Fry the zucchini until crispy brown and flip over continuing frying until brown.
- Remove the patties to a warm platter.
- Serve on slider buns of choice.

Portobello Mushroom Sliders

Ingredients - Makes 4 Sliders

- 4 portobello mushroom caps, washed and dried
- 1/4 cup Worcestershire sauce
- 1 clove garlic, minced
- 1/4 cup low sodium soy sauce
- Pepper to taste
-
- Suggested Toppings
- Grilled slice of green pepper
- Grilled slice of Onion
- Sliced Tomato
- Slider bun of choice

Method

- Place the Worcestershire sauce, garlic and soy sauce in skillet and heat.
- Add mushrooms and cook for 2 minutes on each side.
- Remove mushrooms from sauce to slider bun
- Top with the sides
- Drizzle some of the sauce over top and season with pepper.

The really nice appeal of this vegetable burger with no cheese, is the fact that the only saturated fat is the oil used to cook the vegetables.

Eggplant Burgers

Ingredients - Makes 4 Sandwiches

- 1 eggplant, peeled and slices into 3/4 inch rounds
- 1 - 2 tablespoon Olive Oil
- Slider buns of choice

Topping
- Grilled green peppers
- Grilled onions
- Sliced Tomato
- Mayonnaise mustard spread

Suggested Toppings
- Grilled slice of green pepper
- Grilled slice of Onion
- Sliced Tomato
- Slider bun of choice

Method

- Wash, peel and slice the eggplant. You can leave the peeling on to help hold the shape during cooking and remove, if desired, when building the slider.
- Place the eggplant on paper towel and sprinkle with salt which helps leach out the moisture. Let the eggplant set for 15 minutes or more. You can pat them gently with the paper towel to gather moisture.
- Place the olive oil in a flat skillet (I prefer using a flat cast iron skillet as it heats evenly and holds the heat).
- Once the oil is heated, add the eggplant slices to the skillet. Cook until brown on each side.
- Remove the eggplant to the slider bun.

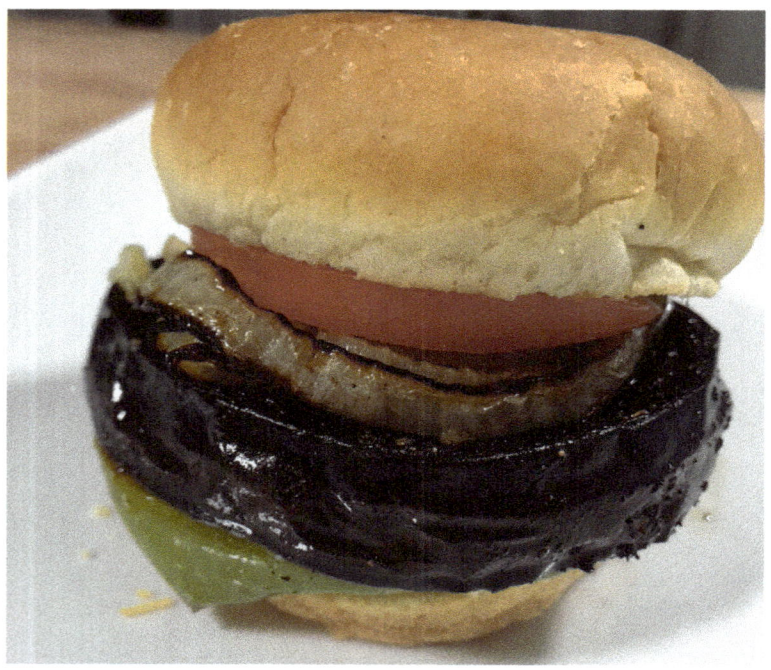

Salmon Burger

Ingredients

- 1 Can Salmon
- 1 Egg, slightly beaten
- 1 Small Onion diced
- 1/4 cup bread crumbs
- 1/2 teaspoon Hungarian Paprika
- Dash of Salt and Pepper
- Slider Buns
- Favorite Toppings

Method

- Drain juice from can Salmon and put in bowl
- Add Egg, Bread Crumbs, Paprika, salt and pepper
- Mix well. If batter seems too soupy, add a few more bread crumbs
- Cover and refrigerate for 15-20 minutes
- Shape the salmon into slider size patties (should make 4)
- Heat a shallow skillet with 1 tablespoon olive oil on medium heat.
- Place the patties in the pan and brown on one side, then turn and brown on the other side.
- While patties are browning, prepare the slider buns and sides and toppings
- Place one patty on each bun and serve.

Suggested toppings for Salmon Burgers

Cajun spicy ketchup
Sriracha mayonnaise
Dill olive oil spread
Old fashioned mustard (with seeds)
Cocktail sauce

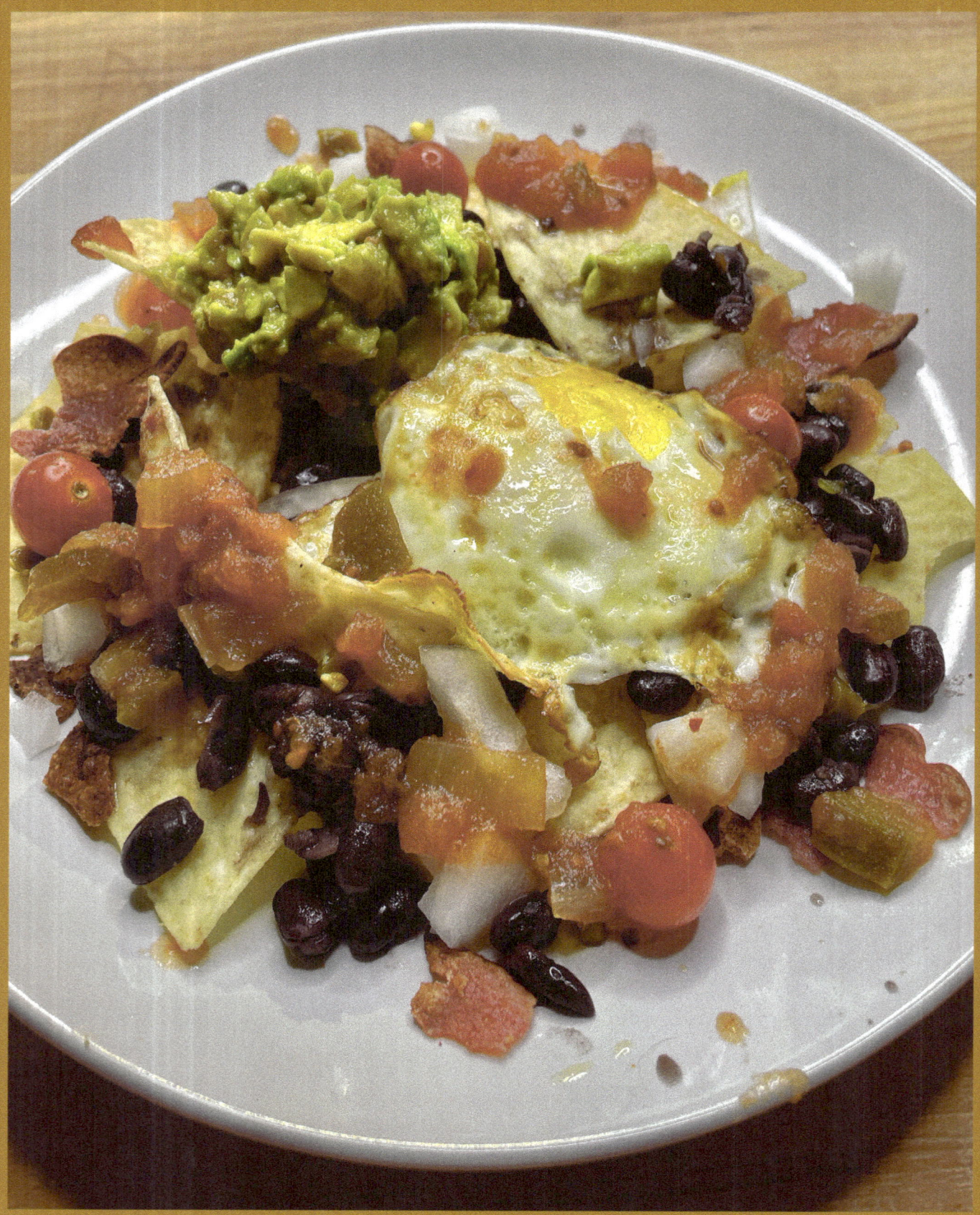

Breakfast

Mammy's Farm Breakfast..................186

Avocado Toast 188

Breakfast Nachos..................................189

Potato Pancake Breakfast Pizza 190

Egg Perfection......................................191

Egg Frittata..192

BLT with Avocado................................193

Mammy's Farm Breakfast

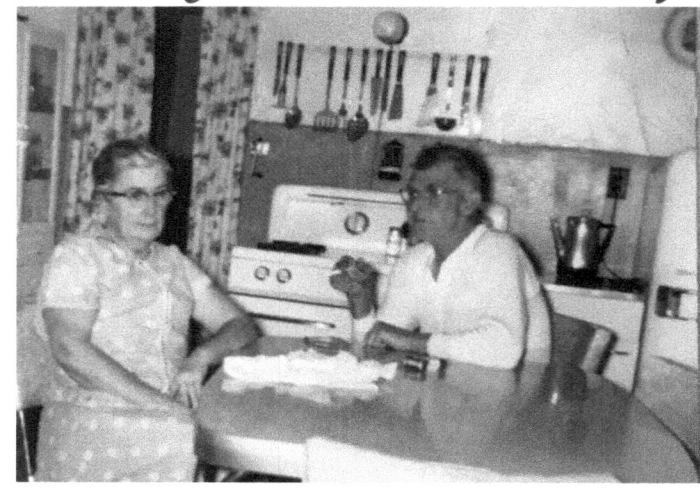

My mammy made a great breakfast and cooked breakfast every morning at 5:00 a.m. for my papaw before he went off to work in the limestone factory. Being a morning person even at a young age, I got to experience the early morning ritual of breakfast with my papaw and mammy before the other kids got up. And I got to drink coffee like a grown up.

For my papaw, there was always plenty of hot coffee and Milnot, the creamer he used. Coffee was made in the electric percolator that sat next to the gas stove. The coffee was served in white cups placed inside a white shallow saucer. My papaw would pour the coffee in the saucer which allowed it to cool quicker and sipped his coffee from the saucer. I learned to drink coffee at 5:15 a.m. just like my papaw.

The menu in the morning was always the same breakfast for my papaw every day, until the day mammy passed away. She would take a can of biscuits from the refrigerator and fill her biscuit tin for baking in the oven. The tin always had some lard in it or she would add some more, melt it and then put the biscuits in the pan. She would heat up the cast iron pot that already had lard in it from the days before, and lay in 4-6 pieces of bacon. Eggs were next and fried in the very hot lard, taking only a minute or two for them to become "not runny". We had eggs two ways, runny and not runny. It was quite some time before I learned the proper terminology was over easy and sunny side up. Anyway, when the eggs were done, she would put a couple tablespoons of flour in the lard, mix it up to create a paste and then pour in the milk. The bacon bits left from cooking the bacon and some of the crispy edges of the eggs that remained in the pan became part of the creamy milk gravy. Biscuits done, gravy in a bowl, eggs and bacon on their plates and sometimes I would join in for a bit of gravy and a biscuit. However, I was waiting for later when the really special breakfast would be cooked.

Coffee was refilled often. There was water and coffee, no juice or milk. These were country farm people, and it was how they ate breakfast every day for most of their lives.

After papaw went off to work, my mammy would start breakfast again with a fresh pan of biscuits. However, only left over bacon and gravy was available, and she didn't add to it. Basically, it was who could grab the left overs first, got them to eat. She made our favorite - - molasses. Hot and runny molasses would cook on the stove and the sweet smell filled the house. We were not allowed to make our own plate of the biscuits and molasses. Mammy had a special touch in the preparation and it made the breakfast taste better. She would tear apart the biscuits on our plate. I ate one, maybe two, but my older cousins could eat 4 or more. Three slices of real butter, would be smeared on the biscuits whether two or 4 on the plate. Then from the stove, mammy would pick up the pot of hot molasses and pour the sweet syrup over the biscuits. We had to keep our hands off the table as she was always fearful we would get burnt if she dripped the hot syrup. She would stir the biscuits, butter and molasses quickly and put in front of one of us to eat, and repeated this process for each of us. Oh, it was a mouthful of sweet heaven! No one else made this breakfast. I tried when I was in college, but it didn't taste the same, and I never made it again. I just couldn't spoil the memory of her molasses with something inferior. Mammy's gift to us all was the memory of her breakfast, and I can still see her tearing those biscuits and pouring on the syrup for us to eat.

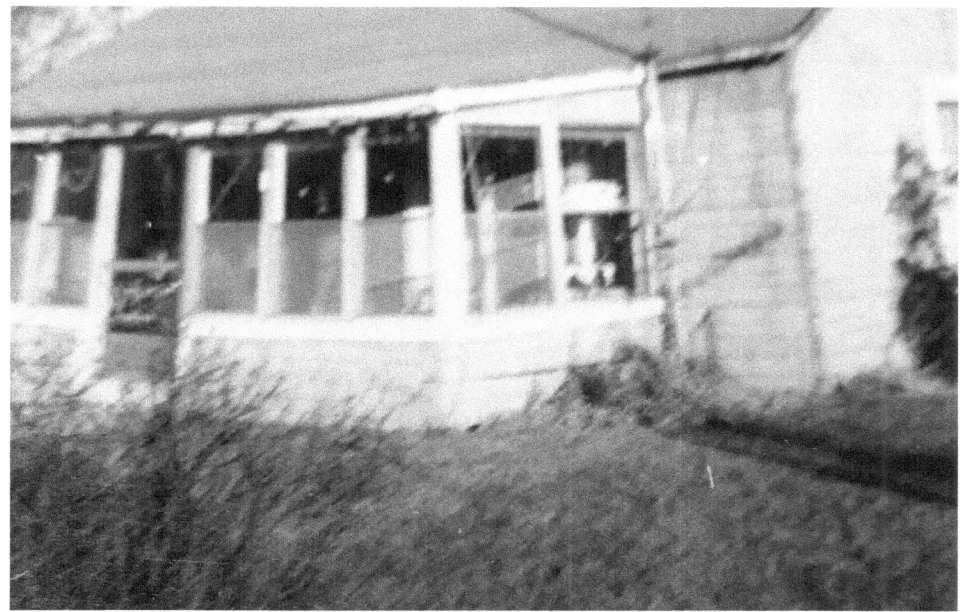

This house was built when my Mammy & Papaw were married in 1928. It was updated periodically, but is the one my mom grew up in, and the one kitchen where I started my cooking instruction.

Avocado Toast

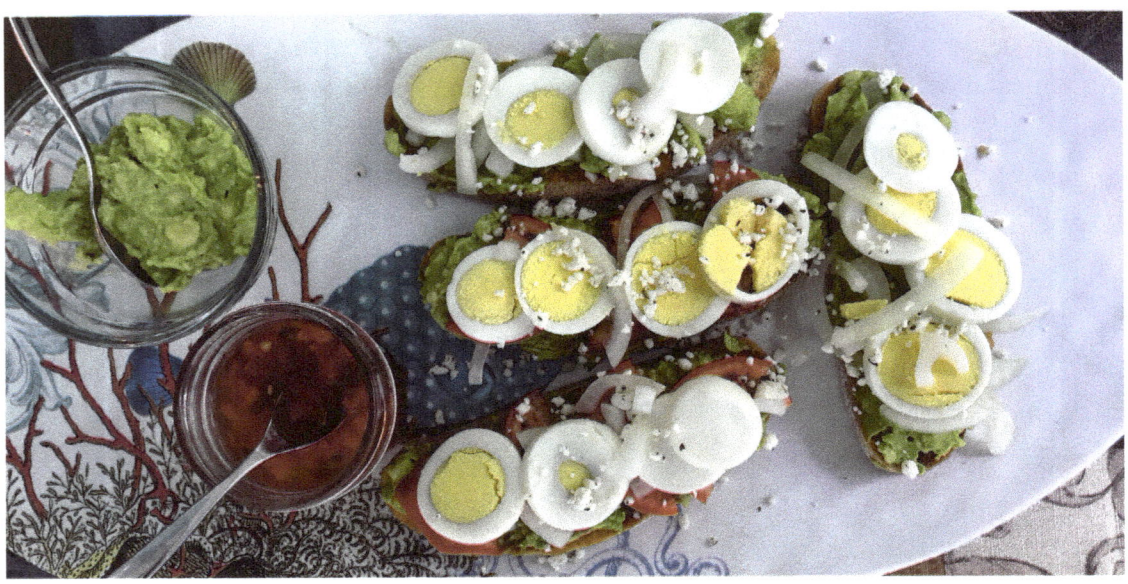

Ingredients (Serves 4)

- Guacamole (see quick recipe below)
- Chopped tomatoes
- Sliced thin white or purple onions
- Non fat cheddar cheese
- 1 sliced tomato
- 2-4 hard boiled eggs (1 per person)
- 4 - 6 strips of turkey bacon cooked in Air/Fryer or Skillet
- 1 Italian long loaf, cut into 4ths and then in half
- Mustard or Hot pepper Jelly for drizzle

Method

- Hard boil the eggs for 5-7 minutes in a boiling pot of water (with lid)
- As the eggs boil, make the Guacamole
- Put cooked eggs in ice bath and peel shells.
- Slice the eggs thin (an egg slicer works quite well)
- When bacon has cooked, chop it into small pieces for sprinkling on sandwiches

Assembly

- Spread the Guacamole on one half of the Italian bread.
- Add the sliced egg, tomato, bacon and onion.
- Sprinkle cheese on top
- Serve with drizzle sauces

Simple Guacamole recipe

- 2 ripe avocados, skin removed and meat put in bowl
- Add dash of garlic powder and black pepper
- Add 1/4 cup red salsa
- Smash and stir until smooth, but still chunky

Breakfast Nachos

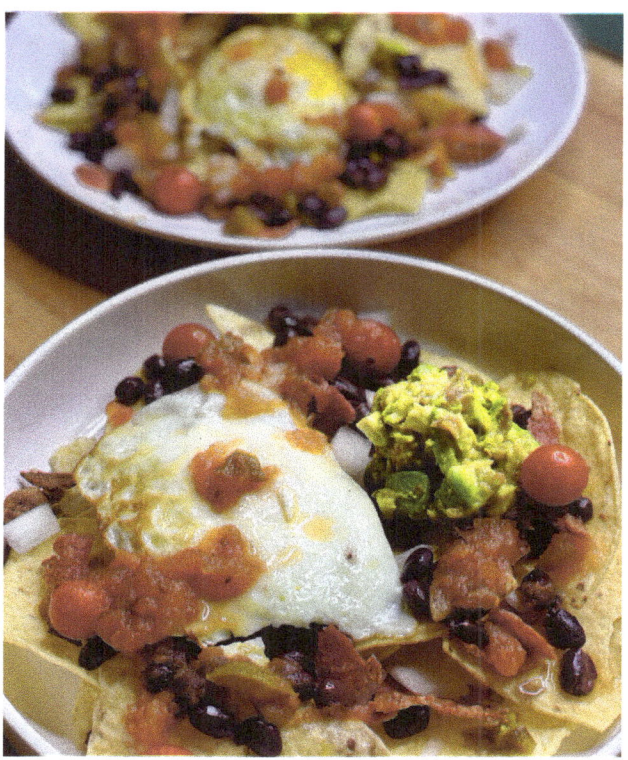

Ingredients (serves 2)

- 2-3 Extra Large Eggs
- Nacho chips - lower sodium and less fat
- Salsa of choice
- Black Beans from a can - or Non Fat Refried Beans
- 1 chopped white onion
- Pickled Jalapeños
- Non Fat Cheddar Cheese
- 1 - 2 chopped Tomatoes on the vine
- Hot sauces of choice
- Olive Oil for frying eggs
- Simple Guacamole

Method

- Heat the beans on the stove or in a microwavable dish.
- Put a handful of nacho chips on the plate
- Add the warm beans on top of the chips
- Add the onion, jalapenos, cheese and salsa.
- Cook 2-3 over easy eggs in a skillet (these will cook quickly so be sure to have all the other ingredients ready)
- Gently place the eggs on top of the prepared chips.
- Add salsa and hot sauce.
- Serve with a scoop of Guacamole

Potato Pancake Breakfast Pizza

Growing up, we always saved our left over mashed potatoes. Wasting food was never an option so we got creative with the left overs. One of my favorites was always potato pancakes. They were fried up crispy and served with a bowl of applesauce. Sometimes, they became a side dish, especially with pork chops. Over the years I added onions and hot peppers to spice them up a bit and serve them not only for breakfast but also at dinner. They are good cooked crispy with an egg on top or alone as a side dish with sandwiches. In this recipe, I used them as the crust for a breakfast pizza.

Ingredients - Serves 4

- 1 cup of left over mashed potatoes
- 1 large egg
- 1/2 cup white flour
- 1/4 cup finely diced jalapeños, optional
- 1 onion sliced thin and pieces separated
- 1/2 red and green pepper, sliced in thin lengths
- 1 medium red tomato, sliced thin
- 6 mushrooms, sliced thin
- 1/2 cup Parmesan cheese

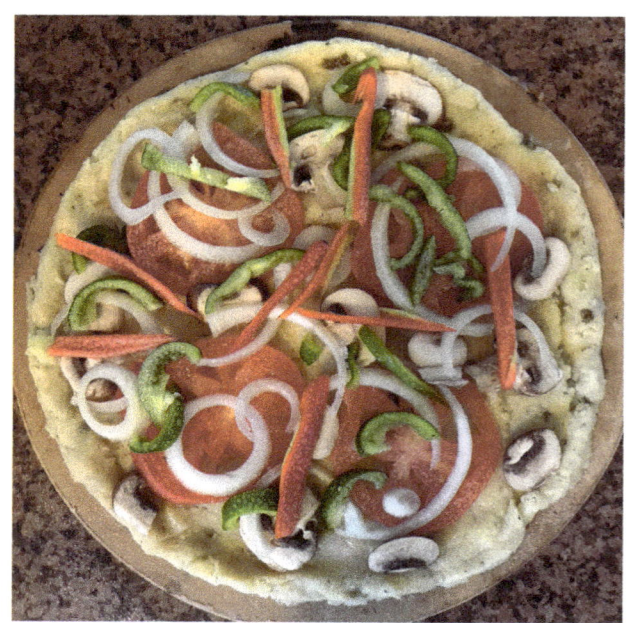

Method

- Preheat oven to 375 degrees.
- Mix potatoes, flour, egg, and jalapeños together to make a batter. If batter is too soft, add a bit more flour to make it manageable.
- Take a flat cast iron or a pizza stone or a fluted tart pan and spray oil on the bottom.
- Press the mashed potato mixture on the bottom to form the crust of the pizza
- Add the onion, peppers and tomato sliced thin.
- Sprinkle with the Parmesan cheese.
- Place in preheated oven and bake until it brown all over (20 minutes).
- When pizza is done serve
- Top with your favorite toppings (chutneys, pepper jams, salsa)

Egg Perfection

Eggs were always available in our house with the price in the 1950's through 1960's ranging from $.50 - $.67 for a dozen. Lucky for us, we had a few farms outside the city where we could get nice brown eggs that sometimes had double yolks. At my mammy's and papaw's house, there were chicken coops down the hill from the house. My job was to gather the eggs daily. Not my favorite job, I think gathering coal in the coal bucket would have been more fun, but as a girl, eggs it was. The chickens hated me for taking the eggs, but I did as was needed.

My first egg dish was scrambled eggs. My mom oversaw the procedure, telling me that perfectly cooked scrambled eggs meant that I would be a good cook one day. It was important for the eggs to be well mixed and cooked with bite size pieces and no scorch marks on them. The only seasoning added to scrambled eggs was a bit of salt and black pepper. No one in those days would dream of putting milk in eggs, but it became popular later. We used fresh eggs, nothing processed through a factory and those eggs would mix up airy and cook fluffy. Nothing else except lots of butter to cook them in was needed.

My second egg lesson was over easy eggs. I debated with dad on this subject to try and understand why eggs were called 'over easy' when they were never turned over! Dad's method was to drop the eggs in a skillet with abut 1/2 inch of hot oil. Taking a spoon or small spatula, he would continuously splash the hot oil over the tops of the egg yolks. As a result, the eggs had a slight coloring of white on top. They were immediately removed from the pan and put on our plate.

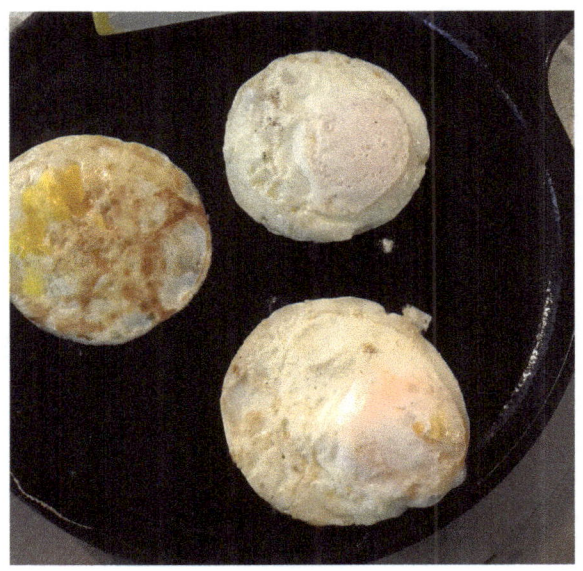

Egg Frittata

Ingredients (Serves 4)

- 4-6 eggs whisked thoroughly
- Chopped red pepper and green pepper
- 6 pieces of turkey bacon, cooked and cut into pieces
- 1 small onion chopped into bite size pieces
- 1/4 cup Parmesan cheese
- Salt and Pepper to taste
- Olive Oil for cooking
- 4-6 Grilled flour tortillas

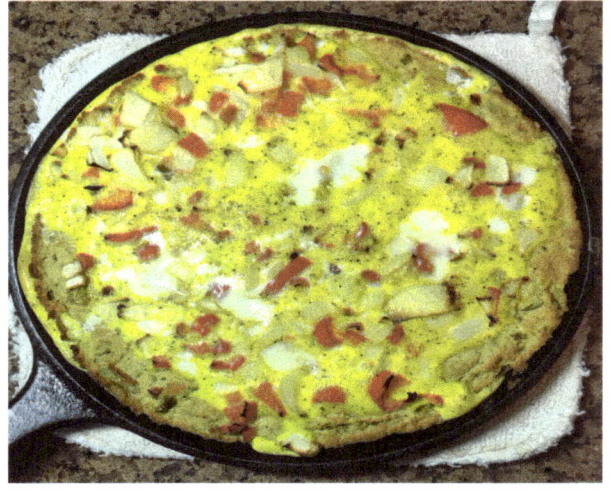

Method

- Preheat oven to 350 degrees
- Using a flat cast iron pan, add oil and heat
- Add turkey bacon and cook until crisp, remove and chop
- To the same pan add the peppers and onions and cook for 2 minutes, stirring as they cook
- Turn off heat and add bacon back to pan
- Whisk eggs with the Parmesan cheese
- Pour egg/cheese mixture over the vegetable mixture
- Place in preheated oven for 15-20 minutes, or until the edges become crispy
- Remove from oven and serve with your favorite toppings and sides

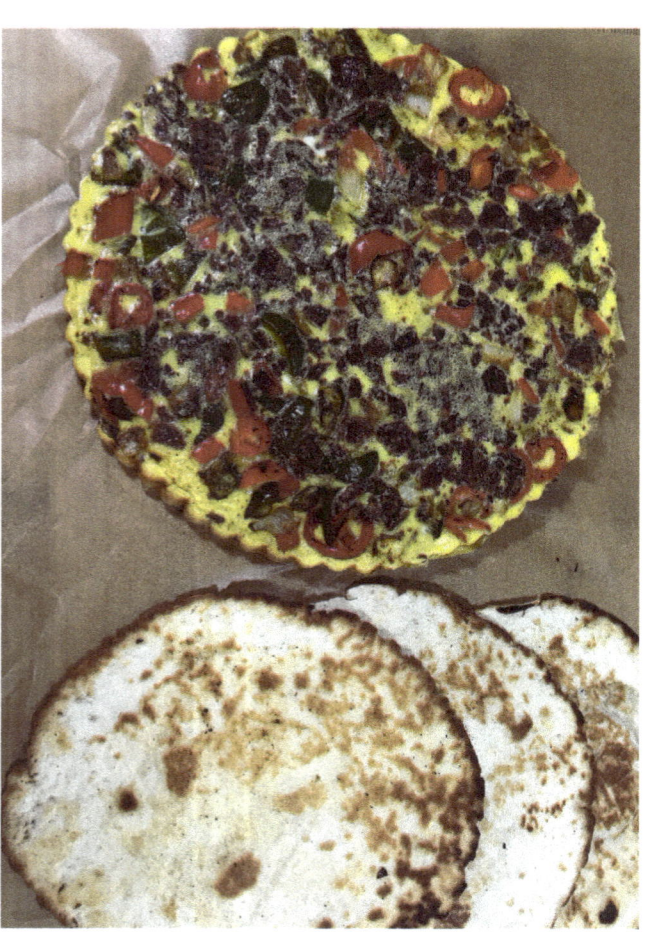

After cooking turkey bacon, peppers and onions, place mixture in a decorative tart pan then add the eggs and cheese prior to baking.

BLT with Avocado

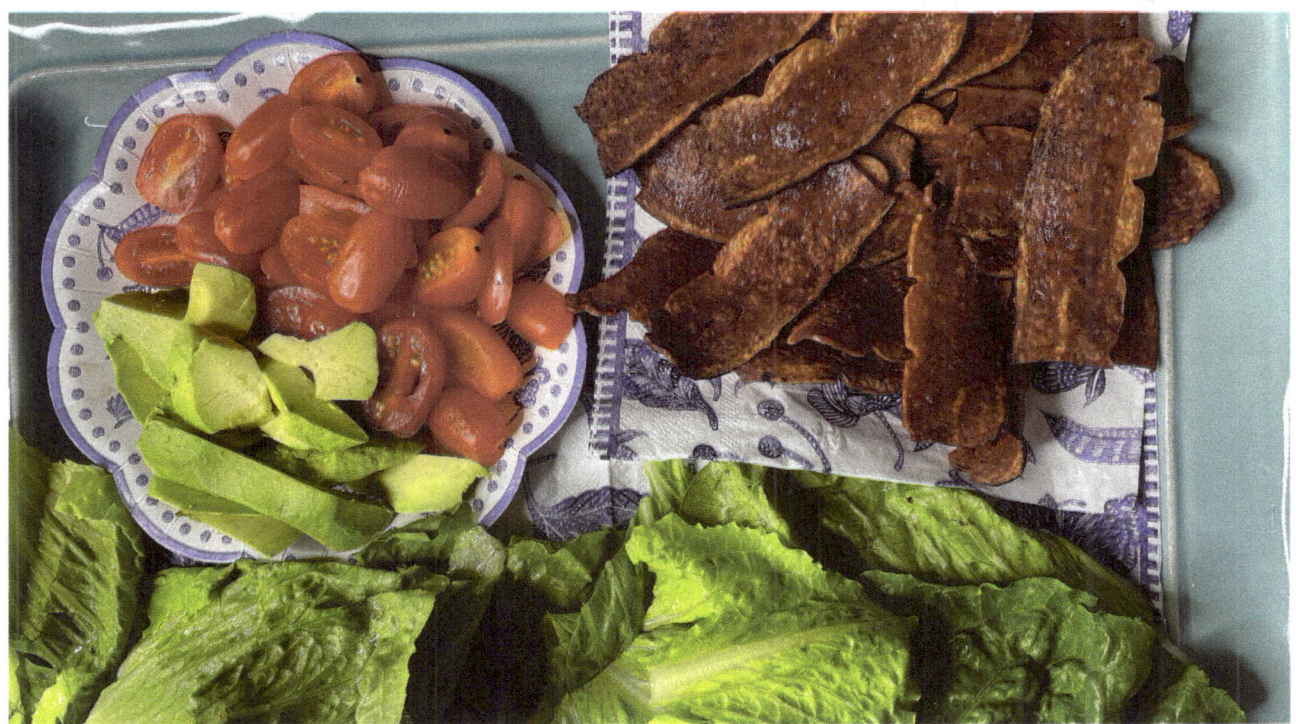

Ingredients (4 sandwiches)

- 8 slices of Turkey bacon cut in half
- Romain Lettuce
- Several cherry tomatoes, sliced in thirds
- 1 avocado peeled and sliced
- Olive Oil Mayonnaise
- Bread of Choice

Method

- Preheat air fryer to manufacturer's recommendation
- Place the 12 half slices of bacon in air fryer
- Set temperature to 380 and fry approximately 15 minutes. During cooking time, be sure to open and check bacon and turn pieces so they all brown evenly.

Serving

- Place all ingredients on a tray and let everyone build their own sandwich.

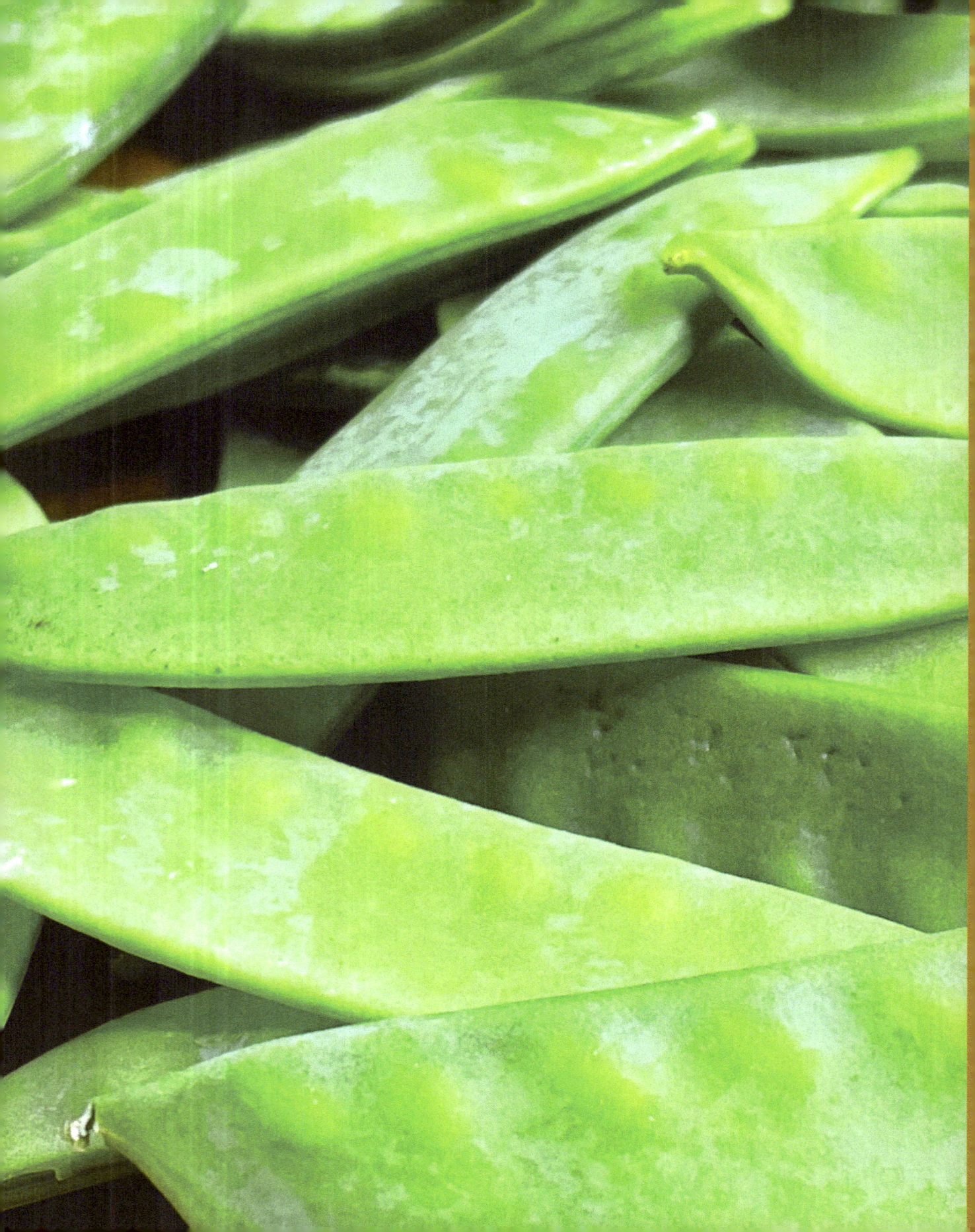

Beans

Mammy's Green Beans 196

Fresh Green Beans 197

Baked Beans 198

Pinto Beans 199

Mammy's Green Beans

Green Beans were grown in my papaw's fields. Huge metal tubs filled with picked beans were brought to the porch where my mammy and I would spend the day snapping beans to prepare for fresh cooking or canning. It was always a treat to spend those days on the porch swing and have conversations with my mammy. She liked me singing songs for her, and we would talk about everything.

Green beans whether cooked by my mom or my grandmothers, even aunts and great aunts were always cooked the same way, same recipe if you can call it a recipe. A large, seasoned pressure cooker was required. These pressure cookers had a heavy lid with seal, one steam release on top and a metal "rocker" that was placed on it to hold the steam in the pot. There were no temperature gauges or pressure gauges back then, just knowledge knowing how much the valve needed to be rocking based on the cooking temperature. Many pressure cookers "blew up" as we called it, when pressure built up too high for the topper to handle. It would fly off and food would come gushing out of the vent hole. Sad as it was for the cook who had to start over, it was rather funny to see.

Beans were always fresh that went into the pressure cooker. They would be washed and broken into bite size pieces. Bacon was the first ingredient - a whole sliced slab of pork bacon, at least one pounds worth. It would be sautéed until brown and all the fat settled into the bottom of the pan. Then the rinsed beans were poured into the pot. The searing and popping of the moisture from the beans was like firecrackers going off on July 4. The pot of beans and bacon would be stirred well, lots of salt added, along with water to cover the beans, and then the top on the pot would be placed. Once some steam started coming out the pressure hole on top, the valve would go on it, heat adjusted so the topper had an even rocking motion, and cooked for at least 20 minutes. Nothing smelled better than those beans cooking!

Fresh Green Beans

Ingredients (Serves 6 or more)

- 1-2 pounds fresh green beans, ends trimmed, snapped in half and washed
- 5-6 slices turkey bacon
- Salt and Pepper
- Olive Oil

Method

- Heat a heavy Dutch oven with 1-2 tablespoons of olive oil.
- With the heat turned to medium high, add the slices of turkey bacon.
- Brown the bacon until crisp.
- Take the freshly washed green beans and put in pot on top the bacon
- Stir very well in the hot bacon and oil for a few minutes to get the beans well coated.
- Add enough water to the pan to cover the green beans.
- Place the lid on the Dutch oven and turn heat to low.
- Cook for 1-2 hours until beans are tender.

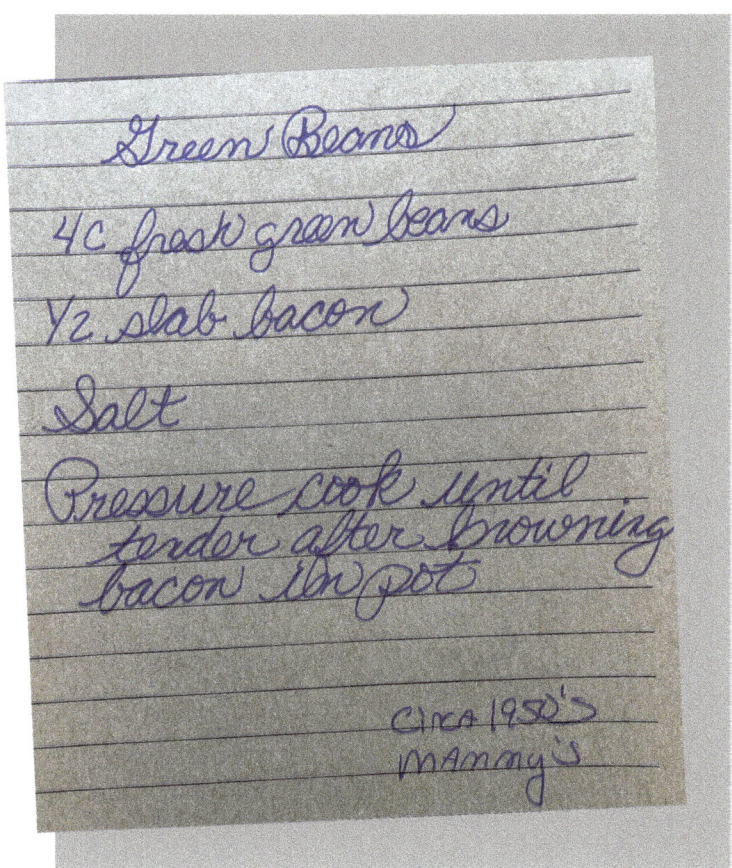

Oh Momma! Where's the Fat?

Baked Beans & Pinto Beans

BAKED BEANS were not just any baked beans, but my Aunt Alberta's baked beans which I still make today and have passed the recipe on to my son and grandchildren.

It was my 12th birthday when our family drove to the upstate to visit my Aunt Alberta, uncle and cousins at their cabin on the lake. It was my birthday and my aunt was making me a cake (3 layers with coconut). While she cooked and I watched her, she shared with me her secret ingredient and method for baked beans. She had me mix the beans that day and walked me through the whole process. It wasn't anything difficult, but her beans were always the best I ate. I still add the ingredients as if Aunt Alberta is standing in front of me directing.

She used canned pork and beans, and in those days there was really a slice of pork fat in the beans. Typically a 16 oz can or more; loaded it up with brown sugar up to 1/2 pound; bottle of ketchup and a lot of chopped white onion. That alone was delicious, but her secret ingredient was yellow mustard. The taste of the mustard in the beans brought all the flavors together. The beans would go into a baking dish and topped with 3-4 slices of raw bacon laid across the top. The beans baked for up to an hour or more until very bubbly, thickened and the bacon edges crisped. They were heaven on a spoon.

From age 12 and onward, I have always made my Aunt Alberta's baked beans. Now, of course, being conscious of lower saturated fat, I use turkey bacon, but they still taste marvelous! My baked beans are always a request when being invited to a family or friends dinner, and I am sure if my Aunt Alberta were around, she would be proud that her recipe has become a family favorite.

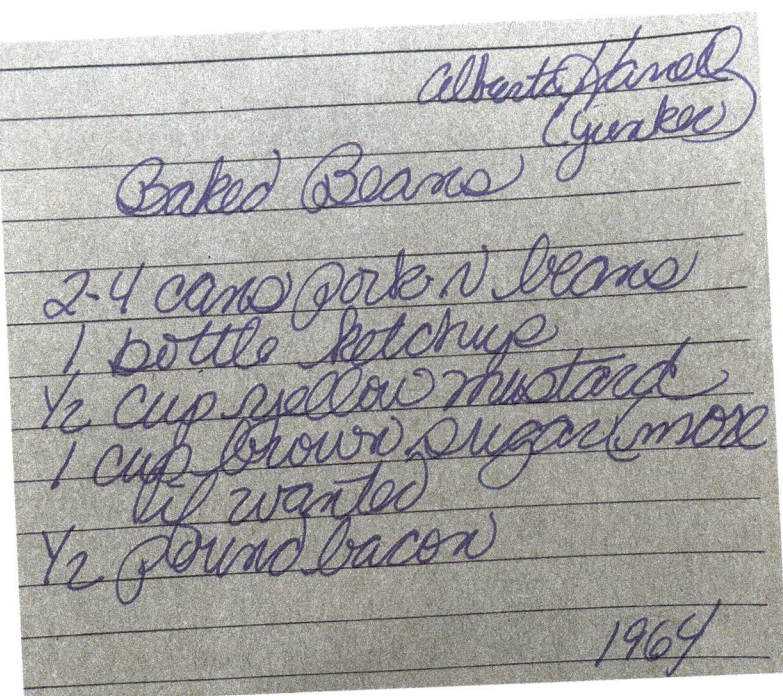

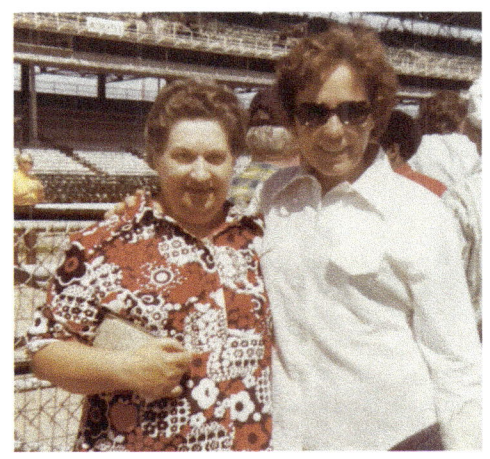

Aunt Alberta & Mom

  PINTO BEANS *were made by my Mammy. Starting with 2 pounds of dried beans and soaking overnight then simmering them for the day, my Mammy would cook them until they were tender, thick gravy from broth and a few tidbits of ham. When I would visit with Mammy and Papaw on school breaks and summers, our lunch would be a piece of white bread on the plate and a ladle of pinto beans poured on top. I didn't think much about the great protein in this dish, just enjoyed the delicious beans. It was filling and all we needed.*

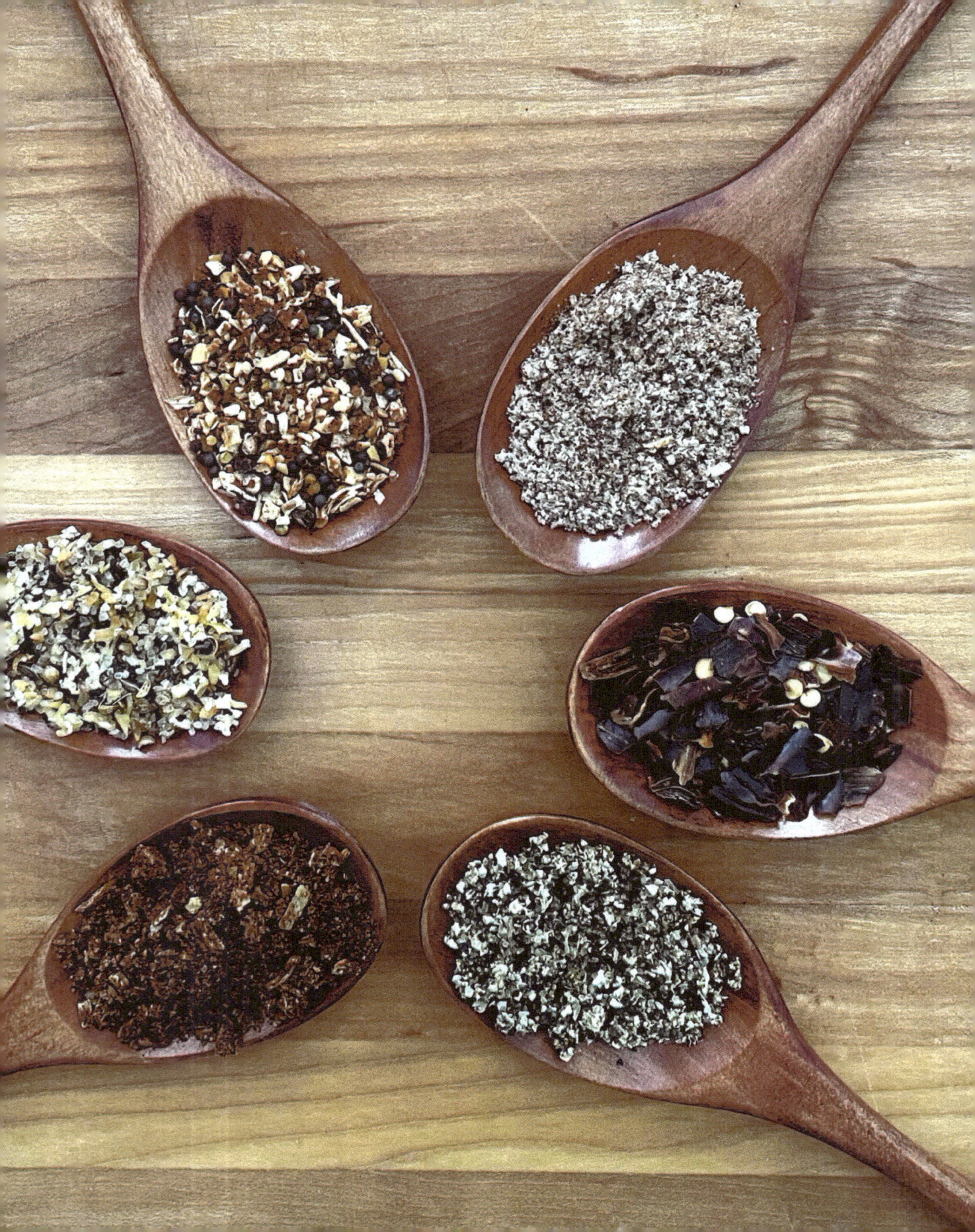

Seasoning, Marinades and Sauces

BBQ Dry Rub 202

Seasoning Salt 202

Blackened Seasoning Rub 203

Cajun Spice Mix 203

Whiskey Marinade 204

Ramen Noodle Sauce 204

Spicy Mayonnaise 205

Mustard Mayonnaise 205

Vinegar Mayonnaise 205

When cooking with less fat, adding rubs and marinades for the meat dishes brings all the flavors together for a delicious dish.

Typically when I make a seasoning blend, I do not measure anything. I add the ingredients based on what I like best. After tasting them, I may add a bit of this or that to the mix. I have, though, taken the time to measure these out , but do not be shy about adding to or taking away an ingredient you may not like.

BBQ Dry Rub

This rub is on the milder side and can stand alone on the meat, or can be enhanced with some BBQ sauce at the end of cooking.

I like using this on chicken and lean pork chops.

Add all these items together in a bowl and mix well: 1 cup red chili powder, 1 tablespoon garlic powder, 1 teaspoon onion powder 1/2 teaspoon cumin; 1 teaspoon salt and 2 tablespoons seasoning salt.

Once mixed well, put in a reused spice jar with new label, or in an air tight container. It will keep fresh up to 6 months. However, mine never lasts that long.

Seasoning Salt

Mix all these ingredients together:

1/4 cup kosher salt, 4 teaspoons ground black pepper, 1 teaspoon regular paprika; 1 teaspoon garlic powder, 1/2 teaspoon onion powder. If you want to make it a bit spicy, add 1/2 to 1 teaspoon ground red pepper or a full teaspoon of Himalayan Paprika. Mix well and put in an air tight container. This seasoning salt is the one used for BBQ Dry Rub.

Blackened Seasoning Rub

This one is great on chicken and fish but I have been known to add a little to a curry

Mix all these ingredients together:

2 tablespoons smoked paprika. 1 tablespoon onion powder, 1 tablespoon garlic powder, 1 teaspoon ground black pepper, 1 teaspoon sea salt, 1/2 teaspoon dried basil, 1/2 teaspoon dried oregano and 1/2 teaspoon dried thyme.

When I use ground black pepper, I measure it out from fresh ground of the pepper mill. I buy the ones from the market spice rack and they come filled and are disposable after use. To measure it out easily, turn the mill upside down making sure the lid is secure, and turn the shaker so the pepper grinds and fills the lid. Then measure out the 1/2 teaspoon from the lid. If any is not used, store it in a small container until you need some more.

Cajun Spice Mix

I love putting this mix on a flattened piece of chicken breast and grilling it, then placing it between a hoagie roll and eating. Makes a great Cajun sandwich.

Mix these ingredients together:

2 teaspoons salt, 2 teaspoons garlic powder, 2 1/2 teaspoons paprika (I like using Himalayan paprika for a bit more heat), 1 teaspoon ground black pepper, 1 teaspoon onion powder, 1 teaspoon cayenne pepper, 1 1/4 teaspoon dried oregano, 1 1/4 teaspoons dried thyme and 1/2 teaspoon red pepper flakes (if you like spicy)

Whiskey Marinade

Blend the following ingredients:

1/2 whiskey, 1/4 cup soy sauce, 3 tablespoons Worcestershire sauce, 2 tablespoons honey, 1/2 juice from fresh lemon, 1/4 cup brown sugar, 1 teaspoon Tabasco sauce for spice

Whiskey Marinade (Using Spiced Whiskey)

Blend the following ingredients:

1/4 cup whiskey, 1/4 cup soy sauce, 1/4 cup Dijon mustard, 1/4 cup finely chopped green onion or shallot, 1/4 cup brown sugar, 1 teaspoon Worcestershire sauce and ground black pepper to taste.

Ramen Noodle Sauce

Remember those packets of Ramen noodles, well I still eat them at lunch time, but I make my own sauce for them. Sometimes I will chop up raw carrots, onions and celery and put on top of the noodles, then add the sauce.

Blend all these ingredients to your personal taste: soy sauce, black vinegar, oyster sauce, garlic, ginger, sesame oil and 1 teaspoon Thai red chili flakes or 1/4 teaspoon Thai red chili paste.
Heat the sauce and pour over the cooked noodles and raw vegetables (if added).

Cook's note. This recipe is based on the flavors I like best. When making a sauce like this, start with a tablespoon and teaspoon of the ingredients. Keep track of what you put in it so you know how much you need to add to bring out the flavor you like best. I like garlic and oyster sauce, so I use more.

Various Mayonnaise Spreads

Just like my husband loves his cheeses and was sad to see most of them fall to the way side, I love Mayonnaise. I like it on ALL sandwiches and I even like to dip my French fries in it.

I first tried the low fat Mayonnaise. It was okay, but the longer I ate it, the more I did not like the consistency and way it felt in my mouth. It was about texture and the lingering flavors. So I switched to Olive Oil Mayonnaise. It is better for me and with some creative blending of other ingredients, I now use it for everything.

Spicy Mayonnaise Spread

I use this one on burgers and egg sandwiches

Mix two tablespoons olive oil mayonnaise with several drops of Sriracha sauce.

Mustard Mayonnaise Spread

I use this one in egg salad and tuna salad

Mix two tablespoons olive oil mayonnaise with Dijon mustard or yellow mustard.

Mayonnaise with Vinegar

I use this to dress a salad

Mix two tablespoons olive oil mayonnaise, one tablespoon apple cider vinegar, 1 teaspoon sugar and a dash of celery seed.

Garlic Mayonnaise Spread

I use this on burgers, ham and turkey sandwiches

Mix two tablespoons olive oil mayonnaise, one minced garlic clove and dash of pepper.

Common Ingredients

Reading Labels

Converting a Recipe

Category	Specific Item	Serving Size	Saturated Fat Per Serving**. This is an estimate	Notes
Ground Turkey	Lean all white	4 oz	2.2 g	This is approximated for 93% lean ground turkey. If making patties for cooking burgers, add the amount of oil used to cook. These cook up well in the air fryer or on the grill.
Turkey Breast	Roasted	3.5 oz	2.1 g	
Turkey Sausage	Breakfast Links	3 links	2.5 g	
Turkey Sausage	Breakfast Patties	2 patties	2.5 g	
Turkey Bacon	Raw for cooking	1 slice	1 g	This bacon is great cooked in the air fryer or used in recipes
Turkey Italian Sausage	Ground/Links	1 link	2 g	I like the ground version incorporated in Italian dishes.
Chicken Breast	Skinless, boneless	3 oz	1 g	
Ground Chicken	White Lean	3 oz	2.6 g	
Chicken Thighs	Skinless, boneless	1 thigh	3 g	
Chicken Italian Sausage	Links	1 link	.5 g	I like this version in slices and browned in casseroles and Italian dishes.
Tuna in a Can	Slip Jack tuna, light and in oil	3 oz	0 g	
Tilapia Fillet	1 fillet	87 g	.8 g	If making a glaze, be sure to calculate the fat in the glaze.
Cod Fillet	Skinless	231 g	3 g	Size of two servings
Tuna Steak	Skin one side	1 fillet 308 g	1.2 g	Size of two servings
Salmon	Wild Alaska, Skin one side	100 g	3.1 g	If making a glaze, be sure to calculate the fat in the glaze.
Pork Roast	Pork Tenderloin Loin, Trimmed	3 oz	1 g	Roasted, fat trimmed
Pork Chop	Boneless, Lean	4 oz	2.5 g	Not cooked in oil. If cooked in 1-2 tablespoons of oil, add to the total grams of fat.
Ground Pork	Lean	3 oz	4.5 g	Not cooked in oil. If cooked in 1-2 tablespoons of oil, add to the total grams of fat.
Pork Sausage	Lean, Sage Flavor	Homemade	4.5 g	I grind pork chop, add seasoning to make it sausage flavor
Beef	Sirloin Tip Steak	100 g	1.5 g	I use these to cut slices for stir fries and stews. Beef is not eaten as often due to Trans Fats.
Beef	Top Loin Steak	3 oz	4.8 g	An alternative when Sirloin Tip Steak is not available.

Category	Specific Item	Serving Size	Saturated Fat Per Serving**. This is an estimate	Notes
Beef	Brisket, Flat Cut	3 oz	2.2 g	I like to roast a brisket and per serving it is low in saturated fat
Lamb	De-boned, fat trimmed	3 oz	8 g	I will use a small cut of lamb to make a stew. Per serving (typically 4 per stew pot) makes it reasonable
Eggs	Raw, Hardboiled, Poached	1 egg	1 g	This varies depending on size of egg. It is packed full of nutrition. Be watchful if cholesterol is an issue
Low Fat Margarine	In a Tub	1 tablespoon	1 g	I do not use low fat margarine for baking, but use it on breads and melt it for glazes and icing or drizzles for rolls.
Margarine	Stick	1 tablespoon	2.5 g	I use stick margarine for baking.
Olive Oil	Extra Virgin	1 tablespoon	2 g	I use Olive Oil most often due to it's loaded with antioxidants more than others. If Total # saturated fats for the day need to be lower, I use Canola Oil
Sesame Oil		1 tablespoon	2 g	I use this oil in stir fries and in sauces for Thai and Chinese dishes
Canola Oil		1 tablespoon	1 g	
Avocado Oil		1 tablespoon	2.5 g	I do not use this as often, but it mixes nicely with flavor for dressings
Grape seed Oil		1 tablespoon	1.5 g	I do not use this oil for stir fry or flat top high heat griddle. It creates a sticky residue on the pans.
Non Fat Mozzarella		Unlimited	0 g	I do not recommend trying to melt the non fat cheeses. They have a tendency to get rubbery. Use raw and sprinkle on food that has been cooled
Non Fat Cheddar				Use raw and sprinkle on food that has been cooled
Non Fat Cream Cheese		Unlimited	0 g	
Parmesan Cheese	Shredded	1/4 cup	4.5 g	When a recipe, like mac n cheese calls for cheese, this is a great alternative since it is strong flavor. The 4.5 grams spread across 4 servings keeps fat down. Use regular, not no fat or low fat.

Oh Momma! Where's the Fat?

Category	Specific Item	Serving Size	Saturated Fat Per Serving**. This is an estimate	Notes
Half & Half		Unlimited	0 g	I use this as a milk/cream substitute. It stands up very well in baking, soups, gravy and even homemade yogurt
Evaporated Milk	Canned	2 tablespoons	1.5 g	Use in baking, works great
Evaporated Milk	Low Fat in Can	2 tablespoons	0	Best option.
Almond Milk		8 ounces	0 g	
Non Fat Whipping Cream	Pre-made in a Can	Unlimited	0 g	
Non Fat Greek Yogurt		Unlimited	0 g	
Tofu	Any	Unlimited	0	
Mayonnaise	Olive Oil Blend	1 tablespoon	1 g	This is a good blend and lower grams of saturated fat than low fat or non fat mayonnaise. I use it for dressings, sandwich spreads and dips.
Peanut Butter	Low Fat	2 tablespoons	2.5 g	I have yet to tell the difference in this compared to full fat. I use it for baking, dressings and just plain peanut butter and jelly sandwiches.
Pasta	All varieties	Unlimited	0 g	
Panko Crumbs		Unlimited	0 g	
Salad Dressing	No Fat, Any flavor	Unlimited	0 g	
Avocado	Haas	1 avocado equalling 1 cup chopped	3.1g	While it is higher in fat than some items, its health benefits are worth working this into a days limit
Walnuts	Shelled, half or pieces	1 cup	4.9g	As a snack at 1/4 cup, these are healthy and reasonable. Use in baked goods like a cake or bread, the 4.9 g is spread out over multiple servings
Pecans		1 cup	6 g	As a snack at 1/4 cup, these are healthy and reasonable. Use in baked goods like a cake or bread, the 4.9 g is spread out over multiple servings

Category	Specific Item	Serving Size	Saturated Fat Per Serving**. This is an estimate	Notes
Almonds	Whole	1 oz (about 20)	1 g	
Cake Mix	Boxed	1/10 piece	3 g	This is an average of most cake mixes in a box. When in a hurry or if baking from scratch is not something desirable, opt for the box mix. Substitute butters with Canola oil and the fat will drop lower.
Banana Nut Bread Mix	Boxed	1/12 piece	0 g	Substitute any butter with canola oil.
Pie Crust	Pre-made in Dairy Dept.	1/8 Pie	2.5 g	This is the best I found to date. Still working on a good homemade version, but butter and lard are not available on this diet. The crust cooks nicely and is flaky for not having butter.
Phyllo Dough	Pre-made in Frozen Food	Unlimited	0 g	Use this for anything pastry - savory pies are very good. I like it for fruit pies, but it gets a bit weak.
Taco Chips		READ THE LABELS	PER SERVING	LOOK AT HOW MANY CHIPS PER SERVING.
Corn Tortilla		READ THE LABELS	PER SERVING	LOOK AT HOW MANY CHIPS PER SERVING.
Flour Tortilla		READ THE LABELS	PER SERVING	LOOK AT HOW MANY CHIPS PER SERVING.

Oh Momma! Where's the Fat?

Reading Food Labels

Remember my original story about being overwhelmed in the market, breaking down and crying as I just didn't know what to buy anymore - - - - Well, it was due to having to read every single nutrition fact label on every single item I picked up in the store. And those were just the regular shopping list items.

With only 15 grams of saturated fat per day, it is important to balance the saturated fat content. While it may be confusing or time consuming in the beginning, I can honestly say that it does get easier. I have already done this for the recipes I cook and present in my cookbooks.

It is important when eating low saturated fat foods to read labels on products that are purchased to use in cooking recipes. I can almost say for fact that most prepared frozen food will be high in saturated fat. So a decision has to be made, "is it worth it and will I have to give up a meal to enjoy this one dish?" Pizza was my downfall. However, I learned to make homemade pizza (very easy) and put on toppings, no fatty cheese, but sprinkling of Parmesan on top (one of the lower fatty cheeses). The Pizzas are flavorful and most of my guests and even kids and grandkids cannot tell it is low saturated fat.

When looking at saturated fat content, look at the total grams (not the percentage). Keep track of those per serving and when creating a recipe, jot down the number. So if the serving size is 1/4 cup with 2.5 grams of saturated fat, and it serves two people then the total saturated fat per serving is 1.75 per person. Typically, I balance the grams of fat between all three meals. However, if I want to have a top sirloin tip cut into strips for my Thai Stir Fry with noodles, I will eat less fat at lunch (maybe salad and/or fruit dishes) so I can enjoy several pieces of the sirloin tip in the stir fry.

It takes time, but surprisingly, it has become a natural process for me to pick up an item, look at the saturated fat content and decide to buy or not to buy.

Center Cut Loin Boneless Chop

Nutrition Facts
For a Serving Size of 219 grams (219g)

Calories 271.3	Calories from Fat 69.8 (25.7%)

	% Daily Value *
Total Fat 7.8g	-
Saturated fat 2.9g	-
Cholesterol 145.4mg	-
Sodium 106.6mg	5%
Carbohydrates 0g	-
Net carbs 0g	-
Fiber 0g	0%
Protein 48.5g	
Vitamins and minerals	
Vitamin A 0µg	0%
Vitamin C 0mg	0%
Calcium 0mg	0%
Iron 0mg	0%
Fatty acids	
Amino acids	

* The Percent Daily Values are based on a 2,000 calorie diet, so your values may change depending on your calorie needs.

Nutrition Facts
Chicken breast
Sources include: USDA

Amount Per 1 unit (yield from 1 lb ready-to-cook ch...

Calories 86

	% Daily Value*
Total Fat 1.9 g	2%
Saturated fat 0.5 g	2%
Polyunsaturated fat 0.4 g	
Monounsaturated fat 0.6 g	
Cholesterol 44 mg	14%
Sodium 38 mg	1%
Potassium 133 mg	3%
Total Carbohydrate 0 g	0%
Dietary fiber 0 g	0%
Sugar 0 g	
Protein 16 g	32%

Vitamin A	0%	Vitamin C	0%
Calcium	0%	Iron	2%
Vitamin D	0%	Vitamin B-6	15%
Cobalamin	3%	Magnesium	3%

Nutrition Facts
Chicken Thighs
Sources include: USDA

Amount Per 1 thigh without skin (116 g)

Calories 206

	% Daily Value*
Total Fat 10 g	15%
Saturated fat 2.6 g	13%
Polyunsaturated fat 1.9 g	
Monounsaturated fat 3.9 g	
Trans fat regulation 0 g	
Cholesterol 157 mg	52%
Sodium 101 mg	4%
Potassium 321 mg	9%
Total Carbohydrate 0 g	0%
Dietary fiber 0 g	0%
Sugar 0 g	
Protein 28 g	56%

Vitamin A	0%	Vitamin C	0%
Calcium	1%	Iron	7%
Vitamin D	2%	Vitamin B-6	25%
Cobalamin	8%	Magnesium	7%

*Percent Daily Values are based on a 2,000 calorie diet. Your daily values may be higher or lower depending on your calorie needs.

Oh Momma! Where's the Fat?

Converting a Recipe

The first step in converting the recipe is to replace the higher fat ingredients. For example if a recipe calls for 6 Tablespoons of Butter, then use 6 Tablespoons of Stick Margarine.

The difference between saturated fat in butter and margarine is:

Butter per tablespoon is 7 grams of saturated fat, plus it has .5 grams of Trans Fats (bad fats)
Stick margarine per tablespoon is 2.5 grams of saturated fat

How did I get those numbers? I read the label on the package, or I look up the value on the official USDA website.

So in this example, the amount of saturated fat for 6 tablespoons of butter is 42 grams and 6 tablespoons of stick margarine is 15 grams. This is almost one third less fat when using margarine.

Typical substitutions include:

- *Cream is replaced with half and half*
- *Yogurt is replaced with non fat yogurt*
- *Milk is replaced with half and half (I do not use low fat or skimmed as it is too watery)*
- *I use oils that are low saturated fat and contain no Trans Fats.*
- *Buttermilk is replaced with non fat half and half with 1-2 tablespoons white vinegar*
- *There is no cheese except Parmesan or non fat cheddar or non fat mozzarella. Parmesan is a strong flavor cheese, so 1/4 cup which equals 4.5 grams of saturated fat is used in a dish where it serves 2 or more, thus reducing fat per serving. Non fat cheddar is really good, but I do not melt it. It melts like rubber, and so I use it after food is cooked as a sprinkling on top.*
- *I do not deep fry anything, but instead use the air fryer or a spray Canola or Olive Oil in a pan to fry.*
- *I use parchment paper on sheet pans instead of oil so I can use oil as part of a marinade on the vegetables or meat that will be cooked on the parchment paper.*

- *I pay particular attention to the cuts and portion sizes of meats.*
- *If I use Beef it is eaten on occasion and in a dish where not a lot is needed to give great flavor.*
- *Meat servings are 4 ounces, while fish is unlimited and chicken is unlimited. However, do not go crazy with tarter sauce and high fat sauces on chicken. Grill, air fry, broil, roast or bake chicken, turkey and fish.*

Eating out can be a challenge and we did not eat out in the beginning until we had a really good understanding of fat content of menu items. A few ideas:

- *We eat pizza without the cheese on the sauce and have shaved Parmesan on top, but lightly*
- *We do not order hamburgers, but order chicken or fish*
- *We order just about any vegetable, except French fries*
- *We watch for items to be prepared with real mayonnaise as it is high in fat, so we opt for something else.*
- *And most importantly, we do not count on the restaurant to know what is a healthy menu since some restaurants think grilled chicken with cheese on top is healthy, not knowing it is full of saturated fat.*
- *We eat a lot of stir fried dishes when we go out.*
- *We eat Mexican food, just hold the cheese*
- *We avoid desserts made with chocolate but look for fruit desserts.*

It takes a little sacrifice, but we know we can enjoy a Splurge day with food we think we miss and realize after a time, we actually do not miss the fatty hamburger and prefer a turkey or chicken burger!

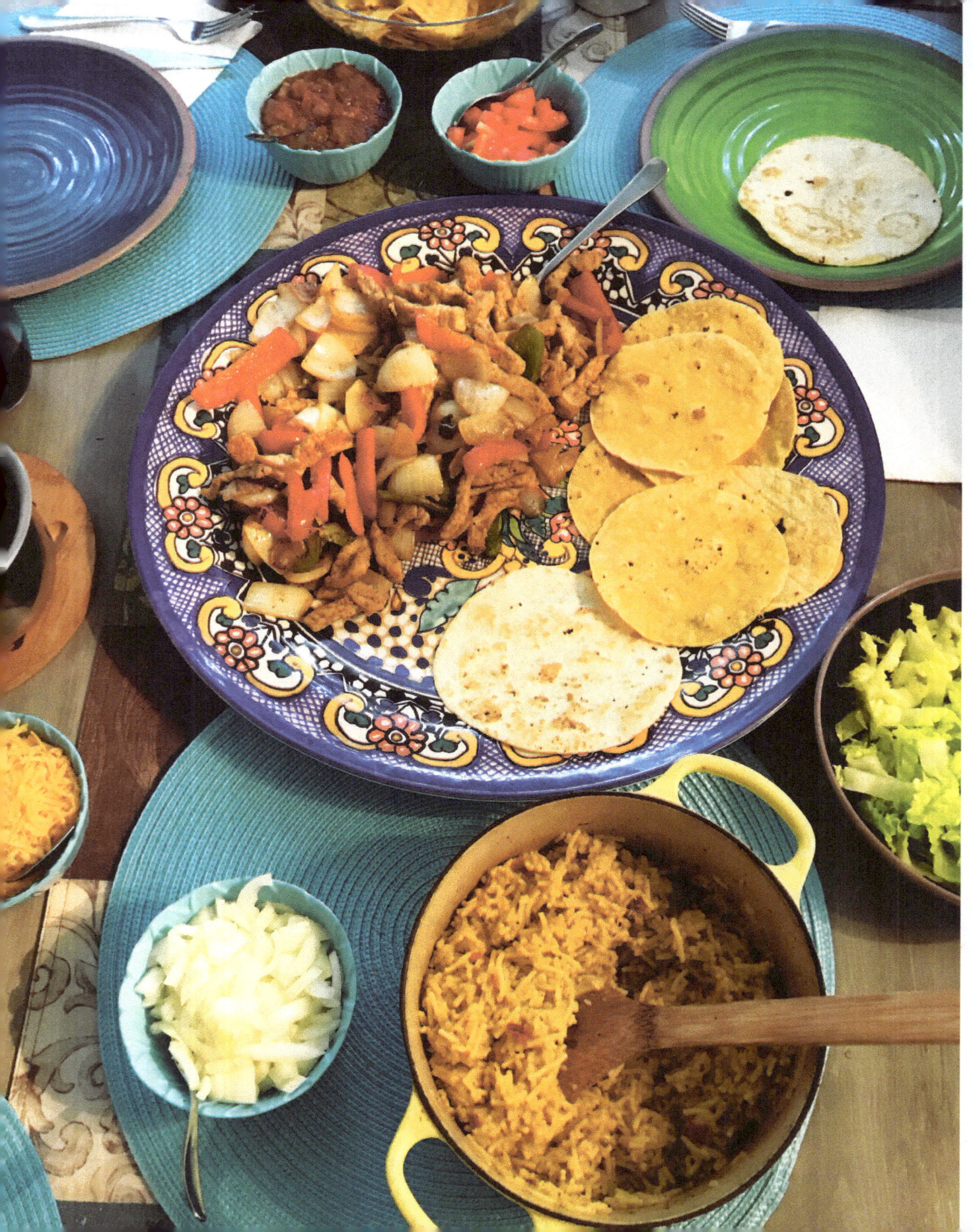

Just the Beginning

Healthy and Tasty Eating

Oh, Momma! is not a book full of diet food. It is food fun to make and fun to eat. But most importantly, it is food that is healthy by reducing the saturated fats.

This book is just an example how delicious recipes and foods can be in our healthy diet and recipes anyone can make, eat, enjoy and eliminate high saturated fats.

I am not a fan of some foods, so why would I want to go on a diet where it makes me eat those foods. That is rubbish to me, so taking my beloved recipes and making them delicious even today, was my goal. The book is a variety of every day foods made healthy. You can change your recipes, too.

I love serving low saturated fat food to family and friend, especially when they do not know. The reaction is amazing, when I reveal to them the new recipe, as most do not realize I have even altered the old recipe to create a healthier version.

When I create or alter a recipe, I evaluate for amounts of saturated fats. I then make the substitutions and cook the recipe. Most times I cook a dish more than once, sometimes more than twice in order to adjust flavors. Then when I think I have it perfect, I cook it again, make note of amounts of ingredients and photograph it afterward. From there, I write up the recipe and file it with the photographs for the next book or next ebook. Then I cook it for others to get their reaction and listen to the comments given. Sometimes, I go back and cook the recipe again, sometimes I leave it as is.

I have spent the last three years evaluating, testing flavors and substituting saturated fats in order to include a recipe in my cookbooks. Today, I have over 400 recipes that I have created from scratch or altered from family recipes.

Hope you enjoy these dishes. I have presented dishes of all ethnic varieties and cooking styles. It's all about keeping close to what you love and being heart healthy for a long time for yourself and for your family!

Social Media Sites

Web Site: www.skinniefats.com
Facebook: https://www.facebook.com/SkinnieFats-101718038101760
Instagram: SkinnieFats

Credits

Outer Cover layout design: Kate Camargo
Outer Cover photographs: Pamela Harrell

Nutritional Information

Nutritional Data: USDA - https://www.usda.gov/

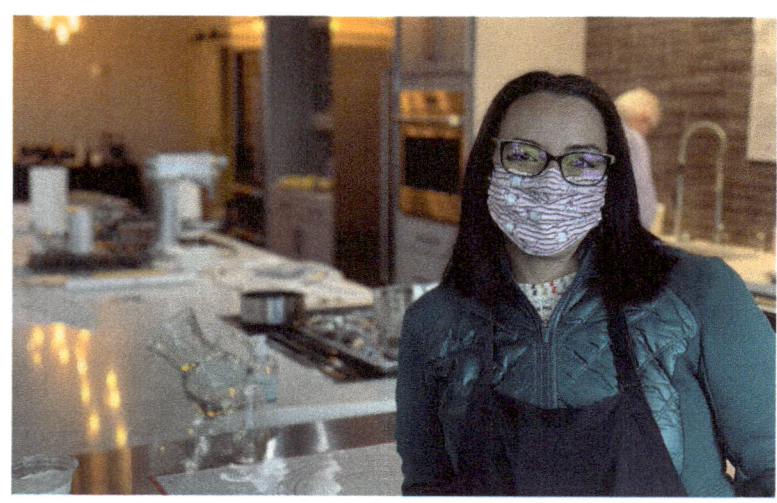

Kate Camargo

Index

Index

A

Asian
  Beef
    Thai Fry 168
  Grilled Chicken 87
  Peanut Coleslaw 24
  Potatoes
    Spicy Fried 119
  Sauce
    Ramen Noodle Sauce 204

B

Beans
  Baked Beans 198
  Carbonara with English Peas 58
  Fresh Green Beans 197
  Island Chili 43
  Mammy's Green Beans 196
  Pinto Beans 198
Beef
  Beef Burgundy 71
  Borscht 174
  Cuts of Beef to Use 166
  Italian Roast Beef 173
  Italian Roast Beef Sandwiches 173
  Old Fashioned Beef Stew 167
  Stroganoff 170
  Thai Fry 168
Beets
  Chicken Salad & Beets 18
Breakfast
  Avocado Toast 188
  BLT with Avocado 193
  Breakfast Nachos 189
  Egg Frittata 192
  Egg Perfection 191
  Potato Pancake Pizza 190
  Vegetables
    Cabbage & Carrot Omelette 125
Broccoli
  Broccoli apple salad 19
Burgers
  Eggplant Burgers 182
  Marinated Ground Turkey Burger 179
  Portobello Mushroom Slider 181
  Salmon Burger 183
  Zucchini Sliders 180

C

Cabbage
  Asian Peanut Coleslaw 24
Chicken
  Asian Griddled Chicken 87
  Black Pepper Chicken 97
  Bourbon Chicken 95
  Chicken Potato Stew 39
  Chicken Salad & Beets 18
  Chinese Chicken & Broccoli 105
  Chinese Chicken Dumplings 106
  Coq au Vin 88
  Fried 86
  Grilled Mediterranean 100
  Italian Meatballs 94
  Kung Pao Chicken 102
  Noodle
    Chicken Ramen Soup 36
  Soup
    Chicken Noodle Soup 35
  Spatchcock Grilled Chicken 104
  Spicy Chicken Meatballs 101
  Tandoori Chicken & Vegetables 90
Chili
  Island Chili 43
  Kielbasa & Turkey 38
  Mom's Chili 32
  Turkey & Beans 33
Chinese
  Chicken
    Black Pepper Chicken 97
    Chicken & Broccoli Stir Fry 105
    Dumplings 106
    Kung Pao Chicken 102

Curry
  Vegetable
    Vegetable & Chick Pea Stew 40

D

Desserts
  Cake
    Apple Pie Cake 140
    Carrot Cake 146
    Lemon Glaze for Cakes 136
    Mom's Rum Cake (funny) 134
    Pistachio Pudding Cake 142

Index

Red Velvet Cake 148
Rum Pound Cake 136
Fruit Filled Coffee Cake 150
Madeleines
  Blueberry 144
  Lemon 144
Pie
  Old Fashioned Apple Pie 152
  Pineapple Chunk Pie 147
Pudding
  Lemon Curd 139

E

Eggs
  Egg Frittata 192
  Egg Perfection 191
  Scotch Eggs 72

F

Fish
  Blackened Tilapia 158
  English Fish & Chips 161
  Fried Cod Tacos 159
  Mediterranean Tuna Salad 160
  Stuffed Tilapia 157
  Tuna
    Nicoise Salad 28

Fruit
  Apple
    Broccoli Apple Salad 19
  Apples
    Apple Pie Cake 140
  Avocado
    Avocado Toast 188
  Pineapple
    Pineapple Chunk Pie 147

I

Indian
  Chicken
    Tandoori Chicken & Vegetables 90

M

Marinade
  Ramen Noodle Sauce 204

Marinades
  Tobasco Whiskey 204
  Whiskey Marinade 204
Mayonnaise Sauces
  Garlic Mayonnaise 205
  Mustard Mayonnaise 205
  Spicy 205
  Vinegar 205–223
Mediterranean
  Chicken
    Grilled 100
Mexican
  Breakfast Nachos 189

P

Pasta
  Beef
    Beef Stroganoff 170
    Bolognese with Meat Sauce 50
    Carbonara with English Peas 58
    Cherry Tomato Spaghetti 50
    Eggplant Lasagnas 60
    Ham & Pepper Rotini 59
    Home Made Pasta 56
    Macaroni, Cheese & Tomato 62
    Mushroom Lasagna 60
    Penne with Vodka Sauce 50
    Vegetable Rigatoni 63
Pork
  Best Pork Chop Ever 67
  Bourguignon 70
  Ham
    Ham & Pepper Rotini 59
  Pork Chop
    Hoosier Sandwich 75
    Soy Seasoning Chops 74
  Pork Roast
    Island Flavored Roast 68
  Sausage
    Scotch Eggs 72
  Spicy Pork & Zoodles 80
  Tacos 78
Potato
  Stew
    Chicken Potato Stew 39

Index

S

Salad
  Asian Peanut Coleslaw 24
  Broccoli Apple 19
  Chef Salad 26
  Cole Slaw 23
  Nicoise with Tuna 28
  Pork Strip 20
  Taco 22
Seasonings
  BBQ Dry Rub 202
  Blackened Rub 203
  Cajun Spice Mix 203
  Seasoning Salt 202
Soups
  Butternut Squash 34
  Chicken Noodle 35
  Potato & Leek 42
Soups & Stews 40
Stews
  Beets
    Borscht 174

T

Tacos
  Pork 78
Tomatoes
  Cherry Tomato Spaghetti 50
Turkey
  Cocktail Meatballs 96
  Ground
    Bacon Wrapped Upside Down Meat Loaf 92
    Spaghetti Bolognese 50
    Turkey & Vegetable Soup 45
  Italian Meatballs 94
  Shepherd's Pie 97

V

Vegetables
  Broccoli
    Chicken & Broccoli Stir Fry 105
    Mediterranean Cauliflower & Broccoli 117
  Butternut Squash Soup 34
  Cabbage
    Asian Peanut Coleslaw 24
    Cabbage & Carrot Omelette 125
    Slow Cooked Carrots & Cabbage 124
  Carrots
    Honey & Thyme Roasted 120
    Slow Cooked Carrots & Cabbage 124
  Cauliflower
    Mediterranean Cauliflower & Broccoli 117
    No Crust Cauliflower Quiche 114
  Corn
    Grilled Corn & Peppers 116
    Momma's Sweet Corn 113
  Eggplant
    Eggplant Lasagna 60
  English Peas
    Carbonara with English Peas 58
  Leeks
    Potato & Leek Stew 42
  Mushrooms
    Mushroom Lasagna 60
  Pasta
    Vegetable Rigatoni 63
  Peppers
    Mediterranean Stuffed 123
  Potato
    Potato Pancake Breakfast Pizza 190
  Potatoes
    Creamy Mashed 115
    Paprika Potatoes 121
    Potato & Leek Stew 42
    Spicy Asian Fried 119
    Spicy Potatoes & Garbanzos 127
  Roasted Sheet Pan Vegetables 117
  Squash
    Stuffed Butternut Squash 128
  Sweet Potatoes
    Air Fries 110
  Tomatoes
    Mac N Cheese with Tomatoes 62
  Zucchini
    Balsamic Grilled 111
    Italian Sausage Stuffed Zucchini 126
    Noodles 81
    Zucchini Lasagna 60

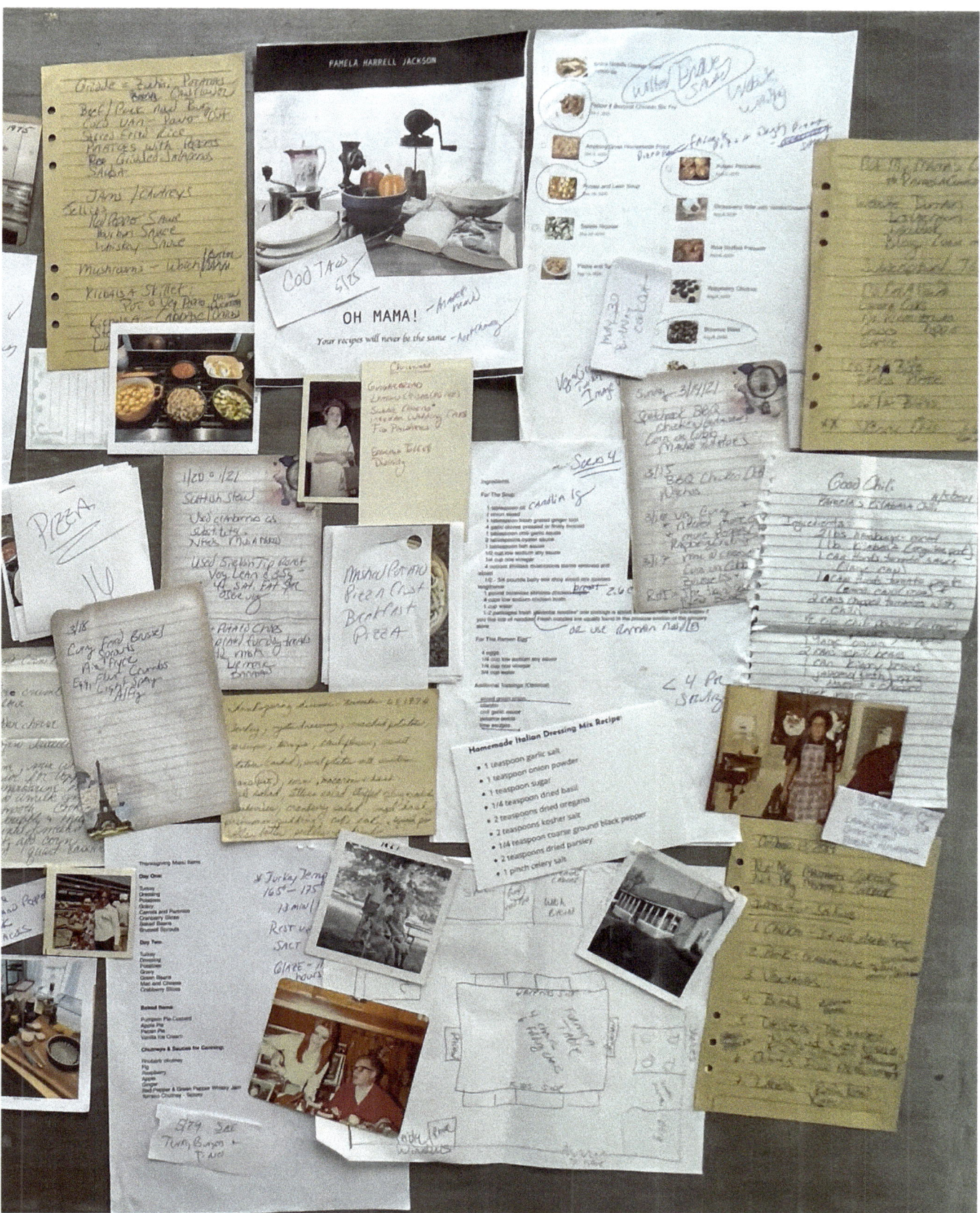

Oh Momma! Where's the Fat?

www.ingramcontent.com/pod-product-compliance
Lightning Source LLC
Chambersburg PA
CBHW061404010526
44119CB00010B/254